The Biology of Tumour Malignancy

The Biology of Tumour Malignancy

G. V. Sherbet

Cancer Research Unit,
University of Newcastle upon Tyne
Royal Victoria Infirmary
Newcastle upon Tyne

1982

ACADEMIC PRESS
A Subsidiary of Harcourt Brace Jovanovich, Publishers
London New York
Paris San Diego San Francisco Sao Paulo
Sydney Tokyo Toronto

ACADEMIC PRESS INC. (LONDON) LTD.
24/28 Oval Road
LONDON NW1

United States Edition published by
ACADEMIC PRESS INC.
111 Fifth Avenue
New York, New York 10003

British Library Cataloguing in Publication Data

Sherbet, G. V.
The biology of tumour malignancy
  1. Cancer
  I . Title
616.99'4   RC261

    ISBN 0-12-639880-1
    LCCN 81-69599

Printed in Great Britain by
The Lavenham Press Ltd., Lavenham, Suffolk

Preface

Cancer has been described as a host of diseases rather than one single ailment. A major cause of cancer deaths is metastatic dissemination of the disease. Primary cancers may be treated successfully by surgery and radiotherapy, but it is metastatic cancer that thwarts the efforts of the surgeon. The aggressive behaviour of tumours is often compounded by cancer-associated or paraneoplastic diseases which are *sensu stricto* a facet of the expression of malignancy.

This book examines the biological aspects of the malignancy of tumours, i.e. their ability to invade and form distant secondary tumours. Since it is directed to a wide readership from undergraduates to researcher workers, I have reviewed in a conventional format the development of the primary tumour and its metastases and hope that readers will find here an up-to-date account of the work being done in the varied areas of this field.

With this background, I have attempted to evaluate the concept of malignancy and to provide a definition of malignancy using an array of criteria of biological behaviour, the state of differentiation and the phenotypic expression of the differentiated state in the form of tumour-associated products such as hormones, peptides of various biological activities, prostaglandins, cell surface glycoprotein/protein components etc. Some attention has been given to the expression of malignancy and its possible modulation by controlling influences exerted by the host in the form of immunological responses. These responses may in certain instances indicate the degree of malignancy of the tumour. The degree of malignancy may also be assessed by means of histological grading techniques and by epigenetic criteria. Several *in vitro* systems have been devised for the purposes of estimating the invasive and metastatic abilities of tumour cells. These have been discussed in some detail since they also provide a device for testing the intrinsic malignant properties of the tumour cell, besides serving as a means for assessing the efficacy of antitumour agents and also for screening suspected carcinogens.

My interest in the amorphous field of tumour biology was kindled by the late Sir Alexander Haddow in the mid 1960s. The strength and vitality of his views have had an enduring influence on me. A second constant source of inspiration, encouragement and help, both at home and in the laboratory, is my wife, Dr M. S. Lakshmi, who has been closely involved in most of my research. I have also had lately much help and encouragement from many colleagues, notably from Professor K. G. M. M. Alberti, Professor A. L. Latner, Professor I. D. A. Johnston and Mr W. M. Ross. I would like to take this opportunity to thank them. I would also like to thank all the members of my research group, past and present, for their assiduous work and for stimulating discussions. I am grateful to Dr G. M. Hodges, Dr M. S. Lakshmi, Professor A. L. Latner, Dr P. A. Riley and Professor Alexander Wolsky for reading sections of or the entire manuscript and making helpful suggestions. My sincere thanks go to Mrs Jean Wake for typing the manuscript with great skill and endless patience. I thank Academic Press for publishing this book. It is needless to say that I enjoyed working with them.

The research work of my group was supported by several agencies over the years. In the past five years, however, financial support has come almost exclusively from the North of England Council of the Cancer Research Campaign to whom I am deeply indebted.

March 1982   G. V. Sherbet

Contents

PART I

PART II

To HiAms

Abbreviations

ACTH	Adrenocorticotropic hormone
ADCC	Antibody-dependent cell mediated cytotoxicity
ADH	Antidiuretic hormone
BCG	Bacillus Calmette-Guérin
BHK	Baby hamster kidney cells
BP	3,4-Benzo(a)pyrene
CAM	Chorio-allantoic membrane
CEA	Carcinoembryonic antigen
CLIP	Corticotropin-like intermediate lobe peptide
DAB	Dimethylaminoazobenzene
DMBA	Dimethylbenzanthracene
DNA	Deoxyribonucleic acid
EBV	Epstein-Barr virus
Ect R	Histogenetic ectodermal response
EGG	Epigenetic grade
End R	Histogenetic endodermal response
EPM	Electrophoretic mobility
FDP	Fibrin degradation products
FSH	Follicle-stimulating hormone
Hak	Hamster kidney cells
HBV	Hepatitis B virus
HCG	Human Chorionic Gonadotropin
HMR	Host mesodermal response
HPF	Hypoglycemia producing factor
HSV	Herpes simplex virus
Ig	Immunoglobulin
i.p.	Intraperitoneal
i.v.	Intravenous
K	Partition coefficient
K	10^3 (e.g. 233K = 233,000)
LAI	Leukocyte adherence inhibition

LH   Luteinizing hormone
LL   Lewis lung carcinoma
LPH   Lipotropin
MAF   Macrophage activating factor
MCA   3 methyl cholanthrene
MD   Morphogenetic displacement
MHC   Major histocompatibility complex
MIF   Migration inhibitory factor
α-MSH   Alpha melanotropin
MSV   Murine sarcoma virus
Mu MTV   Murine mammary tumour virus
NANase   Neuraminidase
NMU   Nitrosomethylurea
PA   Plasminogen activator
PEG   Poly(ethylene glycol)
PG   Prostaglandin
PHA   Phytohaemagglutinin
pI   Isoelectric point
pIE   Isoelectrophoretic point
PML   Progressive multifocal leukoencephalopathy
POA   Pancreatic oncofoetal antigen
PTH   Parathyroid hormone
poly I:C   Copolymer of inosinic acid and cytidylic acid
PyBHK   Polyoma virus transformed BHK cells
RES   Reticuloendothelial system
RNA   Ribonucleic acid
RSV   Rous sarcoma virus
s.c.   subcutaneous
SV-40   Simian virus 40
SV-BHK   SV-40 virus transformed BHK cells
SV-3T3   SV-40 transformed 3T3 cells
3T3 cells   Balb c/3T3 mouse fibroblasts
TAF   Tumour angiogenesis factor
TRES   A BHK-21 hamster kidney fibroblast line transformed by histone
TSH   Thyroid stimulating hormone
TSTA   Tumour specific transplantation antigen

PART I

Development of the
Primary Tumour and its Metastases

General Introduction

உற்றுன் அளவும் பிணியளவும் காலமும்
கற்றுன் கருதிச் செயல்

திரு வள்ளுவர்

Assess the patient and the state of the disease,
Gauge the suffering, and set forth to treat*

Thiru Valluvar
(Tamil Poet, second century, India)
Thirukkural, ch. 95, v. 949

Malignancy may be described in biological terms as the ability of a group of cells to divide progressively, free of homeostatic control, invade, form distant metastases, and eventually kill the host. In behavioural terms, and on the basis of clinical outcome, malignant tumours can be distinguished from the benign ones which are essentially localized, encapsulated and slow growing. These extreme groups may be considered to represent either end of a broad spectrum of tumours differing from one another in their degree of "innocence" or malignancy. Willis (1967) has argued cogently that a clear distinction between benign tumours and malignant tumours cannot be made. A consideration of tumours which are on the borderline between the benign and malignant groups, and also of the known progression of several benign tumours into frankly malignant neoplasms, has provided ample support for the view that it is neither practical nor desirable to attempt to draw a hard and fast line between the two groups.

Foulds (1969) has stated that "malignancy" is an abstract concept designed for the use of the clinician; a concept which has been moulded from cumulative knowledge of the behaviour of tumours in the clinical management of patients. According to Foulds, malignancy is neither an intrinsic property nor a biological feature of the aberrant cell, and Willis

*Translation by courtesy of Dr M. S. Lakshmi.

3

appears to hold the view that the distinction between benign and malignant tumours is a "convenient but arbitrary separation of members of any particular histogenetic series into two sections according to those biological characters which are of greatest significance to prognosis" (Willis, 1967). One may legitimately pose the question, therefore, whether these parameters of biological behaviour or the "biological characters" could be attributed to one or more discrete cellular components, determined and expressed under genetic control? In posing this question, one might naturally recall the observation of Harris (1971) that acquisition of malignancy may occur by a process of generation of cell variants, and a selection of types, out of these variants, that can grow progressively and kill the host. This view has lately been revived and discrete macromolecular changes have been shown to be associated with a proportion of an aberrant cell population, which could progressively become selected for a specific biological characteristic, such as the ability to metastasize, for example. The emphasis on the progressive nature of this process is deliberate, since the acquisition or loss of one more cellular component may not be an all-or-nothing phenomenon in relation to the phenotypic and behavioural alterration. This view may indeed be compatible with the notion that the borderline between "innocence" and malignancy cannot be delineated with any degree of certainty, and indeed compatible with the vast accumulated knowledge of small yet discrete differences in the degree of innocence or the degree of malignancy of tumours.

Thus, despite beginning with a discussion in general terms of the concept of malignancy in its widest implication and abstraction, one is led to talk about degrees of malignancy. It is now almost an adage that the mode of treatment of a malignant tumour is closely linked with an accurate assessment of the state of its progression. In other words, it is imperative that the degree of innocence or malignancy of a tumour can be assessed accurately in order that appropriate treatment can be determined.

My major objective is to assess our current ability to answer the question, concisely composed by Willis (1967): "How innocent or malignant is this tumour?" Therefore the book begins with a review of the natural history of neoplastic disease and a discussion of various stages of its development using the now conventional plan originally adopted by Foulds (1969). The passage through these stages is often characterized and contributed by specific biological properties of the component tumour cells. These properties are discussed as appropriate to the particular phenomenon, as well as to the general picture of malignancy. Although I regard and treat malignancy as an intrinsic biological property of the tumour cell, I recognize that the expression of malignancy may be modified and/or controlled by an interplay of intrinsic tumour factors and extrinsic factors such as the host immune system. Therefore, I endeavour to discuss in some detail the inter-action of the tumour cell with the immune system, the nature and extent of host cell responses, and the possible mechanisms by which the disseminated cell may evade immune destruction and seed out as a secondary deposit. In reviewing these aspects, I have, by design, avoided the complexities of tumour immunology, since there are excellent accounts of this elsewhere.

In Part II, the epigenetic aspects of tumour malginancy are considered. Essentially, this involves treatment of neoplasia as aberrant differentiation. I discuss several features which neoplasia shares with differentiating embryonic systems, and how certain concepts of embryology can enable one to understand paraneoplastic syndromes of ectopic endocrinopathy and the production of other polypeptide and protein markers by neoplastic cells. I attempt to show how the detection of these and the extent of their production could be related to the degree of malignancy. Here, too, I discuss the conceptual and practical problems relating to the use of histotypic differentiation as an indicator of malignancy, and the possibility of employing epigenetic criteria for the purposes of refining the currently available techniques and perhaps for the development of new techniques and assay procedures. I would like to think that, in the course of the book, I have formulated some new concepts, and modified and restated others in order to unite the strains of uniformity running through the processes of cell differentiation and neoplasia.

Development of the Primary Tumour

The most insidious aspect of neoplastic disease is the dissemination of the primary tumour and the formation of secondary growths or metastases at sites distant from the primary tumour. The development of disseminated neoplastic disease, which is dependent upon an interplay of intrinsic features of the neoplasm and the host factors, can be described in several progressive stages: (a) development of the primary tumour, (b) vascu-larization of the primary tumour, (c) detachment of tumour cells and invasion of lymphatics and blood vessels, (d) transport of the malignant cells, (e) attachment of cancer cells to vascular endothelium, (f) extra-vasation or the penetration of the endothelium by the tumour cells, and (g) host organ/malignant cell interactions and the growth of the secondary tumour (Fig. 1). These various stages have been described in detail in older publications by Weiss (1967) and Foulds (1969) and more recently in the scholarly and authoritative reviews by Fidler (1978), Fidler *et al.* (1978) and Carter (1978a, b). In the following pages the various factors operating at the different stages of development of metastases will be discussed briefly, since they play an important part in determining the metastatic capability of the neoplasm.

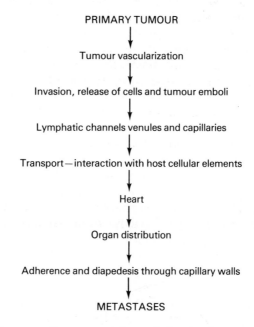

Figure 1 A diagrammatic representation of the development of the primary tumour, its dissemination, and the development of metastases.

Aetiology

The causation of cancer has been attributed to one or more of several neoplastic stimuli emanating from viral, environmental or occupational sources. The process of neoplastic transformation, whether caused by viruses or by chemical carcinogens, has been found to be a heritable change.

Several observations have implicated viruses in the neoplastic process. Of these, the association of the Epstein-Barr virus (EBV) with certain human cancers appears to be highly significant. The EB virus which causes infectious mononucleosis is known to be closely associated with two tumours of man (Epstein and Achong, 1977). There is strong evidence that one of these, the Burkitt's lymphoma, may be caused by EBV (Epstein, 1978a; De Thè *et al.*, 1978; Epstein and Achong, 1979). The second human tumour with which the EB virus is associated is the nasopharyngeal carcinoma (Epstein, 1978b). The cells of this tumour have been shown to carry the viral DNA (Wolf *et al.*, 1973) and as a result EBV coded nuclear antigens are expressed in these cells (Huang *et al.*, 1974; Klein *et al.*, 1974). Also, patients with this tumour have been found to show antibodies to EBV antigens and the antibody response appears to be related to the events associated with the disease (Henle *et al.*, 1973; Henle and Henle, 1976). However, high titres of antibody against EBV have not only been found in infectious mononucleosis (Henle *et al.*, 1968) but also in several other non-neoplastic conditions such as sarcoidosis (Hirschaut *et al.*, 1970), hepatitis (Corey *et al.*, 1975), systemic lupus erythematosus (Evans, *et al.*, 1971) and leprosy (Papageorgiou *et al.*, 1971).

Padgett and Walker (1976) reported the isolation of viral particles from progressive multifocal leukoencephalopathy (PML). These viruses have been found to resemble the well-known SV-40 and polyoma viruses of the papova group (see below) in inducing the characteristic T-antigen which has been shown to be immunologically similar to the T-antigen induced by SV-40 (Dougherty, 1976). The virus isolated from PML has been reported to produce tumours in Syrian hamsters (Padgett and Walker, 1976; Padgett *et al.*, 1977). The association of papova viruses with human tumours has not yet been satisfactorily demonstrated. A. F. Weiss *et al.*, (1975) and Scherneck (1979a, b) reported their occurrence in some human meningiomas and a glioblastoma, but others (Becker *et al.*, 1976; Cikes *et al.*, 1977) have failed to detect any evidence for their presence in association with human brain tumours.

Gardner *et al.* (1971) isolated a human papovavirus (BKV) from samples of urine from an immunosuppressed renal transplant recipient. Takemoto *et al.* (1974) isolated it from brain tumours of patients with immuno-deficiencies. This virus appears to be obtainable exclusively from human sources, grows preferentially in human cells in tissue culture and certain human populations have been found to contain anti-BKV antibodies (Gardner, 1973; Shah *et al.*, 1973; P. J. Brown *et al.*, 1975). It has been shown further that BKV can cause neoplastic transformation of hamster, rodent and monkey cells (Major and Di Mayorca, 1973; Van der Noordaa, 1976; Shah *et al.*, 1975; Portolani *et al.*, 1978). Portolani *et al.* (1978) have also demonstrated the specificity of transformation by the presence of the BKV-T antigen and by rescuing the virus from the transformed cells by fusion with permissive cells by the agency of the Sendai virus.

Another human neoplasm, Hodgkin's disease, which is a neoplasm of the lymphoreticular system, has often been suspected to have a viral aetiology. Some forms of herpes virus have been implicated in its causation (Stevens, 1973; Sikovics and Györkey, 1973).

Among other reported instances where viruses may be implicated in the causation of human cancers is the demonstration of sequence homology between nucleic acids of the MCF-7 human mammary adenocarcinoma and murine mammary tumour (Mu MTV) virus and the Mason-Pfizer monkey virus. Although sequence homology between the viral DNA and MCF-7 RNAs appears to be convincing, that with MCF-7 DNA has not yet been demonstrated beyond doubt (Das and Mink, 1979).

Further evidence, albeit circumstantial, has been reported by Witkin *et al.* (1980). These authors have shown that a higher proportion of sera from breast cancer patients contained IgGs that could react with Mu MTV, as compared with sera from women with benign breast disease or from normal subjects. Also IgM and IgA from some sera bound the virus. Earlier, Witkin *et al.* (1979) found that a greater proportion of breast cancer sera lysed Mu MTV *in vivo*, and also that antibodies raised against envelope glycoproteins gp52 or gp34 could successfully block the reaction of the sera with the virus.

McDougall *et al.* (1980) have recently published data from some preliminary experiments which show that RNA complementary to Herpes simplex 2 virus (HSV-2) ³H-DNA molecular probe could be detected in human cervical cells undergoing premalignant change but not in fully developed squamous cell carcinoma. The significance of this observation is still unclear in relation to aetiology. But the possibility of the involvement of HSV-2 is further indicated by the demonstration of HSV-2 specific DNA-binding antigen in 36% of patients with severe cervical dysplasia and in 40% of cases of carcinoma *in situ* and in the invasive carcinoma (Dreesman *et al.*, 1980).

HSV-2 *ts* mutants have been shown to transform rodent cells *in vitro* and these can produce tumours *in vivo* (Boyd and Orme, 1975; Darai and Munk, 1976; Macnab, 1974; Rapp and Duff, 1973). As far as human cells are concerned, there are some reports which have demonstrated such transformation in embryonic cells (Kucera and Gusdon, 1976; Munk and Darai, 1973; Takahashi and Yamanishi, 1974). However, Marczynska *et al.* (1980) found no transforming effect of HSV-2 on human uterine cervical cell cultures. Cassai *et al.* (1981a, b) investigated dysplasias of the cervix and five genital tumours for HSV-2 DNA. None was detected. Several cell cultures of labial tumours were examined for the presence of HSV specific antigens, but none was detected.

Integrated hepatitis B viral (HBV) DNA has been demonstrated in a human hepatocellular carcinoma cell line, viz. the Alexander cell line derived from a hepatoma obtained from a Mozambican male, which is known to accumulate hepatitis B surface antigens in the medium. The synthesis of three RNA transcript molecules containing HBV-specific sequences has been reported (Chakraborty *et al.*, 1980; Edman *et al.*, 1980; Brechot *et al.*, 1980).

A number of animal tumours is known to be induced by viruses. Thus several oncogenic RNA viruses are known which can induce either leukemias or sarcomas, such as the avian leukemia virus, murine and feline leukemia viruses (MuLV, FeLV), murine mammary tumour virus, the Rous sarcoma virus and the murine and feline sarcoma viruses. These viruses not only produce tumours in their natural hosts, but also in a wide range of other vertebrates, and produce cellular transformation *in vitro* (*see* Benyesh-Melnick and Butel, 1974). Another class of virus, viz. the DNA viruses such as the SV-40, polyoma virus, etc. have been shown to transform cells into the neoplastic state. In the case of SV-40, there is much work which indicates that the transformation occurs as a result of the intercalation of the viral DNA into the genome of the cell being transformed. The viral DNA has been shown to be covalently linked to host cell DNA (Sambrook *et al.*, 1968). This has been confirmed by Wall and Darnell (1971) using DNA-RNA molecular hybridization technique. Not only can non-permissive cells be transformed, but the transforming virus can also be rescued from the transformed cells. Thus, SV-40 virus can be rescued from transformed cells by fusing the latter with permissive cells (Gerber and Kirchstein, 1962; Sabin and Koch, 1963; Watkins and Dulbecco, 1967). The rescued virus has been found to be identical to that used for achieving transformation (Takemoto *et al.*, 1968). Boyd and Butel (1972) showed that infectious virions can also be rescued by injecting permissive cells with high molecular weight DNA prepared from transformed cells.

Certain mutant forms of transforming viruses have been isolated. Among these are temperature sensitive (*ts*) mutants. These induce cell transformation that is conditional upon the temperature to which the virus is sensitive (Ishikawa and Aizawa, 1973; Robb *et al.*, 1972; Tegtmeyer, 1972; Yamaguchi and Kuchino, 1975). Several lines of SV-3T3 cells which show transformed characteristics *in vitro* at 32 °C but not at 39 °C have been isolated (Renger and Basilico, 1972, 1973). Such *ts* variants have also been described in the polyoma virus (Eckhart *et al.*, 1971).

The molecular mechanisms involved in the induction of the neoplasia by viruses have been investigated intensively in the past few years. Oncogenic RNA viruses (retroviruses) not only contain genes which are necessary for the induction and maintenance of the neoplastic state (proto-oncogenes), but also the genetic information required for the replication of the retrovirus. It is believed that the proto-oncogenes are derived from normal vertebrate cells. Both the viral and the proto-oncogenes are introduced into the cell, but the expression of the oncogenes is controlled by the viral genes (*see* Hayman, 1981; Bishop, 1981). Retroviruses that do not transform cells in culture apparently possess only the genes necessary for virus replication. In these viruses, the transforming effect is believed to be produced by cellular genes which become oncogenic under the influence of the DNA copy of the retrovirus integrated into the host cell DNA (Payne *et al.*, 1981; Neel *et al.*, 1981).

In DNA viruses, the viral DNA intercalated into the cell genome appears to alter the expression of certain cellular genes. This is suggested by recent observations that certain host cell-coded proteins, e.g. the 55K and 32K, are expressed in transformed cells (Rundell *et al.*, 1980; May *et al.*, 1980; Linzer *et al.*, 1980). Linzer *et al.* (1980) showed that a 54K protein of cellular origin is expressed in SV-40 infected and transformed murine cells and some uninfected embryonal carcinoma cells. This protein is present in normal 3T3 cells (used for transformation by SV-40 virus), but only to 1-2% of the levels found in the transformed cells. Crawford *et al.* (1980) found a 53K protein not coded for by the virus in SV-40 transformed murine cells. A significant proportion of this protein occurred as a complex with the large T antigen and this, Crawford *et al.* suggest, may have the effect of shifting the 53K protein from the nucleus to the cell membrane.

In the light of these recent developments, I cannot but recall with some gratification that in 1975, I presented a paper at the International Symposium on Molecular Basis of Medicine held in Vienna, in which we described the detection of a species of transformation-associated antigens on the surface of SV-40 and polyoma virus-transformed 3T3 mouse fibroblasts. We raised an antiserum against SV-3T3 cells, absorbed the antiserum fully with untransformed 3T3 cells and quantitated the binding of this absorbed antiserum to SV-3T3 cells, polyoma virus-transformed 3T3 (Py3T3),SV-40 transformed Chinese hamster kidney and rabbit kidney cells (SV-CHK and SV-TRK, respectively). The absorbed antiserum bound SV-3T3 and, to a lesser degree, Py3T3 cells but not SV-CHK or SV-TRK cells. We concluded from this series of experiments that the species of surface antigens detected were host-cell coded and that their expression was controlled by the virus (Sherbet and Lakshmi, 1976; Sherbet, 1978; Sherbet *et al.*, 1974).

Whether carcinogen-induced mutations of DNA may similarly activate the proto-oncogenes already present in the genome has recently been investigated. Shih *et al.* (1981) have shown that DNA from methylcholanthrene-induced transformant cells can be used to transform recipient cells of the same species or of other species. This transfection phenomenon has also been demonstrated with spontaneous tumours.

Functional heterogeneity and progression

The event of neoplastic transformation of cells or the initiation of an incipient neoplastic state is only a prelude to a complex and often protracted process of neoplastic development and progression. Foulds (1949, 1954) proposed that the development of a neoplasm involved "progression" through qualitatively different stages of irreversible change in one or more characteristics of the tumour. This is the concept of "independent progression of characters". Foulds also proposed that progression occurred independently in different tumour characters. Such progression could conceivably result in a functional heterogeneity of a tumour, i.e. result in the evolution of subpopulations of cells with specialized biological characteristics, such as invasive ability or metastatic potential. It is inevitable also that, dependent upon the degree of progression undergone by the various cellular components, there will exist variant lines of cells displaying a spectrum of a given malignant attribute. For instance, it would be reasonable to suppose on the basis of the concept of tumour progression not only that some component cells will have, say, the ability to metastasize, while others will not, but that even this subpopulation with metastasizing ability will possess a spectrum of metastatic potential. Such a clonal evolution of metastatic potential would appear to be a distinct possibility in view of the recent experiments of Fidler and his colleagues. Fidler (1973a) showed that it is possible to obtain tumour lines with increasing "metastatic" potential by subjecting the cell population to a selection procedure involving successive transplantation and intermittent *in vitro* culturing. Fidler injected viable cells of the B16 melanoma into the tail vein of C57BL/6 mice, isolated the tumour nodules which had formed in the lungs of these animals and grew the cells in tissue culture. These cells were designated B16-F1, being the result of first *in vivo* selection for lung colonization. The B16-F1 cells were then injected back into syngeneic mice, and subsequently the pulmonary colonies were isolated and adapted for culture (B16-F2). This procedure was continued ten times to obtain the B16-F10 line. at each stage of the selection process, the ability of the cells to survive and form colonies in the lungs was found to increase (Fidler, 1973a, 1975; Fidler and Nicolson, 1976). Such an outcome is compatible with the view that the original unselected primary tumour contained a number of variant lines that differed widely in their potential for lung colonization. If, on the other hand, the original tumour had contained a proportion of the cell population with comparable proclivity to lodge and form tumour nodules in the lung, there would have been no scope for a gradual and progressive selection process to operate, and such a selection would indeed have taken place in one step. The heterogeneity of tumours with regard to metastatic ability has also been demonstrated by using procedures of *in vivo* selection (Chambers *et al.*, 1981). Tumours are heterogeneous also with regard to other features, for instance, the expression of cytoplasmic steroid receptors, and this has been demonstrated using *in vivo* selection procedures (Risely and Sherbet, 1981).

Although the experiments of Fidler and colleagues do demonstrate the heterogeneity of the B16 melanoma, the relevance or relationship of the process of "colonization" to the complex processes of spontaneous metastasis is uncertain. Liotta *et al.* (1980) found that increased colonizing abilities of these variants corresponded with increases in the incidence of spontaneous metastasis of the corresponding primary tumours. Stackpole (1981) has reported, however, that the F1, and F10 and BL6 variants of the B16 melanoma all show low spontaneous metastasis. His experiments have demonstrated, none the less, the existence in the B16 line of two distinct populations, viz. one with colonizing ability and the other with ability to metastasize spontaneously.

In a recent series of experiments, Fidler and Hart (1981) have changed their approach to the problem. They infected Balb/c mouse embryo fibroblasts *in vitro* with MSV, and cloned six cell lines from the transformant cell population. When the cells were introduced into mice either subcutaneously or intravenously (i.v.) they invariably produced tumours, but the tumours differed considerably in their ability to metastasize to the lungs. Cells derived from these cloned tumours were also found to be heterogeneous. Therefore the heterogeneity of component cells of a primary neoplasm can not only be accepted as an accomplished fact but there is also experimental evidence that this heterogeneity is built into the tumour during its development and progression.

Vascularization of the Tumour

For the successful establishment, growth and dissemination of a tumour, it is essential that the tumour has adequate vascularization. It was known for some time that hyperemia occurs in association with subcutaneously implanted tumour. Implantation in like manner of normal tissue does not induce hyperemia, but syngeneic embryonic tissue can induce a transient hyperemia. This suggested the possibility that actively dividing tumour and embryonic cells were capable of inducing hyperemia (Coman and Sheldon, 1946). Since then it has been demonstrated in a variety of systems that malignant tumours induce vascularization in adjacent host tissue. Greenblatt and Shubik (1968) showed that the Fortner melanoma transplanted into hamster cheek pouch could induce neovascularization.

Tumours implanted into other sites, such as the anterior chamber of the eye of the guinea-pig and rabbit (Greene, 1941; Gimbrone *et al.*, 1973, 1974), have also demonstrated the ability to induce angiogenesis. Gimbrone *et al.* (1974) implanted tumours into rabbit cornea, in which no blood vessels or lymphatics are present, at a distance of about 6 mm from the limbus of the cornea, i.e. the edge of the cornea where it joins the sclera which is supplied with blood vessels. A variety of tumours implanted in this way induced new vessels to grow from the limbus and through the corneal stroma towards the tumour.

Folkman (1974a) showed that tumours implanted into chicken embryos also successfully induced angiogenesis in the host tissue. Earlier, Sherbet *et al.* (1970) and Sherbet and Lakshmi (1971) implanted Morris minimum deviation hepatomas into chick embryos and described the induction of blood islands from chick embryonic tissue by the implanted hepatomas. Sherbet and Lakshmi (1971) demonstrated further that the ability to induce formation of blood islands was largely associated with an extra chromosome in the group 4-10 of the karyotype. The occurrence of an extra chromosome in this group is a highly signficant feature of these tumours. About 76% of minimum-deviation hepatomas have been reported to contain alterations in the chromosome complement of group 4-10 (Nowell and Morris, 1969; Nowell *et al.*, 1967). It appears likely, therefore, that such an alteration may be closely involved with the neoplastic changes undergone by the liver tissue. The association of the ability to induce angiogenesis with alteration in the chromosome complement of the same group may indicate, therefore, that the ability to induce angiogenesis is also closely associated with the neoplastic state. However, recent work (see below) shows that induction of angiogenesis is probably a property shared by tumour cells and actively dividing normal cells. Folkman (1975) identifies two distinct phases of tumour growth, viz. the avascular phase and the vascular phase. The avascular phase is self-limiting. This is because while the tumour volume increases by the third power, the surface area increases only by the second power, and as a consequence a tumour volume is soon reached where the surface area is inadequate for the diffusion of nutrients and catabolic products. Under the circumstances, a steady state is reached with cells at the periphery proliferating but those in the centre of the tumour undergoing death and necrosis, thus producing a dormant population. Folkman cites carcinoma of the cervix *in situ*, and metastatic retinoblastomas as examples of avascular growths. The vascular phase, on the other hand, is characterized by rapid and exponential growth.

Historically, although the association of neovascularization with tumours has been known for well over a hundred years, only recently was it suggested that angiogenesis may be humorally mediated (Greenblatt and Shubik,

1968). Folkman (1974b, 1975) showed that tumours induced the proliferation of cells of proximal capillaries by secreting a substance which has been termed the tumour angiogenesis factor (TAF). This factor, which was isolated by Folkman *et al.* (1971), appears to be produced by tumours both *in vitro* and *in vivo* (Klagsbrun *et al.*, 1976; Brem *et al.,* 1977).

The mode of action of TAF is not fully understood, but it appears to involve the stimulation of endothelial cells to proliferate (Gimbrone and Gullino, 1976; Ausprunk and Folkman, 1977). *In vivo*, TAF may act in conjunction with platelets and factors released by platelets to stimulate endothelial proliferation. Other factors, such as the involvement of collagen of the endothelial basement membrane, have also been envisaged (Schor *et al.*, 1979). Schor *et al.* (1980) found that endothelial cells growing *in vitro* on a native collagen-coated substratum responded to an angiogenesis factor obtained from rat Walker 256 carcinoma. This TAF failed to stimulate endothelial cells growing on plastic Petri dishes or on denatured collagen films.

The limiting factor in the study of the angiogenesis factor is the requirement of an *in vivo* assay for assessing the migration and subsequent proliferation of capillary endothelium. Suddith *et al.* (1975) described an *in vitro* assay. They cultured endothelial cells derived from the umbilical veins of human umbilical cords, and tested their growth characteristics in the presence of culture medium previously "conditioned" by the growth of tumours. They prepared media conditioned by the growth of a number of glial tumours and neuroblastomas, and demonstrated that these conditioned media produced between 25-100% increase in the thymidine labelling index of the endothelial cell cultures. Zetter (1980) has recently reported an *in vitro* assay which employs clonal cell lines of bovine capillary endothelium which can be maintained in culture media "conditioned" by tumours. Clonal epithelial cells, of bovine and human origin, not only proliferate in media conditioned by the growth of tumours, but also form capillary tubes in a complex three-dimensional organization which closely resembles, in light as well as in electron microscopy, capillary beds formed *in vivo* (Folkman and Haudenschild, 1980). Zetter showed, using this *in vitro* assay, that factors derived from tumours stimulated the migration of capillary endothelial cells while these same factors had no effect on aortic endothelial cells.

The tumour angiogenesis factor(s) was once believed to be secreted almost exclusively by tumour cells; it is now known that lymphocytes are able to induce angiogenesis (Sidky and Auerbach, 1976), and activated macrophages seem to synthesize a factor which is similar to TAF (Polverini *et al.*, 1977).

Tumour Cell Detachment and Invasion

Cell locomotion

A reliable indicator of possible dissemination of a tumour is local invasion, which is often also the first step in tumour cell detachment and transport. Benign neoplasms are usually fully encapsulated. Invasion may occur by the locomotive behaviour of individual cells (Trinkaus, 1976; Sträuli and Weiss, 1977) and the adherents of this view have found support in the reports that tumour cells are endowed with adequate locomotive machinery, such as actomyosin filaments, in the form of microfilaments (Franks *et al.*, 1969; Malech and Lentz, 1974). Cancer cells stain strongly for actin as compared with normal cells. Pronounced staining has been described in invading cells of squamous cell carcinoma and also mammary carcinomas (Rungger-Brändle and Gabbiani, 1980). Much circumstantial evidence in the form of association of increased microfilament activity with increased immunofluorescent labelling of actin has been reported (Gabbiani *et al.*, 1976; Schenk, 1975; McNutt, 1976). According to Rungger-Brändle and Gabbiani (1980), the bundles of microfilaments extend into cytoplasmic protrusions, with these protrusions being in direct contact with surrounding tissue. None the less, the evidence for actin content being directly related to the invasive ability of a tumour must yet be considered as circumstantial. Further support may be cited from the observations by Ambrose and Easty (1976a) of considerable pseudopodial activity in the invading zones of the tumour cell (*see also* p. 156). However, the occurrence of pseudopodial activity cannot be regarded as irrefutable evidence of invasive ability (Easty and Easty, 1973). Also, it is not clearly understood how the actomyosin filaments may participate in cell locomotion, in spite of the fact that Isenberg *et al.* (1976) have demonstrated an ATP-induced contraction of bundles of microfilaments isolated from a rat mammary adenocarcinoma.

The infiltration of organs by leukemic cells may be considered as an example where infiltration takes place by individual cell locomotion. Locomotion is also involved in the infiltration of sheets or cords of cells. This means of penetration may be more common than infiltration by individual cells (Sträuli and Weiss, 1977; Tickle *et al.*, 1978).

The locomotion of tumour aggregates has been suggested as another possibility (Leighton *et al.*, 1960; Enterline and Coman, 1950; Easty and Easty, 1974). Tumour detachment may occur in sub-lethal cytolysis and necrosis of tumour cells, by the agency of lysosomal enzymes (Weiss and Holyoke, 1969; Weiss, 1977, 1978; *see* p. 88). The detached emboli may disseminate by direct extension—or be mobilized. Sträuli and Weiss (1977) have made the distinction that detached tumour pieces may not necessarily be in a mobilized state, but that mobilization may involve freeing the cell masses from constraints such as contact-mediated inhibition of locomotion.

The locomotion of cells is dependent to a large degree upon the ability of the cells to form transient adhesive bonds either with other cells or the solid substratum. In either case, the interacting surfaces need to be at a certain optimum distance from each other so that adhesive bonds can be formed. Since biological surfaces bear net negative charges under physiological conditions, it would be reasonable to assume that the closeness of approach of the charged surfaces will be determined by the total magnitude of the electrostatic forces of repulsion and the van der Waal's-London dispersion forces. Such considerations also apply to tumour cell interactions leading to their adhesion to endothelial surfaces, subsequent diapedesis and their lodgement in the parenchyma of the organ.

Surface charge

It could be argued that a high surface charge would aid the locomotion of and invasion by tumour cells. Bosmann *et al.* (1973) examined the surface charge of the low and high malignancy variants of B16 melanoma lines of Fidler (*see* pp. 11-12) and reported that the high malignancy variants showed a greater electrophoretic mobility (EPM) than did the low malignancy variants. A review of electrokinetic data relating to a variety of tumour types appears to suggest that higher surface charge density is not invariably associated with malignancy, but could be a reflection of higher rate of growth often shown by tumour cells (Sherbet, 1978). Measurements of surface charge by the isoelectric equilibrium method have shown that normal liver cells of the Chester Beatty strain of rat possessed a surface charge density nearly equal to twice the density on cells obtained from hepatoma induced in the same strain of rat by the administration of di-methylaminoazobenzene (DAB) (Sherbet and Lakshmi, unpublished work; *see* Sherbet, 1978). The net charge density on the surface of SV-40 transformed 3T3 mouse fibroblasts is marginally lower than that on the surface of untransformed cells (Sherbet and Lakshmi, 1979).

On the other hand, the net surface charge showed no correlation with malignancy as judged by the survival times of patients, and histological and epigenetic grading of a series of human astrocytomas of a spectrum of malignancy and the non-malignant meningiomas, and a line of cells derived from foetal brain. The relevant data summarized in Table 1 allows one to conclude that the net surface charge may be related more closely to the rate of tumour growth than to its malignancy.

High surface charge may help tumour cell dissemination but would not be conducive to the adhesion of cells to endothelial surfaces and subsequently

Table 1

Relationship between surface charge density, rates of growth and malignancy of some human intracranial tumour cell lines

Tumour	Malignancy rating			Net negative[c] surface charge $\times 10^{-4}\ \mu m^{-2}$	Mean[c] doubling time (h)
	Average survival times (months)	Histological[a] grade	Epigenetic[b] grade		
Astrocytoma	2-6	III, IV	10-12	20·05	165 ± 18
	7-10	II	7	15·91	249 ± 24
	10	I	5	14·72	
Meningioma	Non-malignant		4	18·06	194 ± 32
Foetal brain cells	Normal cell line			20·84	66.0

[a]Kernohan grade (Kernohan *et al.*, 1949).
[b]Epigenetic grading obtained from Sherbet and Lakshmi (1974d, 1978).
[c]From Sherbet and Lakshmi (1974a).

to the cells of the parenchyma of the organ being invaded. Recently, the surface charge status of metastasizing (ML) and non-metastasizing (NML) forms of a homotransplantable lymphosarcoma (Carter and Gershon, 1966) maintained in Syrian cream hamsters has been examined in the author's laboratory. The differences in the malignancy of these tumours are well documented. The NML tumours grow as highly localized and fully encapsulated tumours. These do not show any local invasiveness. None the less, viable NML cells have been detected in the blood of tumour-bearing animals (Carter, 1978b). Possibly these are destroyed by the host's immune system. The metastasizing form, on the contrary, forms numerous secondary deposits in the liver, and less frequently in kidney and lung (Guy, 1979; Sherbet *et al.*, 1980). These differences in malignancy are also clearly detectable in epigenetic grading tests (Sherbet *et al.*, 1980) (*see* pp. 185-186).

The electrokinetic measurements reported by Turner *et al.* (1980a) have shown that, in agreement with Bosmann *et al.* (1973), the ML cells had a greater electrophoretic mobility than NML cells, i.e. that at physiological pHs, ML surface carried a greater net negative charge density than did the NML cells. When charge measurements were made using the isoelectric equilibrium method (Sherbet *et al.*, 1972; Sherbet and Lakshmi, 1973), the charge status was found to be reversed. The latter experiments showed that the pI of ML cells was higher than that of NML cells, i.e. the surface charge density on NML cells was greater than that on the ML cells. The EPMs of the cells were measured at various pH values from 4 to 10 and pH-mobility curves were constructed for the two cell types. These curves crossed over at pH 4·8 and the isoelectrophoretic points (pIE) extrapolated from these curves gave a pIE value for ML which was higher than that for NML; thus consistent with their true pI values. From these observations Turner *et al.*

(1980a) have suggested that the apparently contradictory results obtained using microelectrophoresis and the isoelectric equilibrium method may be due to differences in the depths of zones probed by the two electrokinetic methods as suggested previously by Sherbet (1978). The electrokinetic data may then be interpreted as indicating that in ML cells a greater proportion of cationic groups are distributed at deeper levels of the cell surface. Viewed in the light of the striking differences in the biological behaviour of the two tumour types and of the observation that the electrokinetic status as defined by isoelectric equilibrium analysis is consistent with these differences, the experiments described above appear to highlight the possibility that an active role may be played by cell surface components situated deeper in the cell surface in the process of tumour cell dissemination and metastasis.

Another surface-related parameter which has been employed in this context is the partition of cells in two-phase aqueous polymers. When a mixture of two immiscible unlike polymers is allowed to stand, it separates into two phases. If a substance is present in solution in the system it tends to become distributed between the phases as a function of its interaction with the polymeric molecules. Cells and particles suspended in the phase mixture also show characteristic distribution, which depends upon the differential affinity shown by the cells to the two phases. This differential affinity reflects differences in the net effect of the interactions between the particle and the polymer molecules. Several factors govern these interactions, such as the cell surface charge, size of the particle, lipid content of the membrane (in the case of partition of cells) etc. (Albertsson, 1971; Walter, 1975, 1977; *see also* Sherbet, 1978). Therefore, although partition behaviour is a highly complex phenomenon, it has been considered as a much more sensitive parameter than cell electrophoresis.

Walter *et al.* (1967) showed that the partition of erythrocytes in the dextran-poly (ethylene glycol) (PEG) system containing phosphate ions was related to their electrophoretic mobilities (EPM). The counter-current distribution patterns of erythrocytes and liver cells showed that cells with lower partition coefficients also possessed lower EPMs (Brooks *et al.*, 1971; Walter *et al.*, 1973b). In other words, a higher partition ratio in a dextran-PEG system with high PO_4: NACL ratio, indicates a greater surface negative charge density.

Bosmann *et al.* (1973) examined the partition behaviour of the low and high malignancy variants of B16 melanomas. In sparse (log phase?) cultures, the high malignancy variant showed higher partition ratios (43% of total cells in the top phase) than the lower malignancy variant (36% of total cells in the system in the top phase). But cells obtained from confluent cultures possessed comparable partition ratios. It would seem, therefore, that these differences in partition behaviour may be related to possible differences in surface properties of cells in density-dependent growth inhibition and those in log phase of growth. The partition behaviour of cells has indeed been demonstrated to change in the various phases of cell division and growth (Walter *et al.*, 1973a; Pinaev *et al.*, 1976). Compatible with this view also are the electrophoretic mobility measurements of sparse and confluent cultures of the two variants (see below). While, admittedly, the cell lines differ in their surface properties, there is little justification for suggesting any relevance to difference in the abilities of the cell lines to implant in the lungs following i.v. inoculation.

Experiments in the author's laboratory on the behaviour of the B16 melanoma variants in two-polymer phase system incorporating an electrostatic partition potential have produced results that are at variance with those of Bosmann *et al.* (1973). These results are summarized in Table 2, from which it may be seen that B16-F1 cells which did not metastasize spontaneously showed greater partition than F10 and BL6 which were more metastatic. However, the latter, which differed in their metastatic ability, showed comparable partition coefficients. One may conclude from these observations that the surface charge, which is one of the factors that dictate the partition in this phase system, may not be related to the metastatic ability of the melanoma variants.

Table 2

The malignancy of B16 melanoma variants in relation to their partition in a two polymer phase system

Variant[a]	Malignancy:[b] incidence (%) of spontaneous metastasis	Partition coefficient[c]
B16-F1	None	37·7 ± 5·6 (5)
B16-F10	30% (within 4 weeks)	20·5 ± 4·7 (5)
B16-BL6	80% (within 4 weeks)	22·2 ± 3·8 (5)

[a]The variants were grown in tissue culture. Cells from sub-confluent cultures were used in these experiments

[b]From Liotta *et al.* (1980).

[c]Partition in 5% dextran-4% poly(ethylene glycol) system in 0·11 M Na_2HPO_4 buffer, with partition potential. Partition coefficient = $\dfrac{\text{No. of cells in top phase} \times 100}{\text{Total cells added to the system}}$.

The number of experiments performed are given in parentheses. (Sherbet *et al.*, unpublished work.)

Increased surface charge density in association with higher metastatic ability has also been reported by other workers. The surface charge density of human astrocytomas has been found to increase with increasing malignancy as indicated in histology (Sherbet and Lakshmi, 1974a). There have been many early reports of similar increases in other tumour systems (Purdom *et al.*, 1958; Ambrose *et al.*, 1956; Cook and Jacobson, 1968). More recently, Bosmann *et al.* (1973) reported that the high malignancy variants of the B16 melanoma had a higher EPM than the low malignancy variants, while Raz *et al.* (1980b) reported an increase in the number of dense anionic clusterings associated with increased metastatic potential.

On the other hand, Weiss *et al.* (1975) and Sherbet and Lakshmi (1979) reported that SV-3T3 cells possessed lower surface charge densities than did the untransformed 3T3 cells. Polyoma virus-transformed 3T3 cells have also been found to possess a lower surface charge density than the untransformed counterparts (Sherbet and Lakshmi, 1976). Sherbet (1978) found that the negative charge density on the surface of malignant cells obtained from a rat hepatoma induced by the administration of dimethyl aminoazobenzene was lower than on corresponding normal cells.

Walter *et al.* (1981) have reported that variants with different metastatic abilities can be fractionated from the murine lymphosarcoma line RAW-117P by subjecting them to counter-current distribution (CCD) on a PEG-dextran two-phase system possessing a partition electrostatic potential. After CCD, the cells from the various extraction cavities were recovered, cultured overnight *in vitro*, and assayed for metastatic ability by injecting them intravenously into mice. They found that cells with greater partition coefficient were more metastatic to the liver than those with lower partition coefficient. This implies a greater surface charge density on the more metastatic cells. Like most investigations dealing with the possible selection of variants with greater metastatic ability, these experiments have relied on the "colonization" potential rather than spontaneous metastasis. The colonization potential may not be predictive of the spontaneous metastatic ability of tumours (Stackpole, 1981). Stackpole has reported that B16 melanoma lines which colonize lungs after i.v. inoculation do not metastasize. On the other hand, those which do metastasize spontaneously produce very few lung colonies after i.v. injection.

We recently examined the partition ratios of several lines of normal and neoplastic cells in dextran-poly (ethylene glycol) (PEG) phase system with a low PO_4:NaCl ratio. These experiments showed that 3T3 mouse fibroblasts and their SV-40 and polyoma virus transformed counterparts possessed partition coefficients (K) of 23, 30 and 35% respectively. BHK-21 fibroblasts and TRES fibrosarcoma cells, which are BHK-21 cells transformed by histone, possessed comparable partition ratios (52 and 49% respectively). On the other hand, a non-malignant ganglioneuroma showed a partition coefficient of 44%, but three malignant astrocytomas showed partition ratios of 30, 18 and 11%.

Reitherman *et al.* (1973) showed that the partition potential, i.e. the potential difference between the phases, was directly related to the ratio of phosphate/NaCl present in the system. In our phase system, this ratio is low and therefore a potential difference between the phases may not be expected. Hence the partition coefficients could not be a reflection of the surface charge composition of the cells.

The cell membrane property known to be related to the partitioning behaviour under these conditions is its hydrophobicity (Shanbhag and Axelsson, 1975; Walter, 1977). Hence changes in partition behaviour could be a measure of the hydrophobic receptors on the cell surface. But the results obtained to date seem to suggest that low hydrophobicity of the membrane, as seen in astrocytomas, is not an invariable feature of neoplastic change.

It is perhaps needless to emphasize here that because of the extreme complexity of the system, great caution should be exercised in the interpretation not only of the behaviour of cells in two polymer aqueous phases, but also of surface charge status of cells as determined by the methods of cell electrophoresis and isoelectric equilibrium. As emphasized by Sherbet (1978), these two electrokinetic methods appear to probe the cell membrane to varying depths. To accept the charge composition determined by either method and to attempt to relate it or to associate it with neoplastic change or to degrees of malignancy would be tantamount to taking a rather restricted view of the situation, for neither method provides adequate information regarding the distribution of the electrical charges.

Lymphatic Dissemination of Tumours

The detached tumour emboli and cells may be disseminated by three major routes. Tumours growing in body cavities, or secondary deposits adjacent to body cavities, may spread by direct extension, i.e. by shedding fragments which are subsequently implanted into serosal and/or mucosal surfaces to form secondary tumours. The spread of lung tumours or those of mediastinal origin to form visceral metastases, and the formation of peritoneal metastases from malignant ovarian tumours are examples of the metastatic process by direct extension (Fidler, 1978).

The second major means of dissemination is via the lymphatic system. Carcinomas tend to be disseminated by this route and, not infrequently, so do melanomas, neuroblastomas and teratomas (Carter, 1978a). Mesenchymal tumours spread more frequently via the bloodstream (Del Regato, 1977). But the two systems are interlinked, hence a demarcation of the pathways of spread may be considered arbitrary. Melanomas, for instance, in the majority of cases, metastasize mainly via the lymphatic channel in the early phases of the disease but haematogenous metastasis may occur in the later phases of the tumour's natural history (Harvin and Smith, 1968).

Access to the lymphatic system is generally by means of small lymphatic vessels. These possess structural features which may allow permeation by tumour cells. The small lymphatic vessels lack a basement membrane and have a high proportion of gap junctions between the endothelial cells. Like macrophages and lymphocytes, tumour cells may enter the vessels through these gap junctions (Carr *et al.*, 1976). Tumour cells may enter thin-walled venules with equal ease. The blood vessels associated with tumours are highly permeable, which may be attributed to the relatively scanty perivascular connective tissue present (Underwood and Carr, 1972; Papadimitriou and Woods, 1975). These cells may subsequently gain access to the lymphatic system via anastomoses between venules and small lymphatic vessels. Wood (1958) demonstrated the occurrence of such anastomoses. Wood also showed by microcinematography that V2 carcinoma cells penetrated the blood vessels of the ear chamber of the rabbit by active locomotion, invaded the connective tissue and infiltrated the afferent lymphatic vessels. There is much later evidence which confirms that tumour cells can pass freely from the bloodstream to the lymphatics and back to the blood, either by venolymphatic anastomoses or via the thoracic duct (Zeidman, 1955, 1957, 1961; Zeidman and Buss, 1952; Fisher and Fisher, 1965, 1966; E. R. Fisher and Fisher, 1976).

Tumour cells or emboli are carried in the afferent lymphatic branches to the regional lymph nodes. Obviously, therefore, the involvement of lymph nodes is dependent upon the site of the primary tumour and its lymphatic drainage. Since the involvement of regional lymph nodes is an indication of tumour spread, the nodal status is one of the criteria assessed in the clinical staging of the diseases (*see* pp. 135-142). Tumour cells may be trapped in the first lymph node encountered, or filter through to more distant sites. The regional nodes may even be bypassed and the tumour emboli may establish distant metastatic foci. The regional nodes may function both as an immunological barrier as well as a filter.

Dissemination of Tumours by the Blood Stream

The importance of adequate vascularization for the development of a tumour was alluded to earlier. The bloodstream also affords a means of tumour dissemination. The process of vascularization precedes tumour cell detachment and penetration into blood vessels as shown by Liotta *et al.* (1974) and Kleinerman and Liotta (1977) in the case of the experimental tumour T-241 sarcoma. These authors found small vessels in the periphery of tumours after 5 days of implantation of tumour cells into C57BL/6 mice; before this no tumour cells were found in the venous effluent. The amount of tumour material escaping into the bloodstream also appeared to be related to the diameter of the blood vessels; the greater the number of vessels exceeding 30 μm in diameter, the greater was the concentration of escaping tumour cells and emboli. Concomitant with the growth of the tumour there was also an increase in the density of vessels exceeding 30 μm. Vessels of this size allow emboli containing more than six cells to be disseminated. Thus vascularizaton of the tumour to a minimum vessel dimension and density may to a certain extent dictate the dissemination and the subsequent formation of secondary deposits. For it is known that upon the size of tumour clumps may depend successful metastasis (Liotta *et al.*, 1976). This is also supported by the observation that tumours such as carcinoma of the cervix *in situ* represent an avascular phase of growth and are not known to be accompanied by metastasis. Metastases appear after the tumour is vascularized (Folkman, 1975; Folkman and Tyler, 1977).

As mentioned before, the entry of tumour cells into the blood may be directly by the invasion of vessels, probably those at the growing edge of the tumour, or indirectly via the lymphatics. The thin-walled capillaries or venules offer little resistance to the invading tumour cells. Arteries are not normally invaded, presumably because the elastin and collagen fibres in the matrix of the walls resist the invasion. Also, it has been suggested that the resistance offered by the arteries may be due to intravascular pressure (Shivas and Finlayson, 1965). Tumour cells may penetrate the thin-walled vessels by a combination of destruction of the vessel wall by hydrolytic enzymes known to be associated with tumours (*see* pp. 85-91) and active locomotion of the tumour cells. Electron microscopy has revealed defects in the basement membrane of the endothelium of vessels in the vicinity of tumour cells (Kellner and Sugar, 1967). Furthermore, tumour cells collected from venous effluent from a primary tumour were found to be able to break down the basement membrane and purified collagen much more efficiently than cells taken from the primary tumour mass (Kleinerman and Liotta, 1977; *see also* pp. 88-89). This is consistent with the observation of Robertson and Williams (1969) that there was increased collagenase activity at the tumour periphery. Kleinerman and Liotta (1977) also suggest that there could possibly be some relationship between the integrity of the new vessels induced by the tumour and the ability of the tumour to release cells. Often the vasculature in the peripheral regions of a tumour is in the form of poorly defined vascular sinusoids. Hellman and Burrage (1969) found that ICRF159 ((±) 1,2-bis(3,5-dioxopiperazin-1-yl)propane) inhibited the metastasis of the murine Lewis lung carcinoma resulting from blood-borne dissemination. Subsequently, Salsbury *et al.* (1970) and Le Serve and Hellmann (1972) reported that in ICRF159 treated tumours, the irregular sinusoids were replaced by properly formed blood vessels. Thus, alteration in, and normalization of, the morphology of the blood vessels may alter the entry of tumour cells and emboli into the bloodstream. Whatever might be the mechanism, the release of tumour cells into the bloodstream seems to be a rapid and highly efficient process. In experimental tumours, cells have been detected in the bloodstream within twenty-four hours of implantation (Romsdahl *et al.*, 1961) and tumour cells appear in large numbers (Butler and Gullino, 1975). Butler and Gullino (1975) examined the dissemination of a mammary carcinoma (MTW9) in the Wistar-Furth rats and reported that from about 3 to 4 $\times$ 10^6 cells were released per gram per day. However, Kleinerman and Liotta (1977) estimated that about 10^3 to 10^5 cells were released per day from the T241 fibrosarcoma of C57BL mice. Although the two tumour models are entirely different, it ought to be remarked that the reported degrees of dissemination are so markedly different as to suggest the possibility that the experimental surgical procedures may have affected the outcome. Liotta *et al.* (1974) themselves have stated that tumour trauma and the rate of perfusion produce marked changes in the density of cells in the venous effluent. Griffiths (1960) and Fisher and Fisher (1967) believe that surgical procedures and even manipulation of tumours for the purposes of diagnosis may result in tumour cell release. Kleinerman and Liotta (1977) have used pressure-controlled perfusion of venous effluent. But the importance of sudden alterations in venous pressure dislodging tumour emboli (Zeidman, 1957) cannot be minimized.

Tumour Cell Lodgement

Haemostasis in the metastatic process

The tumour cells or clumps of cells that have entered the bloodstream may be carried passively to distant capillary beds where they may lodge, extravasate into the parenchyma of the organ and give rise to secondary growths. Several factors may be involved in the events leading to tumour cell arrest and lodgement.

One of the earliest observations indicated that tumour cells were organized into emboli which adhered to the capillary wall with subsequent penetration of the endothelium by the cells (Iwasaki, 1915) or plugging of minute capillaries (Baserga and Saffiotti, 1955). Wood (1958) found that V2 carcinoma cells infused into the ear chamber of rabbits adhered to the endothelium and were fixed in a thrombus consisting of fibrin and platelets. The formation of fibrin clots around tumour cells was also demonstrated by Jones *et al.* (1971) in the case of the Walker carcinoma 256, using immunofluorescence techniques. O'Meara (1958, 1964) had earlier suggested that the growth of the tumour cells depended on the formation of fibrin around the cells and that this was attributable to the secretion by the tumour cells of the so-called "cancer-coagulative factor" with properties of thromboplastin. An enzyme resembling thromboplastin was isolated by Laki *et al.* (1966), and has been reported to be associated with many tumours (Boggust *et al.*, 1968; Holyoke and Ichihashi, 1966; Holyoke *et al.*, 1972a).

Although the formation of a thrombus around a clump of tumour cells may aid the survival of the cells in the bloodstream, thrombus formation may not be an invariable event in the process of metastasis. Ogura *et al.* (1970), for instance, found no correlation between the extent of metastasis and the levels of fibrinogen in the lung. On the other hand, fibrin may disappear from the tumour emboli while it is still in the bloodstream (Chew and Wallace, 1976). Jones *et al.* (1971) and Dingemans (1974) found that fibrin disappeared within a few hours.

The available experimental evidence on this score is also conflicting. A pretreatment of the host with heparin and other sulphated polysaccharides which mainly act by inhibiting thrombin generation, reduced the incidence of metastases of some tumours (Berkarda *et al.*, 1974; Kiricuta *et al.*, 1973; Ivarsson and Rudenstorm, 1975) but not of others (Hagmar, 1970). Retik *et al.* (1962) had examined the effects of prolonged adminstration of heparin to mice which had been inoculated with sarcoma cells. They reported nearly two decades ago that such treatment appeared to increase markedly the number of metastases. Chan and Pollard (1980) examined the effects of heparin on spontaneous metastases in PA-111 rat prostate adenocarcinoma cell line. They reported an increased metastatic distribution by ipsilateral lymphatics to the lungs. They found also that the draining lymph nodes increased in weight as the incidence of lung metastases increased. Boeryd (1965) reported similar effects on mice into which chemically induced rhabdomyosarcomas had been implanted. Consistent with these was the observation that if fibrinolysis is induced by the administration of plasminogen the occurrence of metastatic deposits could be increased. On the other hand, antifibrinolysis appeared to decrease metastasis (Lang *et al.*, 1975). This is supported by the reported decrease in the numbers and weight of metastatic deposits of Lewis lung carcinoma inoculated into C57Bl/6J mice rendered hypofibrinogenemic by the administration of batroxobin accompanied by the removal of the primary tumour (Donati *et al.*, 1978). This effect was also seen if batroxobin was administered on the eleventh day after the inoculation of the animals and the primary tumour was not removed. The experiments of Donati and colleagues indicate the lodgement of disseminated tumour involving fibrin in the process. None the less, a continuous defibrination beginning with tumour implantation actually increased the metastases.

Since assessing effects of this drug on the "artificial" implantation of intravenously introduced cells would be preferable to the spontaneous metastatic development of the LL tumour, Chmielewska *et al.* (1980) examined the effects of batroxobin on the implantation of the sarcoma cells in the lungs of Balb/c mice. They reported a decrease in the metastatic deposits in lungs of animals which had been defibrinated, indicating that fibrin indeed was involved in the process of implantation of the tumour cells. However, in contradiction with their experiments with the LL tumour, with the JW sarcoma, Chmielewska *et al.* (1980) found a reduction also in spontaneous metastasis, if the host had been depleted of fibrinogen in the initial phases of tumour growth and dissemination.

These inconsistencies in the effects may be because fibrinogen plays different roles in the different phases of tumour cell dissemination and lodgement. Nevertheless, Chmielewska *et al.* (1980) have themselves pointed out that batroxobin also has an immunosuppressive effect. If this is confirmed, the picture of lung implantation of spontaneously metastasizing tumours and lodgement in the lung of intravenously introduced tumour cells in animals depleted of fibrinogen by batroxobin administration may need to be completely redrawn.

Hagmar (1972a) tested the effects of arvin, a component of Malayan pit viper venom, which has a thrombin-like action, on the metastasis of MCG-1SS sarcoma and the B16 melanoma. In neither system did the effects produced suggest any role for fibrin. Chew and Wallace (1976) found a reduction in metastasis if the tumour cells (Walker 256 carcinoma) were pre-treated with fibrolysin before implantation into the host animal.

Anticoagulants such as ancrod and coumarin derivatives have been reported to reduce the arrest of cells in the lungs and subsequent formation of tumour cell colonies, following their introduction intravenously (Hilgard and Thornes, 1976). Thus anticoagulation by coumarin not only reduces tumour colonies by intravenously injected cells (Wood *et al.*, 1956; Agostino and Clifton, 1962; Poggi *et al.*, 1978) but also spontaneous metastases of experimental solid tumours (Hilgard *et al.*, 1977; Brown, 1973a; Hoover *et al.*, 1976). The formation of metastasis from intestinal carcinomas induced by azoxymethane can be inihibited by the administration of Warfarin (Williamson *et al.*, 1980). However, the work of

Hilgard and Maat (1979) seems to suggest this antimetastatic effect could be due to other pharmacological effects than anticoagulation, such as the vitamin K deficiency induced by the drug for example. Hilgard and Maat (1979) found that although coumarin derivatives reduced tumour colonies, the effect was independent of the clotting mechanism; a restoration of coagulability by the administration of human factor IX did not affect the antimetastatic action of coumarin. Besides, a dietary deficiency of vitamin K also had an antimetastatic effect. It is also known that administration of vitamin K can negate the antimetastatic effect of Warfarin (Brown, 1973a). Williamson *et al.* (1980) found that the sensitivity to Warfarin could be increased in rats by performing distal small bowel resection, and they add a rider that this resection itself causes partial anticoagulation, presumably caused by malabsorption of vitamin K.

On the other hand, antimetastatic effects of Warfarin could be mediated by the stimulation of macrophages (Piller, 1977, 1978; Dunn *et al.*, 1977). This is suggested by the work of Maat (1980) in which he demonstrated that the Warfarin-induced decrease of tumour metastasis could be abolished by silica and carrageenan, which is a high molecular sulphated galactan obtained from seaweed. Both silica and carrageenan are known to inactivate macrophages (Allison *et al.*, 1966; Ishizaka *et al.*, 1977).

Neither does an examination of the evidence dealing with the association of fibronolytic activity with tumours allow one to draw any firm conclusions. The association of fibrinolytic activity with a number of tumour models, including virus-transformed cells, has been demonstrated (*see* pp. 86-88). But equally weighty is the evidence that points towards the lack of any correlation between fibrinolytic activity status and the malignancy of a variety of human tumours (Wilson and Dowdle, 1978) and the low and high malignancy variant lines of the B16 melanoma (Nicolson *et al.*, 1976a; *see also* p. 90). Wang *et al.* (1980), however, published evidence which completely contradicts the findings of Nicolson *et al.* (1976a). Wang *et al.* (1980) examined the plasminogen activator activity associated with the B16 melanoma (wild type) cell line, a tissue culture line (B16 mets) derived from metastatic nodules in lung of the B16 wild type, the low malignancy F1, and the high malignancy F10 variants. The plasminogen activator activity was reported by Wang *et al.* (1980) to be higher in B16 mets cells than in the B16 wild type, and also higher in the F10 variant than in the F1.

The reduction in metastases noticed following the administration of polyanionic compounds could be due to direct effects on the cell surface and consequent interference in the interactions between tumour cells and the endothelial cells. It has been shown for instance that substances such as heparin, dextran sulphate, etc. increase the net negative surface charge borne by the cells (Hagmar, 1972b; Kuroda, 1974). Such an increase in the negative charge density may enhance the repulsive forces and reduce the chances of cell arrest on the endothelial surface. An increase in surface charge density may also alter homotypic interactions of the tumour cells. The surface potential generated by the electric charges present on the cell surface is known to be involved in homotypic cell interaction and aggregation. Polyanionic compounds have been shown to inhibit homotypic aggregation (Wilkins *et al.*, 1962; Kuroda, 1974). On the other hand, polycationic compounds may promote such aggregation (Deman and Bruyneel, 1974). Thus high surface charge density could inhibit the formation of tumour cell aggregates and thereby reduce the chances of successful metastases. Successful metastases may depend both on tumour emboli of the optimal size and the numbers of tumour emboli. In comparison with cell clumps, single cells have a much slimmer chance of success at producing metastasis (Fidler, 1973b; Liotta *et al.*, 1974, 1976).

The adhesion and lodgement of individual tumour cells or cell clumps may not be such a non-specific process as this discussion might suggest. Murray *et al.* (1980) have found that cells derived from pulmonary metastatic deposits of the T-241 murine fibrosarcoma show preferential adhesion to type IV collagen rather than to type I or to plastic substratum. It would appear, therefore, that metastatic cells or cells with the potential to metastasize may possess the unique property of preferentially adhering to type IV collagen, which forms the major structural component of the basement membrane. It may be significant also that recently Liotta *et al.* (1980) have demonstrated that cells with greater metastatic potential also possess higher amounts of neutral proteinase activity which preferentially degrades types IV collagen (*see* 35-36).

It is hardly surprising, however, that some tumour cells and emboli may become fixed in a thrombus containing fibrin and cellular elements of the blood. It is indeed a well-documented fact that tumour cells interact with blood platelets while being carried in the bloodstream. When a "foreign" particle appears in the blood, a series of interactions is initiated which involves the platelets and a number of factors ordinarily present in the blood, which results in the production of thromboplastin which converts prothrombin into thrombin. In its turn, thrombin is involved in the conversion of fibrinogen to fibrin. Tumour cells may initiate these events of blood coagulation, and one result is that thrombi with the tumour cells enmeshed in the fibrin network along with the cellular elements of the blood may become established.

Circulating tumour cells are known to become involved in heterotypic interactions with platelets (Gasic *et al.*, 1973a; Warren, 1976; Warren *et al.*, 1977; Chew and Wallace, 1976) and lymphocytes (Fidler, 1974a). A possible clinical manifestation of the involvement of platelets could be a lowered platelet count, possibly as a result of platelet consumption in thrombus formation in association with tumour cells. Gasic *et al.* (1973a) found that thrombocytopenia occurred in mice following intravenous injection of tumour cells and that this was due to platelet aggregation in the capillary bed of the lungs, which are the site of metastasis. Besides, the ability of tumour cells to induce platelet aggregation appeared to correlate with their ability to induce thrombocytopenia. According to Hara *et al.* (1980), the platelet aggregating activity of the tumours resides in the plasma membrane of the cells. They showed that medium conditioned with tumour cells contained the platelet-aggregating factor, and that the component was not in solution but bound to particulate matter. A sialolipoprotein which has the ability to aggregate platelets has been extracted from SV-40 transformed Balb c/3T3 fibroblasts (Karpatkin *et al.*, 1981). This material can cause aggregation in platelet-rich plasma at a concentration of $2 \cdot 5$ μg ml^{-1}. Similar extracts made by non-transformed 3T3 cells apparently have no measurable activity at concentrations as high as 40 μg ml^{-1}. Furthermore, Karpatkin *et al.* (1981) have reported a highly significant correlation between metastatic potential and the activity of platelet aggregating material associated with them.

The ability to aggregate platelets is not an invariable attribute of tumours and only a small proportion of disseminated cells may be involved in the formation of platelet-tumour cell aggregates. Therefore it seems reasonable to suggest that factors associated with platelets may also determine, in part, the ability of a tumour to cause platelet aggregation. Bastida *et al.* (1981) have suggested that differences in aggregation responses may be one of the possible explanations for the metastatic behaviour of certain tumour types in one individual but not in others. Using a variety of tumour cell lines and platelets from a number of donors, Bastida *et al.* showed that the donors differed in the ability of their platelets to aggregate in response to the tumour cells.

Earlier, Gasic *et al.* (1968) had shown that the induction of thrombocytopenia by the injection of heterologous anti-platelet serum lowered the incidence of metastasis, but a transfusion of platelets reversed the effect. But according to Winterbauer *et al.* (1968), the association of thrombus material with tumour does not occur extensively. Of 366 carcinomas investigated, Winterbauer (1968) found embolization in less than 26% of the cases, although association of thrombus material with tumour cells was not noticed in a majority of these cases.

The adhesion of the cell complex formed of platelet, tumour and possibly also other elements such as lymphocytes to the endothelium may be an initial event in the process of lodgement and establishment of the embolus containing the tumour cells into a secondary focus of tumour growth.

Size and deformability of tumour emboli

It is reasonable to expect that homotypic interactions of circulating tumour cells, and also heterotypic interactions of the latter with cellular elements and other intrinsic factors of the blood, will play an important part in tumour cell survival and metastasis, merely by increasing the size of tumour cell clumps. Although the larger the tumour embolus the greater is the probability that it will block the tiny capillary through which it is traversing, Zeidman (1961) believed that passage of cell clumps through the capillaries is not related to the size of the clump.

Fidler *et al.* (1977) found that the high (F10) and the low (F1) malignancy variants of B16 melanoma became lodged in the lungs within 2 min after intravenous injection. Associated with the injection of tumour cells was leukopenia, which was noticed within 5 min and this accompanied the accumulation of leukocytes in the lungs. Leukopenia was also observed following the injection of tumour cells, viable or dead, but not after normal cells were injected. These observations would suggest the possibility that the melanoma cells were trapped in the capillary of the lungs as a direct result of the interactions with host cell elements and presumably leading to changes in embolus size and subsequent blockade of the capillaries (*see also* pp. 24-29). But, if the arrest of emboli did depend upon their physical trapping in capillaries, it may be expected that vasoactive compounds will affect experimental metastasis. Increases in the numbers of pulmonary colonies of intravenously injected tumour cells have been reported to occur if the target organs were exposed to x-irradiation before introduction of the cells (Withers and Milas, 1973; Brown, 1973b; Van den Brenk and Kelly, 1973, 1974). Increased clonogenic growth of intravenously injected tumour cells also occurs following the administration of vasopressor substances like epinephrine (adrenaline), and other β-adrenergic agonists (Van den Brenk *et al.*, 1976). It would appear, therefore, that vasoconstriction may produce marked effects on the arrest of tumour emboli.

Quite obviously, therefore, the deformability of tumour cells or emboli will be a factor that could affect the pattern of distribution of tumour cells. The cell surface groups are known to affect the deformability of cells. Gottschalk (1960) suggested that the charged carboxyl groups of the terminal sialic acid residues may confer structural rigidity on the underlying protein core. Weiss (1965) found that sarcoma 37 and Ehrlich ascites cells treated with neuraminidase (NANase) were more easily deformable than before treatment. At the same time, he also demonstrated that the surface charge on the cells had been reduced by the enzymic treatment, suggesting the possibility that the excision of the terminal sialic acid residues may have reduced the original rigidity of the cell membrane. That sialic acid contributes to membrane rigidity has subsequently been confirmed by Ray and Chatterjee (1975) and Wakely and England (1978). Bretscher (1973) has suggested that the stability of the erythrocyte membrane could be attributed to the glycophorin (sialoglycoprotein) molecules which interact with one another and form a lattice over the membrane. It is conceivable that the removal of the sialic acid moieties interferes with these interactions and contributes to the deformability of the cell.

It follows, therefore, that the pattern of cell arrest is liable to be altered by prior treatment of the malignant cells by NANase. Weiss *et al.* (1974) indeed reported such an effect of NANase on MC1-fibrosarcoma and the Gardner lymphosarcoma. The arrest in the lungs of both these tumours was reduced, though not in statistically significant amounts. But their localization in the liver was found to have increased significantly. Presumably the greater deformability of the cells after NANase treatment may have enabled the treated cells to escape arrest in the capillary bed of the lungs. This conclusion may be a simplistic one, since an alteration in the cell surface components would change not only deformability but also the homotypic interactions as well as heterotypic interactions with other cellular elements of the host. On the other hand, additional indirect evidence may be cited from data relating to the malignant behaviour of B16 melanoma variants and their surface charge and sialic acid content. Fidler and Nicolson (1976) reported that the initial distribution of the low malignancy (F1) and high malignancy (F10) variants of the B16 melanoma depended upon the route of injection. Thus, soon after intravenous injection more B16 cells were found in the lungs and fewer in other organs, unlike when introduced by the intracardiac route. But one day after injection, arrest of cells in lungs was independent of the route. The F10 were arrested in greater number than the F1, whereas the F1 variants also showed some extrapulmonary arrest. Bosmann *et al.* (1973) reported that the F10 variants showed greater electrophoretic mobility than the F1 variants. They also showed that this was associated with increased amounts of sialic acids in the cell membrane. Such a distribution could be expected if the surface sialic acids had the effect of rendering the F10 variants less deformable than the F1 variants.

Tumour cells may secure a foothold on the endothelium by strong active adhesion or indirectly by interaction with cellular elements of the blood, if the capillary walls are structurally imperfect or damaged. In an experimental investigation with Walker 256 carcinoma, Warren and Vales (1972) found that in areas where the endothelium was intact an embolus composed of tumour cells and platelets was formed and adhesion to the endothelial plasmalemma was by pseudopodial activity of the tumour cells. In zones of endothelial damage, fibrin formed the adhesive bond between the embolus and the capillary wall. Also, Warren *et al.* (1977) suggest that the normal variations in endothelial structure such as those described by Bennett *et al.*

(1959) may play a part in influencing the adhesion of tumour cells and cell clumps to the endothelial wall. There may be temporary gaps in the normal physiological event of shedding of endothelial cells.

These various factors which may be involved in tumour cell arrest may be summarized as shown in Fig. 2 (after Warren *et al.*, 1977).

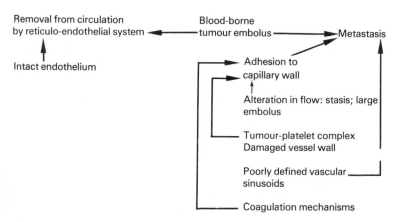

Figure 2   Factors involved in tumour cell arrest (modified after Warren *et al.*, 1977).

Diapedesis of Neoplastic Cells

Active permeation of the endothelium (diapedesis)

Facilitated in its adhesion either by imperfections in or structural damage to the endothelial wall, the tumour cells may extravasate into the extravascular space either by active diapedesis or by destruction of the endothelial basement membrane. One of the earliest investigations cited in this connection is the description by Wood (1958) of the arrest of the V2 carcinoma cells infused into vessels of the rabbit ear chamber by means of fibrin deposition around them, and the migration of the tumour cells through the basement membrane into the extravascular space. These observations were made cinematographically. The penetration of the endothelial fenestration by cellular processes has been described (Sindelas *et al.*, 1974; Dingemans, 1974). Also the discontinuities in the structure of the wall, either inherent or temporary as part of the physiological process of cell turnover, and areas of damage in the endothelial wall may afford ports of extravasation into the extravascular space. The endothelial wall may indeed be destroyed by large scale extravasation of tumour cells (Chew *et al.*, 1976; Chew and Wallace, 1976).

Using monolayer cultures of endothelial cells, Nicolson (1981) has shown that attachment of the tumour cell to the apical area of the endothelial cell stimulates a rupture of cell junctions of the endothelial monolayer and a retraction of the endothelial cell. The tumour now adheres to the exposed basal lamina and may be overlapped by the endothelial cells, thus effectively trapping the tumour cell between the endothelial surface and the basal lamina. Nicolson has also reported that the tumour cell causes a breach in the basal lamina. This could result in the release of structural components of the basement membrane such as fibronectins, glycosaminoaminoglycans, collagen, etc.

The process of extravasation will naturally be affected by factors that may contribute to changes in the permeability of the vascular endothelium. The circulating tumour cells are known to interact with blood platelets which appears to lead to their activation and aggregation (Gasic *et al.*, 1973a). Activated platelets release vasoactive compounds which alter vascular permeability. Platelets are known to contribute to the inflammatory response which normally accompanies tissue injury by releasing intracellular components (Peckham *et al.*, 1968; Mustard *et al.*, 1965). Nachman *et al.* (1970) reported that extracts, cationic in nature, made from human platelet granules could increase vascular permeability in mouse and rabbit skin via histamine release from mast cells. The active component, presumably of lysosomal origin, appears to be a basic protein of mol. wt ~ 30 000. This component produced a biphasic effect. In the acute phase (15 min), the increase in permeability caused was blocked by prior treatment with antihistamine, and involved histological oedema of perivascular tissue and dilatation of capillaries and venules. The delayed (3 h) phase was unaffected by antihistamine and characterized by leukocyte infiltration (Nachman *et al.*, 1972). Serotonin and histamine release may lead to retraction of endothelial cells forming gaps in the capillary wall, thus increasing its permeability. An increase in vasopermeability can conceivably facilitate the exit of the tumour cells from the vascular system, although neither histamine nor bradykinin appear to have much influence (Ozaki *et al.*, 1971). On the contrary, Ozaki *et al.* (1971) seem to subscribe to the view that a chemotactic factor may be involved. They have described the isolation of a substance from several human and animal tumours which apparently induces circulating tumour cells to extravasate and form metastatic deposits. The work of Ozaki *et al.* also claims that this component acts specifically on tumour cells and not on polymorphonuclear leukocytes. In consonance with this, other workers (Yoshida *et al.*, 1968; Yoshinaga *et al.*, 1971) reported the isolation of a factor chemotactic to polymorphs which had no influence on tumour cells. It is not clear, however, if a large number of these factors exist, for the establishment of metastatic deposits is a non-random event. If the factor reported by these workers were merely inducing the extravasation of tumour cells, the metastatic process should turn out to be a random event. This does not appear to be true (*see* pp. 36-38). This will then leave us to postulate why, if tumour cells extravasated randomly, successful metastases may be formed only in some organs and not in others. Essentially this would imply a specificity of interaction between the tumour cell and the target metastatic organ. This indeed fits in with the current thinking in some laboratories.

Endothelial permeability

Another factor which has been suggested to be implicated in the regulation of permeability of the endothelium is α-2-macroglobulin (Becker and Harpel, 1976; Stein-Werblowsky, 1978). Stein-Werblowsky (1980) has proposed that a thick α-2-macroglobulin layer may retain circulating malignant cells in the bloodstream, and that a thin or defective macroglobulin layer may be conducive to relatively easy extravasation. This suggestion appears to be based largely on the combination of two observations, viz. that α-2-macroglobulin is produced by mononuclear cells and that monocytic infiltration reduces haematogenous metastasis (Eccles and Alexander, 1974a). There are no experimental data which may be interpreted to support the view held by Stein-Werblowsky (1980). She has described certain experiments in which tumour cells pretreated with aprotinin apparently showed a reduced ability to metastasize. It is difficult to see how such a pretreatment would alter the permeability of the endothelium. Admittedly aprotinin may and has been shown to adhere, although not in substantial quantities, to the cell membrane. When such a cell or cell clump is arrested, the permeability may be lowered locally by the prevention of the breakdown of α-2-macroglobulin and prevent the cell from permeating the endothelium. Aprotinin is also known to be endocytosed into the cells. Possibly it may be subsequently liberated and exert its antiproteolytic activity.

   It may be that the aprotinin-treated cells are destroyed in greater numbers in the vascular system. In the author's laboratory, complex changes have been shown to occur in the expression of surface proteins and glycoproteins following aprotinin treatment. In particular, we detected greatly altered amounts of surface components of molecular weight of approximately 115 000 daltons following aprotinin treatment (*see* pp. 62-63). This could conceivably render the cells more antigenic. In any case, the evidence available to date does not indicate that α-2-macroglobulin is produced by or even associated with endothelial cells of human blood vessels (Marynen *et al.*, 1981).

Destruction of capillary walls

In a previous section, the possible role played by proteolytic enzymes known to be associated with certain neoplasms in the processes of invasion was discussed. It has in fact also been suggested that these enzymes may actively destroy the endothelial lining and the basement membrane and enable the tumour cell to escape into the extravascular environment. Kleinerman and Liotta (1977) found that malignant cells being disseminated, i.e. those found in the venous effluent from the tumour, possessed significantly greater ability to break down basement membrane and purified collagen than did the cells taken from the primary tumour mass. Once these tumour cell clumps are arrested at a distant endothelial site, the collagenolytic activity which they possess may aid in destroying the basement membrane. Chew *et al.* (1976), investigating the experimental metastases of Walker 256 carcinoma, noticed that a tumour embolus often was fixed in a fibrin clot and adhered to a small vessel. This was followed by a destruction of the endothelium and the basement membrane. The local dissolution of the basement membrane in contact with tumour cells has also been described by several other investigators (Vlaeminck *et al.*, 1972; McKinney and Singh, 1977; Babai, 1976).

The active destruction of the vessel wall to provide a port of exit is indeed a distinct possibility, but studies with the high and low malignancy variants of the B16 melanomas have provided much conflicting evidence. Bosmann *et al.* (1973) reported that *in vitro* the high malignancy variants showed greater trypsin-like and cathepsin-like activity and also higher levels of glycosidase activity. Nicolson (1977), however, was unable to confirm the differences in trypsin-like and cathepsin-like activity reported to be associated with the high malignancy variants grown in a variety of conditions. On the contrary, Liotta *et al.* (1980) found that type IV collagen degrading enzyme activity was greater in F10 variants than in the considerably less malignant F1 variants of the B16 melanoma. The line B16-BL6, which is a variant of F10 and which is more invasive *in vitro* and *in vivo* than the F10, also showed enzymic activity nearly twice as great as the F10. In addition, Liotta *et al.* (1980) also found that the cell line PMT, which is derived from pulmonary metastasis from the T241 murine sarcoma, not only possessed the highest type IV collagen degrading activity, but also the greatest metastatic potential. Earlier, Liotta *et al.* (1979a, b) had reported that neutral proteinase activity preferential to type IV collagen could be isolated from metastatic tumour cells and that this enzyme did not degrade other types of collagen or fibronectin.

When these observations are considered in conjunction with the reported absence of any type IV collagen degrading activity in association with normal adult mouse fibroblasts and their transformed but non-metastatic counterparts (Liotta *et al.*, 1980), and the presence of type IV collagen as a major structural component in the basement membrane of blood vessels (Kefalides, 1971, 1973), the active destruction of the membrane would certainly appear to be involved in both the tumour cells' entry into and their exit from the vascular system. The basic structure of basement membrane from whatever source is similar, but important differences in the organization may be found in membranes derived from different sources. Changes may also be found with ageing. In view of this, an intensive investigation into the structure and organization of basement membranes of tumour vasculature and also possible changes in their structure following treatment of tumour-bearing animals with agents such as ICRF 159 and tranexamic acid could yield useful information.

Pattern of Metastatic Distribution

Organ specificity of the metastatic process

The distribution of metastatic deposits and the mechanisms which may be involved in the organ specific deposition of metastatic cells have intrigued clinicians for several decades. While it is recognized that the mode of spread, e.g. by the lymphatic system or haematogenous, will contribute to the pattern of metastatic deposition (Willis, 1967; Del Regato, 1977), certain types of tumour do show preferential localization in certain tissues and organs, e.g. melanomas, plasmacytomas, reticulum cell sarcoma, histiocytoma and others (Kinsey, 1960; Potter *et al.*, 1957; Parks, 1974; Dunn, 1954). The demonstration of organ-specific homing of experimental tumours by Kinsey (1960) and Sugarbaker *et al.* (1971) requires a special mention. Kinsey used the Cloudman melanoma and Sugarbaker *et al.* used a murine fibrosarcoma; both tumours metastasized into the lungs when implanted into their respective hosts subcutaneously. If pieces of lung were also implanted subcutaneosly, the tumours not only metastasized into the lungs of the host animal but also into the implanted lung tissue. It is known that patients with carcinoma of the breast develop a disproportionate number of metastases in the bones compared to other tissues (Abrams *et al.*, 1950; Hoffman and Marty, 1972). Chorio-carcinomas produce a high incidence of metastases in brain and spleen but metastases in the bone are said to occur only infrequently (Willis, 1967). Another instance of organ specific metastasis is the higher risk of developing metastases in the liver borne by patients with melanomas. It would seem, therefore, that the development of metastatic deposits is a non-random event.

An involvement of mechanistic factors such as the degree of vascularity of an organ in relation to the incidence of metastasis was once advocated until Paget (1889) proposed the "soil" hypothesis; this stated in essence that the distribution of metastatic deposits largely depended upon the target organ providing optimal conditions for the survival and growth of tumour cells. None the less, the selective lodgement of tumour cells in certain organs may involve cellular specificity in terms of recognition and selective adhesive interactions between the tumour cell and the parenchymal tissue of the organ. Also, tumours may produce substances that might create the right conditions in certain organs for localization of the tumour cells leading to metastatic growth.

The B16 melanoma and its selected metastatic variants described earlier (*see* p. 11) have been extensively used as an experimental model in the investigation of the various aspects of interaction between tumour cells and metastatic target tissues. The B16-F1 and F10 variants which have been selected respectively for their low and high ability to form lung metastases, do show considerable differences as regards arrest in the lungs. The F10 cells show greater arrest in the lung than do the F1 variant cells. Furthermore, these differences in arrest occur irrespective of whether the cells were introduced intravenously or through the intracardiac pathway. Since, if introduced by the intracardiac route, the melanoma cells have to pass through the capillary beds of extrapulmonary organs before entering the lungs, unlike in the introduction into the tail vein, where the capillary bed of the lungs is first encountered by the cells, the higher pulmonary arrest of F10 than F1 would suggest that the process of arrest in the lungs is not a non-specific event (Fidler, 1975; Fidler and Nicolson, 1976). As further evidence of this organ specificity, Hart and Fidler (1980) have shown that when BL6 cells, which are a more malignant variant of F10, are introduced i.v. into animals which had subcutaneous or intramuscular implants of lungs and ovaries, they implant also in these ectopic tissues. The organ specificity of the metastatic process is also supported by the observation that long term arrest or localizaton of tumour cells does not necessarily lead to the development of clinical metastases. Hart *et al.* (1981) introduced the murine reticulum cell sarcoma M5076 into compatible hosts by the i.v. route. These were rapidly arrested and remained in the lungs for 3-4 days, after which they became detached, recirculated and finally formed definitive metastatic nodules in the liver, which is the preferential metastatic site of these tumours.

The association of the preferential metastatic ability as a property of the tumour cell membrane has been suggested by Poste and Nicolson (1980). The B16 melanoma variants have been shown to shed plasma membrane vesicles into the culture medium. Poste and Nicolson (1980) harvested the vesicles shed by the F10 variants, which are highly metastatic to the lung, and fused them with F1 cells, which are only lowly metastatic to the lungs. Such fusion is reported to have changed the metastatic pattern of the F1 to resemble that of the F10 cells. But the fusion of vesicles derived from F1 cell cultures with F10 variants did not alter the metastatic behaviour of the F10 variant.

Heterotypic adhesion

One factor which could be involved in bringing about such selective localization of circulating tumour cells is enhanced heterotypic adhesion of the tumour cells. This was demonstrated for the B16 variants using the cell capture assay technique of Walther *et al.* (1973). Nicolson *et al.* (1976c) found that the rates of adhesion to endothelial monolayers in the decreasing order were: F13 > F10 > F5 > F1.

In the author's laboratory, the adhesion behaviour of two forms of a hamster lymphosarcoma (Carter and Gershon, 1966) has similarly been studied. In this investigation unicellular suspensions were prepared from the lymposarcomas (Guy *et al.*, 1977), labelled with ^{51}Cr as described by Greaves *et al.* (1969) and added to fully confluent monolayers of hamster kidney cells (BHK and HaK) and Chang human liver cells, and the kinetics of adhesion of the lymphosarcomas to these cell monolayers were examined. The metastasizing lymphosarcoma (ML) cells adhered to the monolayers in greater numbers than did the non-metastasizing lymphosarcoma (NML). The rates of adhesion of the ML cells were greater than the NML. The highest rate of adhesion was shown by ML cells to liver cell monolayers (Guy *et al.*, 1980). Interestingly enough, liver is the major site to which the ML tumour metastasizes (Sherbet *et al.*, 1980). It may be more than coincidental that the ML cells show the highest rate of adhesion to liver, albeit of human origin. Such organ-specific adhesion has also been described for B16 melanoma cells. It was reported by Nicolson and Winkelhake (1975) and Nicolson (1977) that the melanoma variants which had been selected for greater potential to metastasize into the lungs (e.g. F13, F10) also showed greater ability to aggregate lung cells *in vitro* than the variant (F1) which has considerably lower potential for the formation of metastasis in the lungs. Such aggregation was also specific for the target organ for which the cells were selected to metastasize. Thus the lung-selected B16 variants also showed greater aggregation of lung cells than liver. There was always less aggregation with cells derived from non-target organs.

The role of cell surface components

Whether such increased and specific adhesion plays a role in organ-specific implantation of tumour cells is yet unclear. But since adhesion and adhesion-dependent phenomena of cellular aggregation are mediated by cell surface components, attempts have been made to discover possible alterations in cell surface components of tumour variants selected for specified metastatic ability. Brunson *et al.* (1978) selected the B16-F1 variant line for specific metastasis into the brain, employing the same method as that used by Fidler (1973a) for selecting B16 variants with ability for lung colonization. They developed three variants of the F1 line with increased ability to form metastasis in the brain. Brunson *et al.* (1978) then labelled the cell surface components by lactoperoxidase-catalysed iodination with ^{125}I and examined the proteins by polyacrylamide gel electrophoresis. They reported that in the brain-selected lines two exposed surface proteins of molecular weight 95 000 (95K) and 100 000 (100K) predominated, as compared with the F1 variant. Also, the degree of expression of the 95K and 100K components was related to the degree of brain selection achieved, the greater the ability of the selected cells to metastasize to the brain, the greater was the expression of these components.

On the other hand, the changes in the surface glycoproteins of variants selected for increased lung metastasis were completely different. There was an increased expression of 97, 84, 74 and 66K glycoproteins in the F10 variant, but these were absent or only weakly expressed in the F1 variant (Yogeeswaran *et al.*, 1978). These observations would require further confirmation, for Hart (1979) examined the surface protein patterns of the F1 and F10 variants and found they were qualitatively similar, although there may have been possible quantitative differences. However, since Hart (1979) has not provided the full data relating to these experiments, it is difficult to judge if any quantitative differences were statistically significant.

F10 were also reported to contain 80% more neuraminidase-accessible sialic acid than did the F1 cells. Differences were also described in ganglioside profile of the variants (Yogeeswaran *et al.*, 1978). The results reported by Raz *et al.* (1980a) contradict part of this statement. Raz *et al.* have indeed stated that the pattern of exposed surface sialoglycoprotein was similar between F1 and F10, except that the quantity of 78K sialoglycoprotein(s) expressed was inversely related to lung colonizing ability. Further, Raz *et al.* (1980b) found that while differences did exist in the clustering of anionic sites on the membranes of F1 and F10 variants, there was no difference between the cell lines as regards the total membrane sialic acid. On the contrary, Yogeeswaran *et al.* (1978) claimed that F10 cells showed a significantly reduced total sialic acid content as compared with the F1 cells.

We subjected the metastasizing hamster lymphosarcoma (ML) to a selection procedure in which secondary tumour cells were isolated from livers of hamsters bearing subcutaneous primary tumours, and injected into another hamster. This procedure was repeated five times. At the end of this selection procedure we compared the surface components of the original unselected ML cells and those of ML cells which had been passaged *in vivo* for five metastatic generations. The surface protein patterns were found to be similar in the selected as well as the unselected cells. The only quantitative difference related to protein components of average molecular weight of 20K which showed a statistically significant decrease in both primary and secondary tumour cells obtained after the *in vivo* selection (Turner *et al.*, 1980b). These investigations revealed interesting differences in their adhesion to substrata with immobilized lectins. Significantly less cells were found to adhere to wheat-germ agglutinin than to Ricin II, but more of the selected cells adhered to Gorse I. Since the lectins used have defined sugar specificities, the differences in the adhesion may be interpreted as suggesting that the expression of N-acetyl glucosamine and D-galactose containing glycoproteins is reduced in the metastatically selected cells, while that of L-fucose containing glycoproteins is increased (Guy *et al.*, 1980). Since this procedure of selection could have increased the potential of the lymphosarcoma to metastasize into the liver (Guy, 1979), it appears possible that metastatic potential may be reflected in the patterns of surface protein/glycoprotein components. Our observation of an increased adhesion of metastatically selected cells to L-fucose specific lectin (Gorse I) coated dishes is compatible with a 6-7 fold increase in fucosyl transferase activity in metastasizing mammary carcinomas as compared with non-metastasizing forms (Chatterjee and Kim, 1978). In this context, it may be mentioned also that the unselected metastasizing lymphosarcoma (ML) also showed a greater adhesion to fucose-specific lectin than did the non-metastasizing form of hamster lymphosarcoma (Turner *et al.*, 1980b). Higher amounts of fucosyl-containing glycoproteins have been reported for tumour surfaces (Van Beek *et al.*, 1973; Warren *et al.*, 1975) but their correlation with metastatic potential is unclear.

Some results reported by Reading *et al.* (1980) may also call into question any exclusive involvement of fucose-containing glycoproteins alone. These authors employed a variant line of RAW117 lymphosarcoma which had been selected *in vivo* for liver metastasis. When these cells were selected for *non*-adhesion to immobilized wheat-germ agglutinin (WGA) the selected cells were found to have lost totally the ability to metastasize into the liver. Similar selection by non-adhesion to immobilized Ricin, peanut agglutinin or Con. A did not result in a loss of metastatic ability. The obvious conclusion was that the subpopulation of cells which were highly metastatic to liver also showed adhesive specificity to immobilized WGA. Reading *et al.* (1980) did not examine the effects of selection on immobilized Gorse I lectin. None the less, it may be pointed out that the experiments performed in our laboratory on lymphosarcoma cells selected for metastasis to the liver had shown a reduction in adhesive specificity to immobilized WGA (Turner *et al.*, 1980b). It may be that alteration in both types of glycoprotein is involved with the process of metastatic selection. In contrast to the work of Reading *et al.* (1980) in which the selected cells were tested for metastatic ability, in our lymphosarcoma system there was no obvious increase in liver metastases although tumour cell yield from liver from tumour-bearing animals appeared to have increased after five selection cycles had been completed (Guy, 1979). Since our lymphosarcoma system may have attained the full metastatic potential, another way of tackling this problem would be to reverse the selection process and look for associated surface alterations.

Recently Yogeeswaran and Salk (1980) examined 32 rat and mouse tumour lines and reported that in the more malignant cell lines (showing 57-100% incidence of metastasis) there was a 1·4 fold increase in total sialic acid, a 2·0 fold increase in surface-exposed sialic acid and an even greater increase in the sialylation of surface galactose and N-acetyl galactose residues than in less malignant cell lines. Although these differences are compatible with the observations of Bosmann *et al.* (1973)—that the F10 melanoma variants possessed greater electrophoretic mobility than did F1 variant cells—not too much significance may be read into these differences. Turner *et al* (1980a), for instance, found that while metastasizing lymphosarcoma cells showed greater mobility than non-metastasizing lymphosarcoma of the hamster, isoelectric equilibrium determinations indicated the opposite. Turner *et al.* (1980a) have indeed pointed out that the distribution of ionizable groups ought to be taken into account rather than attaching too much importance to mobility in free electrophoresis, which involves only the surface electric charges residing in the outer 1 nm of the cell surface.

From this often contradictory and somewhat confusing mass of data one may perceive the emergence of a trend which would tend to suggest that the surface glycoprotein patterns of the variant lines selected for colonizing in (metastasizing to?) specific target organs may vary greatly. Whether the occurrence of specified surface components could be causally related to the organ-specific metastatic process will remain in the realms of speculation, in spite of the recent report by Shearman *et al.* (1980) on the presence of a cell surface antigen(s) detectable by monoclonal antibody correlated with organ-specific metastasis.

Shearman *et al.* used a liver-specific metastatic variant of a lymphoma cell line transformed by Marek's disease virus (MDV). They produced antitumour cell hybridomas by fusing spleen cells derived from mice injected i.v. with MDCC-AL2 cells, which are a liver-specific metastatic variant, with 315·43 myeloma cells. Several antibody producing clones were obtained, of which one (1·20) reacted specifically with the AL2 cells. The 1·20 antigens appeared to be associated with specific metastasis to liver, for pretreatment of AL2 cells with 1·20 antibody blocked the ability of the cells to colonize embryonic liver *in ovo* tests. Another monoclonal antibody, the 1·5 antibody, similar in specificity to the 1·20 antibody, could not inhibit formation of liver foci by AL2. The 1·5 antibody, which directly agglutinates AL2 cells, significantly enhanced the number of foci on the chorioallantoic membrane. This is interpreted as indicating that the homing of the AL2 cells to liver is not a non-specific process of trapping of tumour cell emboli. Shearman *et al.* (1980) found that about 20% of AL2 cells carried the 1·20 antigen and also a strong correlation between the expression of this antigen and the ability of the cells to form liver metastasis.

Other mechanisms could also be postulated. For example, adhesive specificities between tumour cells and target organ tissue could be achieved by differences in the distribution of surface components accompanied by differences in the fluidity of the membrane of the cell.

Prostaglandins and Tumour Metastasis

A few years ago it was reported that experimental metastases can be inhibited by the administration of aspirin, this action of aspirin being related to decreased platelet aggregation *in vivo* (Gasic *et al.*, 1972; Kolenich *et al.*, 1972). Wood and Hilgard (1972), however, were unable to confirm the antimetastatic effects of aspirin. These authors found that no statistically significant reduction in the metastasis of V2 carcinoma of the rabbit was caused by aspirin, even though the ability of platelets to aggregate had been reduced demonstrably. Powles *et al.* (1973a) suggested that the effect of aspirin could be due to an inhibition of release of lysosomal enzymes. For they found that Walker tumour cells injected intra-aortically developed deposits in soft tissues and in the bone with associated hypercalcaemia. However, if the animals were treated with aspirin and indomethacin, tumour deposits were seen only in the soft tissues. Although this continued deposition of tumour cells in soft tissues in spite of aspirin administration again contradicts the role of platelet aggregation, there are common links in these observations.

It is known that prostaglandins, which are naturally occurring cyclic metabolites of unsaturated fatty acids, are osteolytic in nature (Powles *et al.*, 1973b) and are also involved in the process of platelet aggregation. Circulating tumour cells have been shown to activate blood platelets, which may then aggregate. This has been shown both *in vivo* and *in vitro* (Gasic *et al.*. 1973; Copley and Witte, 1976; Warren, 1974), and activated platelets are also a source of prostaglandin (Santoro *et al.*, 1976).

Drugs such as aspirin and indomethacin inhibit the synthesis of prostaglandins from arachidonic acid. Tumours are known to produce prostaglandins and it appears that they may be involved in the metastatic process. It would be worthwhile, therefore, to describe briefly this group of compounds which subserve numerous physiological functions.

Prostaglandins are cyclic metabolites derived from the C_{20} fatty acids, arachidonic acid and ecosatrienoic acid. The series 2 and 1 prostaglandins are derived from these precursors respectively. The mobilization of arachidonic acid from phospholipids by the action of phospholipases is the first step in the synthesis of prostaglandins. The arachidonic acid is metabolized to the endoperoxides, viz. PGG_2 and PGH_2, which are themselves precursors for PGI_2, PGE_2, $PGE_{2\alpha}$ and the thromboxanes A_2 and B_2 (Fig. 3).

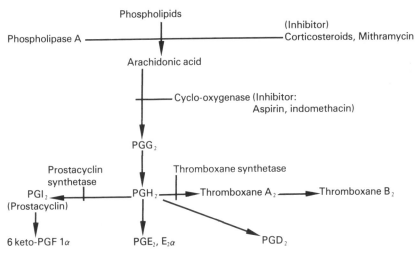

Figure 3 Metabolism of arachidonic acid and the biosynthesis of prostaglandins and thromboxanes.

The synthesis of prostaglandins can be inhibited by inhibiting the mobilization of arachidonic acid by using corticosteroids and mithramycin, or by inhibiting the action of the cyclo-oxygenase, which can be achieved by aspirin and indomethacin.

In the past few years, numerous reports have appeared which indicate that, both in experimental neoplasms as well as human tumours, greater amounts of prostaglandins may be extracted from the tumour than from the corresponding normal tissue (Powles *et al.*, 1973; Tashjian *et al.*, 1974; Galasko, 1976; Galasko and Bennett, 1976; Levine *et al.*, 1972; Bennett *et al.*, 1975, 1976, 1977; Powles *et al.*, 1976; Atkins *et al.*, 1977). Tumour cells also produce prostaglandins *in vitro* (Goldyne *et al.*, 1978; Humes and Strausser, 1974; Plescia *et al.*, 1975). The biosynthesis of prostaglandins appears to be enhanced in neoplastic cells, as demonstrated by Trevisani *et al.* (1980) for the Yoshida ascites hepatoma AH130. When incubated *in vitro*, these hepatoma cells produced PGE_2 to the same level as in normal hepatocytes during the first two hours in culture. Subsequently, however, the rate of biosynthesis increased rapidly to approximately a four-fold increase after six hours in culture. These authors also demonstrated that the biosynthetic process could be enhanced by supplying sodium arachidonate; such an increase could be blocked by the action of indomethacin or L8027, which is also a prostaglandin synthetase inhibitor.

The induction of tumours by chemical carcinogens may also be influenced by prostaglandins. Lupulescu (1978) found that the induction of squamous cell carcinoma by 3-MCA could be enhanced by the injection of PGE_2 and PGE_{2a}. The addition of carcinogens or tumour-promoting phorbol diesters to *in vitro* cell cultures appears to stimulate the release of prostaglandins into the culture medium (Hong *et al.*, 1976, 1977; Levine, 1977; Levine and Hassida, 1977). Ashendel and Boutwell (1979) showed that the ability of various phorbol esters to raise PGE levels correlated with their tumour promoting activity. It may be worthwhile pointing out, however, that prostaglandins may also be associated with host stromal and inflammatory cells rather than exclusively with neoplasms themselves (Bennett *et al.*, 1980). The increase in prostaglandin-like activity in primary and metastatic squamous carcinoma of the neck appeared to bear no relationship either to tumour size, site or the degree of tumour differentiation. Rolland *et al.* (1980) have reported to the contrary. In a study involving 91 cases of carcinoma of the breast selected to reflect natural histological distribution, they found greater amounts of prostaglandins in stage T1 and T2 tumours than in T3 and T4 (*see* pp. 135-138 for TNM classification) with the more cellular the tumours and the more adherent the cells were to one another, the higher was the PG content. Although the tumour size may be accepted as showing some relationship to PG content, claims of an association between histological differentiation and PG content may be deemed as unsubstantiated.

None the less, the association of prostaglandin with the establishment and growth of metastases has been demonstrated by Kibbey *et al.* (1978) in a series of rat mammary carcinomas. They reported that the carcinoma SMT-2A which was metastatic contained less PGE_2 and prostaglandin synthetase than tumours MTW9A and MTW9B, neither of which can form metastases. The hypercalcaemia associated with certain non-metastatic cancers of murine origin has been attributed to the production of PGE_2 by the tumours (Tashjian, 1978; Tashjian *et al.*, 1972).

Fitzpatrick and Stringfellow (1979) and Stringfellow and Fitzpatrick (1979) have reported an inverse correlation of PGD_2 with metastatic potential. According to these reports, PGD_2 is the principal arachidonic acid metabolite produced by the high and low malignancy variants (F10 and F1 respectively) of the B16 melanoma cells, and the F1 variants produced greater amounts of PGD_2. Stringfellow and Fitzpatrick (1979) found that a pretreatment of F10 and F1 variants with indomethacin resulted in an increase in the occurrence of metastatic colonies in the lungs. The involvement of the prostaglandins in the metastatic process was further confirmed by the observation that the increased metastatic effect of indomethacin could be reversed by exogenous administration of PGD_2. Stringfellow and Fitzpatrick (1979) interpret these results as suggesting that the PGD_2 inhibition of metastasis is produced by the suppression of platelet aggregation. PGD_2 has been shown to inhibit platelet aggregation in several species (Smith *et al.*, 1976; Nishizawa *et al.*, 1975). Although these investigations do appear to suggest that PGD_2 plays a direct role in regulating the formation of metastatic deposits in the lung, they also imply that the prostaglandin is produced exclusively by the tumour cells.

A second uncertainty about these and similar experiments is in the context of the tumour models themselves. Experiments of the type which involve the introduction of the tumour cells into the tail vein at best indicate the arrest of the cells at the first capillary bed encountered, and this process is far removed from the process of spontaneous metastasis. Since platelets themselves can synthesize PGE_2 (Smith and Willis, 1971), it would be somewhat speculative at this stage to attribute to prostaglandins a role in the regulation of the metastatic process by interfering with platelet aggregation. On the other hand, the investigation of Rolland *et al.* (1980), while also indicating an involvement of PG in the metastatic process, shows a direct correlation. In 91 breast cancer patients, they recorded higher PG contents in tumours which had already disseminated into the lymphatics and blood vessels. They also claimed that the PG content of metastatic cells in the lymph nodes was greater than that of the primary tumours. These authors appear to believe that PGs occur early in the development of breast cancers and that there is an elevation of PG levels at the time of active invasion by the tumour. In the experience of other investigators, e.g. Bennett *et al.* (1975), the greater the PGE_2 content of human breast carcinoma, the greater was the likelihood that it would metastasize to bone. Consistent with these observations is the reported reduction in the incidence of metastasis by the administration of aspirin and indomethacin (Gasic *et al.*, 1973b; Kolenich *et al.*, 1972; Giraldi *et al.*, 1980).

The possibility still exists that osteolysis may favour the osteotropic behaviour of certain tumours. As discussed earlier, the work of Powles *et al.* (1973a) indicates the association of osteolysis with the deposition of Walker carcinoma cells in the bone. Another study which may be cited in this context is that of Strausser and Humes (1975). These authors showed that injection of the Maloney sarcoma virus into Balb/c mice induced tumours in the leg. However, treatment of the animals with indomethacin at the time of tumour induction appeared to reduce tumour growth, and inhibit invasion of the bone and osteolysis. In a short series of human breast cancers, the presence of bony metastases at the time of examination or subsequent development of such metastases has been reported to correlate with the ability of the primary tumours to induce osteolysis *in vitro*; such *in vitro* osteolytic activity being inhibitable by indomethacin (Powles *et al.*, 1976), though not fully characterized. However, the possibility that other humoral osteolytic factors may be involved in the osteotropic behaviour of breast carcinomas cannot be excluded (Bockman and Myers, 1977). Besides, osteolysis may also be produced by enzymes such as collagenase and trypsin (Powles *et al.*, 1977) which are known to be associated with tumours (*see* pp. 85-90).

A third possibility is the indirect stimulation of osteoclastic activity. Horton *et al.* (1972) detected an osteolytic substance (the osteoclast-activating factor, OAF) from media in which peripheral blood leukocytes were cultured, subsequently shown to be released by the leukocytes (Trummel *et al.*, 1975). OAF may be released by lymphocytes following antigenic stimulation (Horton *et al.*, 1974).

A further complication is the known immunosuppressive action of certain prostaglandins. Prostaglandin E is known to inhibit lymphokines (Gordon *et al.*, 1976; Lomnitzer *et al.*, 1976), which are factors produced by sensitized lymphocytes, and inhibit also the production of antibodies by the B-lymphocytes (Bray *et al.*, 1974; Morley, 1974; Quagliata *et al.*, 1973) and mitogen-induced proliferation of lymphocytes (Smith *et al.*, 1971). It has been postulated, therefore, that at least in so far as PGE is concerned, its excessive production by tumours may produce immune suppression and thus allow tumour development and metastasis to take place (Humes and Strausser, 1974).

Plescia *et al.* (1975) showed that two murine tumours which produced large amounts of PGE_2 may be immunosuppressive *in vivo*. The probable immunosuppression mediated by the tumour, of course, was demonstrated using *in vitro* assay of rosette formation by sheep RBCs and mouse splenocytes. This suppression could be partially abolished by indomethacin and other inhibitors of prostaglandin synthetase (Plescia *et al.*, 1975; Grinwich and Plescia, 1977). Although Plescia *et al.* (1975) have attributed the retardation of tumour growth in some mouse tumour models by indomethacin and aspirin to a reversal of prostaglandin E-mediated immunosuppression, the evidence may be considered as being circumstantial. Admittedly, however, the major targets of locally produced prostaglandins are the lymphocytes and/or macrophages. These are known to contain PGE-sensitive adenylate cyclases. After cyclic AMP increases are achieved, these cells are known to become less sensitive to various stimuli. The tumour may produce increased amounts of PGE_2 as a response to an immunological assault by the host. This is indicated by the increased PGE_2 production response by tumour cells in the presence of lymphocytes (Owen *et al.*, 1980). Owen *et al.* (1980) state in no uncertain terms that the contribution to PGE_2 levels by the lymphocytes themselves was minimal.

Much of the preceding discussion has considered the tumour cell as an exclusive source of prostaglandins. The immunosuppressive function may be mediated by prostaglandin-producer non-specific suppressor cells (*see also* pp. 71-73). Humes *et al.* (1977) showed that activated macrophages were producers of prostaglandins. The PGE_2 produced by macrophage subsets has been found to control lectin-mediated lymphocyte proliferation. If the prostaglandin production is inhibited, mitogen-induced proliferation increases, but the proliferation levels return to normal on the addition of extraneous PGE_2 (Goodwin *et al.*, 1977, 1978).

Tumour Cell Interactions with the Immune System

Introduction

The presence of circulating tumour cells has often been demonstrated in human as well as experimental cancers (Griffiths and Salsbury, 1965; Salsbury, 1975; Carter, 1978a). Fidler (1976) found that when tumour cells are introduced into animals intravenously, less than 0·1% of the original number of cells survives, implants successfully and forms metastatic deposits. It may be expected that a proportion of the cells is subjected to mechanical damage and that a majority of the circulating cells is destroyed by humoral factors and/or cell-mediated cytotoxicity. The malignancy or innocence of tumours essentially implies the ability of certain tumours to form metastatic deposits and the lack of it in certain others. This ability may lie in cells of some tumours being able to escape from the immune surveillance of the host, while others are completely destroyed by it. In this section, therefore, an attempt will be made to examine the interaction of the tumour cell with the host's immune mechanism, with a view to establishing possible differences between non-metastasizing and metastasizing tumours.

It was believed in the early decades of this century that neoplasms were freely transplantable into allogeneic recipients. The compatibility between the tumour and the host was presumed to be due to the loss of histocompatibility antigens. However, in the 1950s it was shown that if a tumour growing in an isogeneic host was ligated and allowed to undergo necrosis, the animal would reject subsequent challenge with the tumour (Foley, 1953), but in similar experiments the inbred hosts allowed the exchange of skin grafts (Prehn and Main, 1957). This firmly pointed towards the involvement of the host's immune system in the development of the tumour. It is now known that a majority of experimental tumours induced by means of chemical carcinogens or transforming viruses carry associated transplantation antigens against which the syngeneic host can be fully immunized and induced to reject the tumour.

One way of assessing the possible prognosis of the disease would be to evaluate the extent and depth of the response made by the host's immune system. Cellular immune response has long been held to be of greater significance than the humoral response in the rejection of tumours (Alexander and Fairley, 1967). Therefore, the degree and nature of infiltration of tumours by cellular elements of the host's immune system could be indicative of the aggressiveness of the neoplasm.

The significance of lymphocytic infiltration

The presence of leukocytes in and around tumours is a common feature. The infiltration of tumours, especially by host lymphocytes, has long been recognized as a prominent feature in the histology of both animal and human tumours (Wade, 1908; Sistrunk and MacCarty, 1920; MacCarty, 1922; Foote and Stewart, 1946).

Sistrunk and MacCarty (1920) reported about a 25% increase in postoperative survival of patients with mammary cancers that showed lymphocytic infiltration. Ioachim (1976) has demonstrated the occurrence of dense aggregates of lymphocytes in various carcinomas *in situ*. Ioachim *et al.* (1976a) also compared the degree of lymphocytic infiltration in relation to the histology of fifty carcinomas of the lung. Cellular infiltration was found to be the greatest in squamous cell carcinoma but there was little or no lymphocytic infiltration in oat-cell carcinomas. Also, the more differentiated tumours produced greater host cell response than did the poorly differentiated carcinomas. This relationship had previously been found by MacCarty and Blackford (1912) in a series of gastric cancers, and is compatible with the observation of Willis (1973) that lymphocytes tend to be more numerous in slow growing well-differentiated tumours than in fast growing anaplastic ones, and in accord with the adage that differentiated function and cell division and growth are mutually exclusive states.

Hamlin (1968) stated that the degree of lymphocytic infiltration of human mammary carcinoma indicated a favourable prognosis. A good prognosis of medullary carcinomas of the breast was indicated by lymphocytic and plasma cell infiltration (McDivitt *et al.*, 1968; Bloom *et al.*, 1970). Also, in Hodgkin's disease a correlation between lymphocytic infiltration and favourable prognosis has been recognized (Keller *et al.*, 1968). Carter (1978a) has generally endorsed the view that tumours with dense and organized host cell infiltration may carry a better prognosis than similar lesions which lack well developed host cell infiltration. Recently, Pagnini *et al.* (1980) have reported that the five-year survival of patients with squamous cervical carcinoma was around 80% in cases where lymphocytic infiltration was moderate to marked, while for patients with no lymphocytic infiltration of tumours, the comparative figure for five year survival was only about 40%. Willis (1973), however, has expressed several reservations regarding the implications for prognosis of lymphocytic and plasma cell infiltrates of tumours. The functional significance of these infiltrates especially is still unclear, although it is believed that the infiltrates could represent cell-mediated and humoral responses made by the host against the tumour (Ng and Atkin, 1973; Van Nagell *et al.*, 1977, 1978).

The majority of lymphocytes infiltrating tumours appear to be T-lymphocytes and have been described as being in the activated form (Haskill *et. al.*, 1975; Jondal and Klein, 1975; Gallili *et al.*, 1979). Infiltration by plasma cells, however, appears to be a distinguishing feature of squamous cell carcinomas. Again, the extent of infiltration appears to be related to the degree of differentiation of the carcinoma (Ioachim, 1976). These infiltrating cells are probably also immunologically active as indicated by the fact that immunoglobulins against tumour-specific antigens have been demonstrated in eluates of both animal and human tumours (Ran and Witz, 1972; Thunold *et al.*, 1973; Watson *et al.*, 1974). In spite of the possible inverse relationship between the degree of infiltration and the clinical aggressiveness of the neoplasm, there seems to be no correlation between the pattern of metastatic spread and the host cell responses. Husby *et al.* (1976) have, however, reported that B-lymphocytes may be associated with metastatic deposits.

The role of macrophages

Most solid tumours have been reported to contain macrophages or cells possessing properties of macrophages (Milgrom *et al.*, 1968; Evans, 1972;

Tønder and Thunold, 1973; Wood *et al.*, 1975; Kerbel *et al.*, 1975). The macrophage content can vary widely. Evans (1972) reported the macrophage content as high as 60% in some tumours. Wood and Gillespie (1975) found murine solid tumours to contain 9-54% large non-malignant cells bearing receptors on their surfaces for immunoglobulin F_c. These cells showed rapid adhesion to plastic, which was relatively resistant to trypsin, phagocytosed latex particles and were lysed by antimacrophage antisera in the presence of complement. Also, using the Fc receptors to distinguish between host and tumour cells, host cell infiltration on a large scale has been demonstrated by Kerbel and colleagues (Kerbel and Davies, 1974; Kerbel *et al.*, 1975; Kerbel and Pross, 1976). Subsequently, Wood and Gollahon (1977) investigated a series of 36 human tumours of various histopathological types. Of these, 22 tumours contained between 2-56% immunoglobulin Fc-positive cells, which they then characterized by means of non-specific esterase staining, phagocytic ability and morphology to be approximately 95% macrophages.

Whether macrophages play a role in the immunity against the tumour is a controversial topic. They are believed to be implicated as effector cells in the immune response made by the host to the neoplasm (Nelson, 1976). The interactions between tumour cells and macrophages are complex, as a consequence of which both cell types are affected. Tumours appear to be able to suppress macrophage activity (North *et al.*, 1976; Saba and Antikatzides, 1975; Snyderman and Pike, 1976; Snyderman *et al*, 1976). An impairment of macrophage function can be achieved *in vitro* by sera from tumour bearing animals (Otu *et al.*, 1977) or by culture media conditioned by tumours *in vitro* (North *et al.*, 1976; Otu *et al.*, 1977). On the contrary, there are several reports that tumours can stimulate macrophages (Meltzer *et al.*, 1977; Poste, 1975; Roblin *et al.*, 1977; Snodgrass *et al.*, 1977; Mantovani, 1978). Thus cocultivation of tumour cells and macrophages may stimulate the latter (Kaplan and Seljelid, 1977).

Macrophages are known to possess tumoricidal activity. Peritoneal macrophages are cytotoxic *in vivo* as well as *in vitro* to tumour cells, allogeneic or syngeneic, against which the animals are immunized (Alexander *et al.*, 1972; Alexander and Evans, 1971; Eccles and Alexander, 1974a, b; Den Otter *et al.*, 1972; Evans and Alexander, 1970, 1972). Macrophages isolated from MSV-induced primary tumours are cytotoxic to tumour cells (Holden *et al.*, 1976; Puccetti and Holden, 1979; Taniyama and Holden, 1979). The cytolytic activity may be enchanced by the use of the immunological adjuvants BCG and *Corynebacterium parvum*, which have been reported to increase macrophage activity and content of tumours (Baldwin and Pimm, 1973; Likhite, 1974; Woodruff *et al.*, 1976). Earlier, Alexander and Evans (1971) had reported that macrophage activation can be achieved *in vitro* by treatment of the cells with bacterial endotoxins, double stranded nucleic acids derived from viruses, and by synthetic polynucleotides such as poly I:C. The naturally occurring tetrapeptide, the so-called Tuftsin (Najjar and Nishioka, 1970; Nishioka *et al.*, 1972, 1973), which is associated with IgG, has been shown to enhance the cytotoxic activity of neutrophils and peritoneal macrophages against human and murine tumour cells (Nishioka, 1979a, b). Activation could also occur *in vivo*. Dextran sulphate and zymosan are also able to stimulate macrophage function (Schultz *et al.*, 1977a, b, 1978).

A distinction may be made that whilst macrophages activated by the immunization of mice with syngeneic tumour cells were cytotoxic to the tumour cells in an immunologically specific manner (Evans and Alexander, 1970), the cytotoxic ability of macrophages activated by means of extraneous agents does not involve any immunological specificity. However, lymphocyte-mediated activation of macrophages appears to involve specificity towards the antigen or tumour employed to sensitize the lymphocytes (*see* pp. 54-56).

If activated macrophages are cytotoxic to tumour cells *in vitro* as well as *in vivo*, it may be expected they will influence the development of the tumour and possibly also the metastatic process. The relationship between macrophage content and tumour dissemination has been examined by several investigators. Eccles and Alexander (1974) reported that the percentage of tumour-associated macrophages was directly related to the immunogenicity of the tumour and inversely to its metastatic potential. An inverse correlation between metastatic potential and macrophage content was also described by Lauder *et al.* (1977). Wood and Gillespie (1975) found that if a tumour cell suspension was depleted of macrophages by taking advantage of their adherence to plastic surfaces and injected into animals, the resultant tumours displayed increased metastatic potential. On the other hand, when mice with established pulmonary metastases were injected with syngeneic macrophages that had been activated *in vitro*, a dramatic reduction was noticed in the lung nodules (Fidler, 1974b). *Corynebacterium parvum* is also able to reduce lung colonization by tumour cells injected intravenously (Bomford and Olivotto, 1974), presumably effected by the activation of macrophages. *C. parvum* is generally regarded as an agent which activates host macrophages (Scott, 1974; McBride *et al.*, 1975; Woodruff *et al.*, 1976; Woodruff and Warner, 1977; Bjornsson *et al.*, 1978), but other mechanisms such as the induction of suppressor cells (Kirchner *et al.*, 1974) or the enhancement (by *C. parvum* and also BCG) of natural killer (NK) cell activity (Oehler and Herberman, 1978; Oehler *et al.*, 1978) have also been suggested. A non-specific stimulation by the administration of BCG before inoculation of the tumour has also been reported to increase the macrophage infiltration of the tumour and lead to a small reduction in the incidence of metastases (Eccles and Alexander, 1974).

Gershon *et al.* (1967a) and Birkbeck and Carter (1972) working with metastasizing (ML) and non-metastasizing (NML) forms of a hamster lymphosarcoma observed that activated macrophages were invariably associated with the non-metastasizing tumour but they were scarce or absent in the metastasizing lymphosarcoma. Schirrmacher *et al.* (1979a) have made similar observations in a methylcholanthrene-induced lymphosarcoma system of which, as in the case of the hamster lymphosarcoma, a metastasizing and a non-metastasizing form are available. In histology, the non-metastasizing (NML) tumour, was found to have been heavily infiltrated by host macrophages. In sharp contrast, the metastasizing (ML) form contained few macrophages. Besides, peritoneal macrophages obtained from hamsters previously sensitized with NML implants and mixed with the tumour cells in the proportion of 1:10 produced no tumours when injected into new hosts. In similar experiments, tumour cells mixed with lymphocytes from spleen could produce tumours in 50% of the animals injected.

Parallel experiments with macrophages derived from animals carrying the ML tumours may be of some value, and could enable a comparison to be made of the functional status of macrophages from non-metastasizing and metastasizing tumours. Recently Mantovani (1978) reported that macrophages from mice bearing the chemically induced non-metastasizing tumour the FS6 sarcoma, were cytotoxic to the tumour cells *in vitro*. But macrophages from mice bearing a metastasizing variant of this tumour, the weakly immunogenic mFS6, enhanced the proliferative activity of the tumour. It could be postulated that these differences in the tumour inhibitory activity are achieved by means of a blocking mechanism such as the incessant shedding of membrane-bound antigen from metastasizing tumours. Davey *et al.* (1976) proposed that an instability or high turnover of membrane-bound antigen could be an integral feature of the metastatic process and that a relationship may exist between the lability of membrane components and the capacity to metastasize.

Much circumstantial evidence, based on the stimulation or the suppression of macrophages activity, for their involvement in the development of metastasis may be adduced. Coumarin derivatives such as Warfarin have been found to have an antimetastatic effect not mediated by blood coagulation factors. Kovach *et al.* (1965) found that Coumarin (5-6-benzo-α-pyrone) increased carbon clearance of the blood. Subsequent work has shown that the administration of this drug enhances phagocytic activity by macrophages (Piller, 1976a, b, 1977, 1978; Dunn *et al.*, 1977). Coumarin administration also increases the total number of macrophages (Piller, 1978). On the basis of these reports, the antimetastatic activity of Coumarin could conceivably be attributed to macrophages. In support, instances may also be cited where macrophage inhibitors have led to the abolition of Warfarin-mediated antimetastatic effects (*see* pp. 26-27). The potentiation of tumour growth as a result of administration of macrophage inhibitors has also been reported by several authors (Thomson and Fowler, 1977; Keller, 1976; Lotzova and Richie, 1977).

Both phagocytic and non-phagocytic mechanisms have been implicated in the destruction of tumour cells. The non-specifically activated macrophage may act via non-phagocytic means such as those involving the release of lysosomal enzymes (Hibbs, 1974a, b). In any case, a discussion of which of these is involved in a major way would be academic, for phagocytosis is a plasma membrane activity in which lysosomes are often involved (Stossel, 1975). Stimulation of macrophages by materials such as zymosan is also known to cause the release of lysosomal hydrolases (Davies and Allison, 1976). But it is unclear how specific killing of the tumour cells can be achieved by this mechanism. Currie and Basham (1975) obtained a soluble factor from endotoxin-treated macrophages which was said to be selectively cytotoxic to cancer cells. If the tumoricidal effect of macrophages is indeed produced by an intermediary toxin, there will be no need for macrophages to be in the close vicinity of the tumour, nor for contact between the two cell types. One may recall, however, that Evans and Alexander (1970) had observed that a close contact between the activated macrophages and the tumour cells is required for cell kill to occur and that phagocytosis of the tumour cell occurs only when the latter has been extensively damaged. This indicates that the membrane surface may be involved in the cytocidal action of the macrophages. Consistent with this is the reported finding that the cytocidal action of macrophages could be altered if their membrane components were deleted by enzymatic digestion (Hakim, 1980).

The arrest of tumour cells and their subsequent development into tumour nodules may be seen simply as a degree of retention of the cells over the rate of their clearance from the organs by the involvement of the reticulo-endothelial system (RES).

The administration of RES stimulants has occasionally led to increased pulmonary metastasis (Pimm and Baldwin, 1975; Proctor *et al.*, 1976, 1977). Stiteler *et al.* (1978) described similar effects of glucan in an experimental tumour of DBA2 mice. In mice undergoing chronic response to bacterial endotoxin and zymosan, the retention in the lungs of i.v. introduced B16 melanoma cells was reduced with parallel reductions in the numbers of tumour nodules in the lungs (Glaves, 1980). Acute response to RES stimulants, on the other hand, facilitates the rentention of tumour cells. Glaves points out that approximately 90% of i.v. injected cells are arrested in the lungs within five minutes. In the following two hours, a majority of these are rapidly cleared. The clearance rate drops sub-sequently, leaving approximately 3% of the injected cells in the lungs after 24 hours. Glaves says that her observations indicate that the RES parti-cipates in a specific step in the metastatic cascade, since this most active (2 h) period of clearance is also the period when maximal changes could be brought about in tumour cell retention using RES stimulants.

A fairly recent report by Evans and Lawler (1980) shows no correlation between the immune status of the host and the macrophage content of tumours. They investigated a series of 33 MCA-induced murine sarcomas. Animals were sensitized by implanting tumour cells and excising the tumours after 10 days. In another method, sensitized animals were sub-lethally irradiated 10 days after extirpation of the tumours. These animals were then challenged with the tumour that had been used for sensitization. The growth of tumours in control mice and in sensitized mice was recorded. These data were then transformed into an immunogenicity ratio which is the ratio of mean tumour diameter of control mice and that of sensitized mice. No relation appeared to exist between the macrophage content of the tumour and the immunogenicity ratio. Although the duration of tumour growth before excision and the subjection of animals to irradiation could have affected the macrophage content of the tumours, an alteration of the immunological status of the host by either method does not seem to have brought about a major change in the macrophage content of the tumours.

In résumé, the participation of macrophages in tumour development and dissemination may be described in terms of (a) their infiltration into the developing tumour, the degree of infiltration probably reflecting prognosis of the disease when assessed in conjunction with other host cell infiltrates; (b) their activation to become tumoricidal—macrophages may be activated by immunization with tumour cells or by the administration of extraneous agents; and (c) the cytotoxic effect which may be specific or non-specific—being presumably dependent upon the mode of activation.

This résumé inevitably directs the discussion to certain allied problems such as: what causes the macrophages to migrate towards and infiltrate into the tumours; what are the mechanisms involved in the processes of activation of the macrophages and the subsequent destruction of tumour cells?

The cell-mediated destruction of tumour cells involves an extensive interplay of and co-operation between lymphocytes and macrophages (Alexander *et al.*, 1972). Sensitized lymphocytes liberate an array of biologically active substances which mediate the processes of cellular immunity. Among these are factors chemotactic to macrophages, lympho-toxins, macrophage activating factors (MAF) and migration inhibitory factors (MIF). It has been suggested on the basis of *in vitro* studies that the chemotactic factor induces the migration of the macrophages towards the tumour (David, 1975). Vassalli *et al.* (1976) have postulated that plasmin production may be involved in the process of migration of macrophages from the bloodstream into neighbouring tissues. As discussed in a later section (pp. 86-87), a higher plasminogen activator content has been described in a variety of malignant tissue (but *see* pp. 87-88) and it is conceivable that an enhanced production of plasmin by tumours may be involved in the directional migration of macrophages. It is unclear how such an effect could be achieved. The findings of Hakim (1980) are that the cytocidal action of PHA-induced macrophages is reduced by treatment of the latter with proteolytic enzymes including plasmin. It is difficult to reconcile this inhibitory effect of plasmin with its alleged ability to induce migration of the macrophages towards the tumour. Neuraminidase, on the contrary, increases the cytocidal effect of the macrophages. All the enzymes used by Hakim not only remove cell surface components or the terminal sialic acid moiety in the case of neuraminidase, but they also may bring about a considerable alteration in the conformation of the membrane components (*see* Sherbet, 1978). Indeed, it has been claimed that enzymes such as trypsin and neuraminidase remain adsorbed to the cell surface (Bernard *et al.*, 1969; Poste, 1971; Sachtleben *et al.*, 1972). Hakim has in no way monitored the effect of his enzyme treatment of the macrophages *per se*. Therefore, apart from suggesting or confirming an earlier view of Evans and Alexander (1970) of a requirement of close contact between the macrophages and the tumour cells, the experiments of Hakim (1980) do not suggest any significant change in our state of knowledge of the cytocidal action.

It is known, nevertheless, that the neutral proteinase, plasmin, can exert a variety of effects such as the generation of inflammatory mediators (Cochrane *et al.*, 1973) and kinins, which are known to increase vascular permeability (Kaplan and Austen, 1971). Plasmin is also said to be able to degrade basement membrane (Lack and Rogers, 1958). These processes could conceivably aid the infiltration of tumour tissue by macrophages.

Plasminogen activator activity is not a universal feature of malignant tumours. Several malignant tumours have been described which appear to have no associated plasminogen activator activity. It would be of some considerable interest, therefore, to see if there was any correlation between the degree of macrophage infiltration of tumours and the level of plasminogen activator activity which may be associated with them. There could also be some mechanism by which the plasminogen activator activity of macrophages themselves could be induced.

The process of activation of macrophages by agents such as *C. parvum*, BCG, etc. can be achieved either with or without the involvement of the cell-mediated immunity of the host. Evans and Alexander (1972) showed that macrophages obtained from immunized animals can be activated by bringing the cells into contact with the same antigen.

Macrophages may be activated by a lymphokine produced by sensitized lymphocytes. Ruco and Meltzer (1977) showed that macrophages could be activated to become tumoricidal by supernatants of spleen cell cultures sensitized by BCG *in vivo*. Papermaster *et al*. (1978) demonstrated that several lymphokines, including MAF, were produced by a human lympho-blastoid cell line. The biological activities of the lymphokines were not species specific.

Kripke *et al*. (1977) found that macrophages activated by MAF produced by lymphocytes of C57BL mice immunized with the B16 melanoma or the syngeneic UV-112 were cytotoxic only to the cell type which had been used to immunize the animals. Obviously also, there should be mechanisms present by which the activated macrophage can destroy the neoplastic but not the normal cell. The work of Kripke *et al*. would tend to suggest such recognition might involve membrane bound components.

Possible mechanisms of evasion of immune surveillance

In spite of the veritable cascade of tumour cells liberated into the blood-stream or the lymphatic channels, metastatic deposits are produced only by a very small proportion of the disseminated cell population. The mani-festation of metastatic disease may be altered by the manipulation of the host's immune system (Gershon and Carter, 1970; Alexander and Eccles, 1975; Stutman, 1975). In other words, the recognition by the host's immune system of the metastatic cell is an essential part of the phenomenon, and such a recognition process must inevitably involve features of the tumour cell itself. The objective of the ensuing discussion is to examine the factors and mechanisms which may confer upon the tumour cell properties which enable it to escape immune surveillance (Fig. 4).

Sneaking through phenomenon
One might appropriately begin the discussion of how the tumour cell evades the surveillance of the host with a brief reference to the somewhat intriguing occurrence which has often been described as the "sneaking-through" phenomenon. It refers essentially to the experience of several investigators that a sub-threshold inoculum of tumour cells is often more successful in the formation of a progressively growing tumour than a large inoculum above a certain threshold. Naor (1979) has collated a number of tumour systems in which the "sneaking-through" phenomenon has been reported

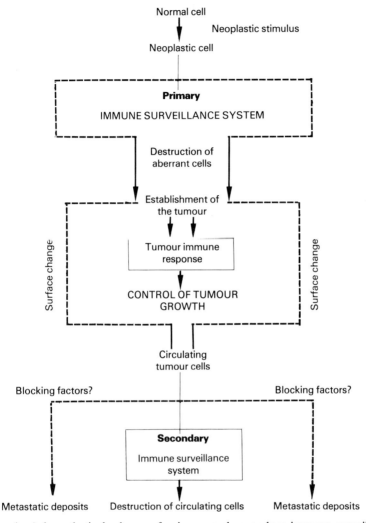

Figure 4 A hypothetical scheme of primary and secondary immune surveillance against neoplasms.

to occur, including the various interpretations provided by the investigators. A well-subscribed view is that "sneaking-through" occurs as a consequence of an insufficient immune stimulation by the tumour cells which, in effect, allows the tumour to grow progressively to a size where the tumour is established beyond immunological control. Obviously, this phenomenon has significant implications for tumorigenicity and for tumour immunology. It is not known, however, if in this "sneaking through" period tumour cells can also sneak through to distant sites of the body and establish foci of secondary tumours. It could be postulated, on the basis of the work of Flannery *et al.* (1973), that this could occur in tumours which metastasize early. Flannery *et al.* found that in a squamous cell carcinoma of rats, the *in vitro* antitumour cytotoxicity of cells from regional lymph nodes reached a peak about two weeks after implantation but declined thereafter to very low levels over the next six weeks. The development of metastases in the animals was concomitant with this latter "inactive" phase. A natural inference is that the reduced cytotoxicity of the lymphoid cells may have allowed lymphatic dissemination. However, recurrence and survival rates in human patients may be independent of lymph node involvement. Fisher and Slack (1970) found the recurrence and survival rates of breast cancer patients with 5-10 negative axillary nodes was similar to that of patients with 25-30 axillary nodes free of tumour. Breast cancer could be one of the systems which do not have an "inactive phase" in the regional lymph nodes.

Naor (1979) has suggested that suppressor cells (*see* p. 71) may be involved in the sneaking through of tumour cells. He has suggested the possibility that a weakly antigenic tumour or an inadequate inoculum may activate suppressor cells which may shut off antitumour immune responses and allow tumour development. If the suppressor cell mechanism were to be involved, this could have repercussions also on the formation of metastatic deposits.

Antigenic adaptation

It follows from the preceding discussion that a differentiation ought to be made between two possibly distinct functions of the host immune system, viz. (a) immunological functions relating to the detection of the initiation and development of tumours (primary surveillance) and (b) those functions of the immune system which may be concerned with the control of the dispersal and arrest of malignant cells leading to metastatic disease (secondary surveillance). Stutman (1975) has in fact argued that the mechanisms by which these two distinctive functions are performed may be different.

The basic tenets of the immunological surveillance theory are that most neoplasms are antigenic and that they provoke immune responses from the host, by virtue of differences in their antigenicity (Burnet, 1964, 1967, 1971). If the aberrant cells have new antigenic determinants, an appropriate immunological response is mounted by the host to detect and destroy the aberrant cells (Burnet, 1970).

In order to evade this surveillance, the neoplastic malignant cell must avoid recognition by a process of adaptation of the antigenic make-up of its surface. In other words, the metastatic cell should show an immune selection, albeit negative, so that it can avoid immune destruction. This implies that not only should non-metastasizing and metastasizing tumours of similar histogenetic origin be antigenically different, but also that metastatic deposits should be antigenically different from the primary tumour. This has been substantiated adequately. We have recently shown that the non-metastasizing NML lymphosarcoma of the hamster is distinctly more antigenic than the metastasizing ML form (*see* pp.61-63). In the same system, several years previously, Gershon *et al.* (1967b) had shown that while the NML tumour grows the animal develops a high degree of immunity as demonstrated by the rejection of a second graft of the same tumour. If this concomitant immunity is abrogated, even the NML tumour is able to metastasize (Gershon *et al.*, 1968). The greater antigenicity of non-metastasizing tumours as compared with related metastasizing ones has also been described by Schirrmacher and his colleagues on several occasions (e.g. *see* Schirrmacher *et al.*, 1979b; Schirrmacher and Jacobs, 1979). Schirrmacher *et al.* (1979b) could produce a local tumour by subcutaneous implantation of 10 cells from the metastasizing ESB lymphoma. But 10^3 to 10^4 cells from the non-metastasizing lymphoma (Eb) were required to achieve this.

Alteration of antigenic profile

One of the ways in which the cancer cell can evade the immune surveillance system could involve subtle alterations in the antigenic profile of the cell surface. One or more of several changes could provide an escape mechanism for the cell. Among these are possible deletion and differential expression of antigens and the modulation of surface antigens.

Instability of surface antigens

The occurrence of freely circulating tumour antigens in the peripheral blood and urine of patients has been frequently reported. There is considerable evidence that these antigens are shed from the tumour cells. Not only has release of antigenic material been demonstrated *in vitro* (Ben-Sasson *et al.*, 1974; Bystryn, 1977), but immunological identity has been established between soluble surface antigens and the material shed from the cell surface (Ting and Rogers, 1977; Stuhimiller and Seigler, 1977).

Currie and Alexander (1974) found that the release of tumour specific transplantation antigens (TSTA) from metastasizing rat fibrosarcoma in culture was far greater than similar release of TSTA from a non-metastasizing fibrosarcoma. Subsequently Davey *et al.* (1976) examined the rate of turnover of surface antigens in a metastasizing and a non-metastasizing form of ascitic lymphoma of inbred DBA2 mice. Again, the metastatic form released histocompatibility antigens both *in vitro* and *in vivo* at a greater rate than did the non-metastatic lymphoma. Kim *et al.* (1975) described electron-microscopic evidence that the cell surface coats of metastasizing rat mammary carcinomas were thinner than those of the non-metastasizing tumours.

One could envisage the possibility, therefore, that an instability of cell surface antigens and their rate of turnover may be an integral feature of malignancy and that there could be a quantitative relationship between the degree of lability of the membrane components and the capacity to metastasize (Davey *et al.*, 1976).

Differential expression of antigens and immunogenicity

The instability of the membrane antigens and the process of shedding of the antigens from the surface could result in differences in the overall make-up of the antigenic pattern of primary tumours and their metastases. It could be expected, therefore, that not only will the antigenic profile of the primary tumour differ from that of the metastatic cells and as a result they will differ in antigenicity, but it also follows that such a differential expression of antigens and differences in immunogenicity may be found between non-metastasizing and metastasizing forms of a tumour.

It was reported several years ago that cells transformed by oncogenic viruses possessed thicker surface coats, i.e. glycocalyces, than did corresponding untransformed cells (Burger, 1969, 1973; Poste, 1971, 1973; Martinez-Palomo, 1970; Martinez-Palomo and Braislovsky, 1968; Vorbrodt and Koprowski, 1969). The transformed cells were in fact reported also to synthesize surface coat material much faster than did the normal cells (Poste, 1971). These data would suggest some correlation between tumorigenicity of cells and the occurrence of surface coat material. The ability of the viral transformed cells to form metastatic deposits was, however, not examined in relation to the occurrence of the surface coat material.

Sherbet and Lakshmi (1974a) reported such a possibility following their investigations of human astrocytomas of various grades of malignancy. We found that the high grade (Kernohan grades III and IV) astrocytomas possessed surface material that could be removed by trypsinization, which could not be detected on astrocytomas of low grades of malignancy, nor on the surface of cells grown from the non-malignant meningiomas, or on foetal brain cells. We postulated therefore that this trypsin-labile surface coat material may be associated with malignancy. The histological assessment of malignancy, however, ought to be distinguished, at least in this case, from the biological definition of malignancy. For astrocytomas are not known to metastasize in the conventional meaning of the term, although they do invade and infiltrate into other parts of the brain.

The occurrence of surface coat material in relation to metastatic ability was examined by Kim *et al.* (1975) using spontaneous mammary carcinomas of the rat. Kim *et al.* (1975) reported that all the spontaneously meta-stasizing tumours which they investigated possessed little or no glyco-calyx. In contradistinction, non-metastasizing mammary carcinomas pos-sessed thick glycocalyces. They also observed that a direct relationship existed between the immunogenicity of the tumour and the amount of glycocalyx present on the tumour cell. The thickness of glycocalyx was inversely related to the metastasizing capacity of the cells.

We recently undertook a detailed investigation of the antigenic profiles of non-metastasizing (NML) and metastasizing (ML) lymphosarcomas of the hamster. Anti-NML antibody raised in rabbits and made tumour specific by adsorption with normal hamster tissues reacted heavily against NML tumour in Ouchterlony immunodiffusion gels, and the antibody was highly cytotoxic to NML cells *in vitro*. On the other hand, tumour specific antibody could not be raised against the metastasizing lymphosarcoma. This indicates that the NML tumour is more antigenic than the ML tumour (Sherbet *et al.* unpubl.). This conclusion is consistent with the observation of Greene and Harvey (1960), who found that anti-NML antibodies may be active in tumour-bearing hamsters. They found that if NML cells were mixed *in vitro* with serum taken from animals seven days after tumour implantation, and these cells were injected as a second graft, they are totally rejected. However, NML cells treated similarly with normal hamster serum result in rejection of only 50% of the implants.

In an attempt to determine the reasons for this reduced antigenicity, we examined the binding of each purified antiserum (anti-NML and anti-ML) to the other heterologous tumour cell population, using cytotoxicity assays and binding of ^{125}I-labelled purified anti-NML and anti-ML immuno-globulins. These experiments have indicated that these hamster tumours possess common tumour antigens, since antibody raised against either tumour reacted with the heterologous tumour cells as judged by immuno-diffusion testing, cytotoxicity and IgG binding assays. It appears, however, that the shared antigens may be expressed to a different degree. The binding of ^{125}I anti-ML IgG to ML cells was reduced by 90% if the IgG was absorbed with the NML tumour. On the other hand, the binding of anti-NML IgG to NML cells was reduced by only 40% following adsorption of the IgG preparation with ML cells. Cytotoxicity testing also revealed that while absorption with NML tumour removed all or most of the activity of anti-ML antibody against ML cells, after absorption with ML cells anti-

NML IgG was still cytotoxic to NML cells. On the basis of these studies, we have suggested that the ML cells possess between 20-40% of the tumour-associated antigens present on the NML cells. We have also suggested as a general postulate that non-metastasizing tumours such as the NML possess some membrane-bound antigens which are common with the metastasizing tumours like the ML, but that the former may also have extra sets of antigens which are immunobiologically unique. This was suggested also by the work of Kim *et al* (1975), although they had not based their conclusions on the degrees of expression of the various sets of antigens.

A simple explanation for this differential expression of antigens is that some of them are shed from the cell surface. Kim *et al.* (1975) stated that the absence of the glycocalyx in metastasizing tumours is due to its dissociation from the plasma membrane, for they detected solubilized surface antigen in the blood of hosts carrying the metastasizing carcinomas.

The deletion of surface antigens could possibly result from the increased proteolytic activity which may be associated with malignant tumours (*see* pp. 85-91). We investigated this possibility using the ML and NML lymphosarcomas, and the TRES fibrosarcoma of the hamster, and employing aprotinin (Trasylol) which is a wide-spectrum antiproteinase. The surface protein/glycoprotein patterns of these tumours were investigated and also the changes produced in these patterns following incubation with the antiproteinase (Table 3). In the TRES fibrosarcoma, which is a moderately malignant tumour, aprotinin treatment resulted in the increased expression

Table 3

Effects of the antiproteinase, aprotinin, on the expression of 115K surface protein(s) on tumour cells in relation to degree of malignancy[a]

Cell type	Malignancy rating	Total recovered count $\times 10^5$	% Incorporation of ^{125}I into 115K		% Increase
			No treatment	After aprotinin treatment	
ML	High	8·5	6·3 ± 0·23		
		4·5		9·95 ± 0·64	58
TRES	Moderate	4·0	7·8 ± 0·57		
		4·2		10·00 ± 1·85	28
NML	Non-malignant	6·8	12·5 ± 1·1	14·7 ± 1·4	18

[a]Cell surface proteins were labelled by lactoperoxidase-catalysed radioiodination (Hynes, 1973). They were then seperated by electrophoresis on polyacrylamide gels (*see* Wildridge and Sherbet, 1981).
(Lakshmi *et al.*, 1982)

(28%) of a surface protein of molecular weight of approximately 115K (K = 1000). Interestingly enough, the 115K protein occurred in greater quantities (+ 58%) on the ML cell surface following treatment of the cells with the antiproteinase. The non-metastasizing NML tumours also showed an increase in the expression of this surface protein following aprotinin treatment, but the level of increase in this case was only about 18% (Lakshmi *et al.*, 1982).

These observations suggest that the differential expression of antigens on ML and NML cells may have been brought about by the dissociation of certain antigens or groups of antigens mediated by proteolytic enzymes associated with the malignant cell. The differences in the reappearance of the 115K surface component may reflect the rate of turnover of the component by each tumour. It may be of some significance that the lowest level of reappearance is seen in the non-metastasizing tumour, a moderate (28%) increase in the moderately malignant TRES fibrosarcoma but the highest level of reappearance (58% increase) is seen in the ML tumour, which is known to possess very high metastatic ability (Sherbet *et al.*, 1980). In other words, the rates of synthesis and deletion from the surface could be related to the metastatic ability of the tumours.

A third point brought to light by this investigation is whether or not a specific antigen, or group of antigens, is involved in the metastatic process. It could not be fortuitous that all three tumour types that we investigated showed changes relating to the 115K. It would be interesting to see if the expression of surface components of this molecular weight range is affected in other tumour systems also.

It may be worthwhile pointing out in this context that the occurrence of a common marker glycoprotein of molecular weight of 100K has been reported (Price and Stoddart, 1976; Bramwell and Harris, 1978a, b; Bowen and Kulatilake, 1979; *see also* pp. 121-125). The component(s) which we found apparently deleted from malignant cells is of a higher molecular weight, but the estimation of the molecular weight is based purely on their electrophoretic mobility on polyacrylamide gels and must be considered as merely tentative estimate of size.

Circulating antigens and immune complexes

Most of the work reviewed here seems to support the postulate of Davey *et al.* (1976) that the degree of lability of membrane components may be directly related to the ability to metastasize. This instability of the membrane components and the resultant constant shedding of surface material could allow metastatic lesions to form.

Two mechanism could be envisaged. Firstly, the reduced antigenic expression may have the effect of making the metastatic cell less immunogenic. Secondly, the antigen shed into the circulation may pre-empt the effects of humoral and/or cell mediated immunity against the tumour. Currie and Alexander (1974) proposed this as a means in the facilitation of the secondary spread of cancer. They reported that the cytotoxic potential of lymphocytes from lymph nodes of rats bearing the non-immunogenic metastasizing MC3 sarcoma could be specifically inhibited by both serum and culture supernatant containing MC3 antigens. But the cytotoxicity of lymph node cells from the immunogenic non-metastasizing sarcoma MC1 could not be inhibited by supernatants of MC1 cultures. Similarly, Kim *et al.* (1975) reported that circulating antigens in the blood of host animals bearing the metastatic carcinoma interfered with the blastogenic capacity of circulating lymphocytes to mitogenic stimulation by lectins. *In vivo* this would lead to an enhancement of tumour growth and a delay in its rejection by the host (Rao and Bonavida, 1976, 1977). Presensitization of animals with tumour antigen may also cause enchancement of tumour growth and delay in rejection (Rao and Bonavida, 1977) by inhibiting cell-mediated immunity, although in this case the occurrence of suppressor lymphoid cells cannot be ruled out. None the less, it may be pointed out that Rao and Bonavida (1977) found that effects of circulating tumour antigens, i.e. the acceleration of tumour growth and delay in rejection, were specific, for these effects were not seen when sensitized animals were implanted with antigenically unrelated tumours. In other words, circulating antigens may abrogate in a specific manner the cell-mediated responses against the growing tumour and the circulating tumour cells.

This process of immune paralysis has also been shown in human cancers. The *in vitro* cytotoxicity of peripheral blood lymphocytes obtained from patients with colonic carcinoma for the carcinoma cells in culture could be inhibited by exposing the lymphocytes to serum from the patient (Nind *et al.*, 1975). Currie and Basham (1972) in fact showed that the factor which abrogates the cytotoxicity of lymphocytes from patients with disseminated melanomas could not only be found in the patient's sera, but could also be detected and eluted from the melanoma cells themselves, suggesting a release of soluble antigen into the systemic circulation. This has received confirmation from the work of Thomson *et al.* (1973a, b, c) and Grosser and Thomson (1976), who found that serum blocking activity seen *in vitro* corresponded with the amount of circulating tumour antigen.

This phenomenon resembles the process of abrogation of the cytotoxicity of sensitized lymphocytes for tumour cells against which they are immunized. Sera from both tumour-bearing animals and patients have been shown to contain factors which inhibit the killing *in vitro* by lymphocytes of tumour cells to which they are sensitized (Bubenik *et al.*, 1970; Hellström, *et al.*, 1969, 1971; Hellström and Hellström, 1970; Jagarlamoody *et al.*,

1971). The factors are known to absorb specifically to the respective neo-plastic cells and subsequently elute from the cells and also from growing tumours (K. E. Hellström and Hellström, 1970; Hellström *et al.*, 1971; Ran and Witz, 1970).

The exact nature of these "blocking factors" is not known, but they are believed to be immune complexes (Sjögren *et al.*, 1971) or tumour antigens themselves shed into the circulation. In either case, the immune mechanisms may be interfered with, and therefore the blocking factors are relevant in the metastatic spread of cancer.

The relationship between the amount of circulating tumour antigens or immune complexes and the extent of metastatic spread is yet unclear.

As a general statement of fact, the expression of immunity against a tumour is evident when the tumour is small but either decreases or is absent with increase of tumour mass (Barski and Youn, 1969; Youn *et al.*, 1973; Thomson, 1975; Grosser and Thomson, 1975; Marti and Thomson, 1976; Flores *et al.*, 1976). Using the leukocyte adherence inhibition (LAI) test, which is based on the inhibition of the adherence to glass of sensitized peripheral blood leukocytes produced by the binding of the appropriate tumour antigen (Halliday and Miller, 1972), Grosser and Thomson (1976) showed that there was an excess of soluble tumour antigen in the case of advanced breast cancer. The peripheral blood leukocytes from patients with Stage I or II breast tumours or malignant melanoma displayed LAI, but leukocytes from patients with metastatic cancer showed no reactivity in the leukocyte adherence inhibition test.

Black (1980) has recently discussed the possible role of immune complexes as "blocking" factors. While it is clear that immune complexes occur at great frequency in sera from cancer patients, the mechanism by which they function is unclear. Also unclear is the possible correlation between the incidence of immune complexes in sera with the incidence of metastases. It may be of significance in this context that the blocking activity of sera from rats bearing metastatic tumours has been found to correlate both with the disappearance of antibody from the serum and the development of metastatic deposits (Currie and Gage, 1973; Currie and Basham, 1972). Theofilopoulos *et al.* (1977) examined sera from over five hundred patients with various types of tumours for immune complexes. Immune complexes were detected in 19% of normal subjects, but the incidence in patients with tumour was between 16-52%. In general, there was an increase in immune complexes with increasing tumour mass and metastatic disease. The spread of values for the amounts of immune complexes is so wide that no specific conclusion could be drawn. For instance, the differences in immune complex content in sera from patients with no evidence of disease and those with metastatic disease were statistically significant. But the differences observed between patients with localized disease and those with metastatic disease did not appear to be statistically significant.

Staab *et al* (1980) have reported a significant correlation of the type attempted by Theofilopoulos *et al.* (1977). Staab *et al.* determined CEA-immune complexes in 363 patients with adenocarcinoma of the gastro-intestinal tract. According to these authors, 89 of the 363 patients contained CEA-immune complexes at the time of resection of the tumour. Seventy-two of these 89 patients had metastatic disease. Another interesting feature was the appearance of the complexes post-operatively. All patients who had CEA-immune complexes post-operatively developed metastatic disease. Patients with local recurrence had no detectable amounts of immune complexes, while those who did show immune complexes had always had distant metastatic spread. The reason for such a clear-cut demonstrable correlation is certainly the availability of well tested radio-immunoassay methods for the demonstration of the free antigen and the complexes.

Immune complexes may regulate cell-mediated immunological function one or more of several ways. In conditions of antibody excess, immune complexes mask tumour-associated antigens (Baldwin and Robins, 1976) or induce antibody-dependent cellular cytotoxicity (Greenberg and Shen, 1973).

In the presence of excess antigen, immune complexes may facilitate binding of the antigen to lymphocytes by an antibody-mediated cross-linking process causing a specific blockade of these cells and low zone tolerance (Diener and Feldman, 1972). Among other suggested means of action are (a) binding to Fc receptors of lymphoid cells and causing direct lysis of the effector cells or indirectly by activating suppressor cells (Gershon *et al.*, 1974); (b) inhibition of lymphoproliferative responses to tumour antigens (Gorczynski *et al.*, 1975; Hatter and Soehnlen, 1974) and (c) by producing lymphocyte sequestration (Stuttman, 1973).

Antigenic modulation

A differential expression of the surface antigens may be caused by an inhibition of the expression of certain antigens and/or an increased shedding of the antigens due to their instability. It is also possible that there occurs an active process of modulation of the antigenic profile.

It has been demonstrated beyond doubt that the rate of acceptance (trans-plantability) of highly antigenic tumours can be improved dramatically by experimental manipulation designed to reduce the density of tumour-specific antigens occurring on the surface of the cells (Fenyö *et al.*, 1968; Ioachim *et al.*, 1974). Ioachim *et al.* (1972) showed that the expression of determinants of the Gross leukemia virus in rat leukemic cells can be experimentally modulated by passaging the tumour cells alternately *in vivo* and *in vitro*. The phenotypic expression of the virus can be lost *in vivo* under immunological pressure but recovered in the *in vitro* phase. Antigenic modulation of the TL antigen from the surface of murine thymus leukemic cells occurring during allotransplantation has been reported by Old *et al.* (1968). They demonstrated the loss of the TL antigen from TL + cells exposed to TL antibody in the absence of complement. In the ascites leukemia phenotype TL1, 2, 3 modulation at 37 °C was rapid, detectable within 10 min and completed within 1 h. The process was inhibited by reducing the temperature to 0 °C, or in the presence of actinomycin D or iodoacetamide. The EB virus is also reported to become expressed when the primary Burkitt lymphomas are established in culture, but they are absent in the primary tumour cells themselves (Gross, 1970). This again could be a result of the removal of immunological constraints.

Can such antigenic modulation be a subtle mechanism of antigenic adaptation involved in the secondary spread of cancer? There is very little work done in this direction. Davey *et al.* (1976) investigated the antigenic modulation occurring in two transplantable ascites lymphosarcomas of inbred DBA/2 mice with different metastatic abilities. They examined the elimination of antigen-antibody complex from the surface of cells exposed to allo-antisera. They noticed that antibody rapidly disappeared from the surface of the metastasizing lymphosarcoma, but no such elimination seemed to have taken place from the non-metastasizing cells, even after incubation of the antibody-coated cells for 6 h after exposure to the antiserum. However, the metstasizing cells seemed to regain the complement of antigens, since these cells could be lysed by the addition of fresh antiserum and complement. *In vitro*, therefore, the metastasizing lymphosarcoma is able to modulate its antigenic profile, while in contrast the non-metastasizing lymphosarcoma is not.

Several years ago, Deichman and Kluchureva (1966) reported that lung metastases of SV-40 induced tumours of the hamster lost certain transplantation antigens from the cell surface. A deletion or loss of antigens from metastatic cells was also reported by Sugarbaker and Cohen (1972) who tested the antigenicity of a primary MCA-induced sarcoma and seven metastases derived from the primary tumour. While the primary remained immunogenic all through the experiment, the metastatic lines differed greatly in their immunogenicity. Cells from two metastases grew without being inhibited in mice immunized with the primary tumour. These metastatic cells were themselves immunogenic. Three other metastatic cells grew in mice similarly immunized with the primary tumour but were not found to be immunogenic.

On the contrary, however, the experiments of Faraci (1974) appear to suggest that the primary tumour and its metastatic cells may share certain antigens but, in addition, new antigens may be present on the latter. This is reported by the more recent work of Pimm and Baldwin (1977) on the immunogenicity of MCA-induced primary tumours and tumour lines initiated from their secondary deposits. Pimm and Baldwin (1977) found that 2 of 4 primary tumours showed little or no antigenicity as assessed by antitumour protection afforded by graft excision or implantation of irradiated tumour tissue. In contrast, the tumour lines initiated from the secondary deposits were distinctly immunogenic and protected the host against challenge with up to 5×10^6 tumour cells. Four metastatic lines which they had initiated were antigenically distinct from the primary tumour.

Fogel *et al.* (1979) also reported marked differences between cell surface antigens of primary tumours and their metastases. They reported that C57BL/6 mouse spleen lymphocytes sensitized against cells of primary Lewis lung carcinoma (LLP) were highly cytotoxic to LLP cells but less so to cells from lung metastases (LLM). Conversely, lymphocytes sensitized against LLM cells were more cytotoxic to LLM cells but less so to LLP cells. Consistent with this is our recent finding of antigenic differences between a hamster primary lymphosarcoma (ML) and its liver metastases (Sherbet *et al.*, 1982). Tumour specific anti-ML IgG was found to be between two and five times more cytotoxic towards primary tumour cells than cells derived from its liver metastases.

In a recent paper, Schirrmacher (1979) has approached this in a different way. He used the ESb metastasizing lymphoma of the DBA/2 mice which is rejected if transplanted into B10/D2 mice. But since the strains have identical H-2 complexes, he transferred spleen cells from B10/D2 mice immunized against the ESb tumour into DBA/2 mice and showed that this protected them against the metastasizing tumour. Unfortunately, protective immunity was demonstrated in these experiments only in terms of tumorigenicity of the ESb cells in DBA/2 mice and only occassionally were the animals subjected to detailed histological investigations for metastases. The experiments would have been more meaningful if the sensitized cells could have been shown to be more effective in animals which had established microdeposits of secondary tumours.

The biochemical investigations into the patterns of proteins expressed on primary tumours and their metastases, which have been described in an earlier section (*see* pp. 38-42), have been inconclusive. This is probably due not only to the inadequate sensitivity of and discrimination by the techniques employed, but presumably also due to the various enzymatic and other treatments required for the preparation of cell suspensions, etc. for cell surface labelling.

Immunological status and metastatic pattern

The question of antigenicities of primary and metastatic cells is probably far more complicated than the simplified premise of looking for generalized differences which runs through most of these investigations would suggest. There could be little doubt that the seeding of secondary cells in distant organs involves the evasion of the "secondary" immunosurveillance system (*see* Fig. 4).

The enhancement of secondary spread of cancer as a consequence of irradiation has been described in human cancers as well as in experimental tumour models, and is thought to be a result of immunosuppression (*see* Stjernswärd and Douglas, 1977). Pimm and Baldwin (1978) have summarized the data available on the increased incidence of metastasis in certain animal tumour models under conditions of immunosuppression induced by procedures such a thymectomy or by the use of antilymphocyte/antithymocyte sera and immunosuppressive steroids such as hydrocortisone.

A study of the kinetics of tumour growth in syngeneic animals shows that the smaller the size of the tumour inoculum, the larger is the metastatic mass. In immunosuppressed animals, on the other hand, the mass of metastatic deposition is independent of the size of the initial tumour inoculum (Segal *et al.*, 1980). North *et al.* (1981) have investigated two chemically induced rat fibrosarcomas which do not metastasize spontaneously if transplanted into syngeneic immunocompetent hosts. But in immune-suppressed animals or in athymic rats, they show active dissemination into the lungs and lymph nodes. Even more remarkable is the observation that cutaneous squamous cell carcinoma, which is known to remain localized for prolonged periods, shows an increased propensity to metastasize in transplant-recipient patients on immunosuppressive regimes (Penn, 1977; Sheil, 1977).

The question becomes more complex when one considers the suggested possibility of altering the metastatic pattern by manipulating the immune system. Weiss *et al.* (1974) found that the pattern of arrest of tumour cells administered systemically changed in animals which had been sensitized to tumour antigen either by the presence of the growing tumour or by exposure to attenuated cells. They examined an MCA-induced sarcoma maintained in syngeneic C3H/HeHA mice and an oestradiol-induced lymphosarcoma passaged in C3H/St Ha mice. Having established that both tumours were capable of evoking humoral as well as cell-mediated responses in their respective hosts, they compared the localization of labelled tumour cells in normal mice and those immunized against the tumour. The patterns of arrest were markedly different. For the fibrosarcoma, considerably reduced amounts of radioactivity were recovered from the lungs of immunized animals as compared with the controls. The radioactivity recovered from the liver was far greater in immunized animals than that from the liver of normal animals. Alterations were found also in the pattern of recovery of radioactivity from the various organs of normal and immunized animals following i.v. introduction of the lymphosarcoma. These were not as dramatic as in the case of the fibrosarcoma, nor were the shifts in the pattern comparable with those detected in the fibrosarcoma. The authors also then showed that the shifts in the patterns occurred only following injection of homologous cells. One may conclude from this that the immunological status with respect to the tumour plays a definite role in determining the pattern of localization of the disseminated tumour cells. None the less, it should be pointed out that one instinctively equates the recovered radioactivity pattern with distribution of the injected tumour cells. Such an equation may not be fully justified.

It would seem, however, that the host's immunological system may not be the sole arbiter of the metastatic pattern. Ioachim and colleagues described specific patterns of metastasis of two kinds of experimental leukemias injected into W/Fu strain rats (Ioachim *et al.*, 1976b, 1977). Whatever the route of injection, lymphoid leukemic cells showed metastases in the thymus and the lymph nodes, but myeloid leukemia cells produced tumour in the spleen and liver without any involvement of the thymus. The same pattern of metastatic distribution persisted in animals which had been immunosuppressed.

Thus, notwithstanding the fact that investigations of a biochemical nature have so far failed to reveal any significant differences in the surface components of primary and secondary tumour cells, or their derivatives selected for specific metastasis to particular organs, one may require to invoke factors intrinsic to the cell membrane as playing a functional role in organ specific metastasis.

The occurrence of specific antigenic components could be envisaged in this process. Shearman *et al.* (1980) have demonstrated a specific antigenic component detectable by monoclonal antibody which may have a functional role in this process. They demonstrated the occurrence of such an antigen in 20% of cells of a tumour line selected for metastasis to liver. A small number of cells of another line selected for metastasis to the ovary also possessed this surface antigen.

An immunological analysis of metastatic dissemination of cancer must inevitably involve also an analysis of the immunogenetics of the process. Segal *et al.* (1980) reported that LL carcinoma grows in allogeneic mice but does not metastasize. This result is contentious (*see* Salomon *et al.*, 1980). None the less, in the system which Segal *et al.* have employed, metastatic dissemination of LL carcinoma cells occurred only when the recipient strain of mice shared with C57BL mice both the background and products of the H-2D region of the major histocompatability complex (MHC).

Feldman and colleagues have followed up these investigations with an analysis of the expression of MHC-encoded determinants on primary tumour cells and their metastatic counterparts (De Baetselier *et al.*, 1980). They used an MCA-induced sarcoma serially transplanted in syngeneic (C_3Heb × C57BL/6) F1 mice (H-2^b × H-2^k). Their major findings were that the primary tumour was composed of a mixture of H-2^k positive and H-2^k negative cells. Of these, the H-2^k positive cells were able to survive in the circulation and succeed in forming metastatic deposits in the lungs. This expression of H-2^k determinant and ability to form lung metastases was found to be stable over 10 serial passages in syngeneic F1 mice. Apparently a process of modulation of histocompatibility determinants could enable a tumour cell to evade the immune serveillance.

Since the MHC may be involved in the control of immune effector cells, such an immune selection of metastatic cells appears feasible. The situation, however, may be more complex than it would appear. It has been reported, for instance, that interferon increases the expression of certain determinants of the histocompatibility complex (Lindahl *et al.*, 1976; Attallah and Strong, 1979) and may make the cells more susceptible to lysis by natural killer cells, although this increased susceptibility has not been demonstrated unequivocally.

Suppressor cells

The process of regulation of the immunological responses is an essential part of the immunological defence. For a conservative use of the system in surveillance against infection, autoimmune and neoplastic disease, the intensity and duration of the immunological response are under delicate cybernetic control. This may take the form of humoral factors neutralizing the components which caused the immunocompetent cells to produce the humoral factors, thus leading to a cessation of further stimulation of the cells. A control of the immunological responses can also be achieved by the mediation of non-specific or specific suppressor cells. Non-specific suppressor cells have frequently been found to be macrophages (Kirchner *et al.*, 1974; Poupon *et al.*, 1976). *In vitro* mitogen-induced lymphocyte blastogenesis and generation of cytotoxic T cells, and *in vivo* production of antibodies may be inhibited in cancer patients and in tumour-bearing animals. This has been attributed to activated monocytes.

Quan and Burtin (1978) investigated the PHA responses of peripheral blood lymphocytes from 170 patients with colorectal and head and neck cancers. These lymphocytes showed a significantly decreased response to PHA as compared with normal subjects or those with benign conditions. In six patients, response to PHA could be increased by the use of carrageenan, which is toxic to macrophages, indicating the involvement of the latter as non-specific suppressor cells. Earlier, Kirchner *et al.* (1974) and Poupon *et al.* (1976) had arrived at a similar conclusion when they demonstrated that the suppressor activity of spleen cell suspensions could be abolished by the removal of macrophages using glass wool or carbonyl iron. Monocytes have been implicated as non-specific suppressor cells also by others (Zembala *et al.*, 1977).

The suppressor activity of macrophages could be mediated by prostaglandins which are known to possess immunosuppressive effects (*see* p. 47). Activated macrophages are known to synthesize and release prostaglandins (Humes *et al.*, 1977). Tumour cells are also known to stimulate, macrophages, presumably to bring about their activation to function as non-specific suppressor cells, presumably also by the same mechanism. Macrophages have also been implicated in the depletion of L-arginine, which is essential for lymphocyte proliferation, by producing the enzyme arginase (Kung *et al.*, 1977). Non-specific suppressor cell activity is not restricted to activated macrophages. Naor (1979) has reviewed a considerable amount of evidence that both B and T cells could also act as non-specific suppressor cells.

The process of regulation of the immune response cannot be solely dependent upon a non-specific mechanism. Suppressor cells whose activities are directed specifically towards the tumour antigen may be envisaged. Several workers have demonstrated the presence of specific suppressor T cells in animals immunized with homologous tumours. Fujimoto *et al.* (1975, 1976a, b) immunized A/J mice against an MCA-induced sarcoma by inoculation of animals and subsequently removed the tumour. The immunized animals could reject up to 10^8 tumour cells. If the tumour inoculum was accompanied by thymus or spleen cells from A/J mice bearing the sarcoma, the rejection appeared to be suppressed. The suppression of rejection was seen even if the thymus or spleen cells were injected five days after tumour challenge. Confirmation of the T-cell nature of the suppressor cell came from experiments which demonstrated that anti-θ antiserum and antithymocyte serum in the presence of complement abolished suppressor cell activity.

The suppressor T cell is described as possessing an associated product of I-J subregion of the H-2 complex (Tada *et al.*, 1977; Pierres *et al.*, 1977), antiserum to which appears to abolish suppressor activity (Greene *et al.*, 1977). The suppressor cells demonstrably antagonize the effector cells (Fujimoto and Tada, 1978; Fujimoto *et al.*, 1978) but the mechanism of this inhibition of effector cells is yet unclear. They are believed to produce a suppressor factor which is an immunoglobulin (Nelson *et al.*, 1975a, b).

We are yet a long way away from understanding any possible implication of the suppressor cell activity in the metastatic process. Suppressor cells seem to be activated rapidly and their generation relies on continuous stimulation by the tumour antigen (Fujimoto *et al.*, 1976a, b). Since primary tumours and their secondary deposits do share antigens one may speculate that suppressor cell activity may also play a role in enabling metastatic deposits to form.

Natural killer cells

In the past few years, naturally occurring cytotoxic lymphocytes have been detected in normal, tumour-bearing and immunodeficient animals. These natural killer (NK) cells have been found to be able to lyse a wide range of target cells from tumours as well as normal tissues (Kiessling and Haller, 1978; Herberman and Holden, 1978). The NK cells form a subpopulation of lymphoid cells thought to be distinct from T or B lymphocytes or macrophages. They were reported to be resistant to the action of anti-θ antiserum and complement, to occur in T-deficient animals and to possess no surface immunoglobulins or Fc receptors. In addition, they are not susceptible to the action of carbonyl iron/magnet or carrageenan, and do not show adhesiveness to nylon columns (Herberman *et al.*, 1975a, b; Shellam, 1977).

Some of these observations have not been borne out by subsequent work and therefore the nature of NK cells is still uncertain. It would seem that NK cells and K cells which mediate antibody-dependent cellular cytotoxicity (ADCC) against tumour cells have several features in common, and may indeed be identical. The various features summarized by Herberman *et al.* (1978) include a possible T cell lineage of both NK and K cells. Both possess low affinity receptors for sheep erythrocytes. Anti-T serum and complement can eliminate both NK and K cell activities. The occurrence of Thy-1 antigen on these cells is suggested both by Herberman and colleagues and Dennert (1980). Both cell types may also possess Fc receptors for immunoglobulin. The view currently being held by Herberman *et al.* (1978) is that NK and K cells are identical except that the former are not dependent upon antibody for their function.

A T-cell lineage may be suggested by the occurrence of Thy-1 antigens on NK cells, although, on account of the expression of this antigen on cells from other tissues as well, its expression *per se* is insufficient evidence for the linkage of NK cells with the pathway of T-cell differentiation. Zarling and Kung (1980) have in fact now shown that monoclonal antibodies which are able to suppress cytotoxic T-cell activity do not affect NK cells or poly I:C augmented NK cell activity. In addition, the recognition of target cells in T-cell cytotoxicity is subject to MHC restriction, while NK cell activity apparently is not.

In summary, NK cells may be characterized as Fc-receptor positive, SIg-negative, non-T cells.

There is still considerable difficulty in understanding the specificity of action of the NK cells. They seem able to recognize the virus-related antigens associated with their target cells (Herberman *et al.*, 1975a, b; Kiessling *et al.*, 1975; Sendo *et al.*, 1975; Nunn *et al.*, 1976; Lee and Ihle, 1977; Shellam and Hogg, 1977). Yet mouse NK cells can function also in a xenogeneic system as shown by Haller *et al.* (1977) using human haema-topoietic and T-lymphoma cells.

Dennert (1980) posed the question: do NK cells recognize common components or structures present on their target cells, whatever may be the origin of the latter, or do NK cells possess a spectrum of recognizant abilities (receptors?) with individual specificities for particular structures occurring on the target cells? Dennert argued that if there was a clonal distribution of specificities, cloned NK cells would show differences in their lytic activity against a given range of target cells from uncloned NK cells. The experiments he described show, however, that the NK cell clones displayed the same specificities as the uncloned cells, which indicates that either the NK sublines recognize a common target structure or they have receptors of several different specificities.

There is some evidence that NK cells might recognize membrane-bound antigens, such as the 140K membrane-extract fraction, which may be common to several types of tumour cells, or the 240K fraction, which is apparently unique to certain tumour cells (Roder *et al.*, 1979). Zaunders *et al.* (1981) have described glycoprotein antigens (120-140K) whose expression is restricted to certain tumour cell types as a possible candidate participating in the processes of recognition between the tumour cell and the NK cell.

The NK cells are thought to play a part in the immunosurveillance against neoplasia. Since they require no prior priming and no immunological memory, such a role seems feasible. Recently it has been shown that the cytotoxicity of NK cells can be enhanced by cocultivation of tumour cells or virus-transformed cells with mouse or human lyphocytes (Trinchieri *et al.*, 1977, 1978; Trinchieri and Santoli, 1978). The view that this effect is due to interferon has been strengthened by the demonstration of similar enhancement of NK cell activity by interferon-inducing agents (Oehler *et al.*, 1978; Herbermann *et al.*, 1978), by purified interferon preparations themselves (Herbermann *et al.*, 1978, 1979; Zarling *et al.*, 1979; Moore and Potter, 1980; Moore *et al.*, 1980) and by inducers of interferon (Zarling *et al.*, 1980). In the mouse, the augmentation effect is seen also *in vivo* (Gidlund *et al.*, 1978). In man, the activation of NK cells following interferon therapy has been reported by Huddlestone *et al.* (1979). The NK cell activity reached a peak (about five times greater cytotoxicity index than before commencement of treatment) approximately 18 h after treatment with interferon. The activity then declined to slightly above pre-treatment levels. The administration of anti-interferon antibodies to *nude* mice can block NK cell activity and allow the growth of xenogeneic cell lines heavily infected with viruses (Reid *et al.*, 1981). An augmentation of NK cell activity can also be produced by other lymphokines such as interleukin-2 (Henney *et al.*, 1981).

Since a variety of tumour cell lines have been shown to be able to induce lymphocytes to produce interferon (Trinchieri *et al.*, 1977), this could conceivably provide a mechanism by which NK cells could be spurred into participation in the immune surveillance process, at least against virus-induced neoplasms.

Attallah *et al.* (1979) reported that interferon caused an increased expression of CEA on human colonic carcinoma cell line WiDr. This and/or expression of other foetal antigens or differentiation antigens may allow the aberrant cells to be recognized by the NK cells. Increases in antigens of the histocompatability complex as a consequence of interferon treatment have also been reported (Lindahl *et al.*, 1976; Attallah and Strong, 1979). Much of this evidence requires to be examined closely or perhaps re-investigated, since athymic *nude* mice, which are known to possess higher NK cell activity than euthymic mice, have been found to allow the growth of human tumours which reportedly can synthesize foetal antigens such as CEA and β-2-microglobulin (β-2m) known to be associated with the HLA complex (Carrel *et al.*, 1976; Tom *et al.*, 1977; Di Persio *et al.*, 1980) (β-2m is also known to be present on the blastocyst, though no H-2 antigens occur). This is incompatible with the finding that susceptibility to NK cells may be related to the expression of differentiation antigens or products by the target cells. Gidlund *et al.* (1981) reported that certain cell types which are induced by extraneous agents to differentiate (i.e. synthesize phenotypic products or acquire features of the differentiated state) show concomitantly a reduction in susceptibility to NK cells.

On the other hand, Moore *et al.* (1980) found that the enhancement by interferon of the cytolytic activity of NK cells was seen only if the target cells had not been pre-exposed to interferon. The pre-exposure of the target cells to comparable amounts of interferon diminished their susceptibility to lysis by NK cells. It is believed that this protective effect could be a result of the modulation of surface antigens (Moore *et al.*, 1980). since the protective effect can be abolished using metabolic inhibitors such a cycloheximide and actinomycin D (Trinchieri and Santoli, 1978).

NK cells have been detected *in vivo* apparently causing no damage to normal tissues, yet *in vitro* these cells will lyse a variety of target cells, including autologous cells. Therefore, one needs to postulate not only specific mechanisms whereby the NK cell can recognize an aberrant cell, but also mechanisms which protect normal cells from destruction. The reported protective effect of interferon has been suggested as a possible means by which NK cells could be stimulated by virus-infected or neoplastic cells into their natural cytolytic activity, while at the same time the interferon synthesizer affords normal tissue cells protection from NK cell activity. It is difficult, however, to see how this could be subsumed as a general rule, since Moore and colleagues have found that the protection action of interferon extends even to cancer cells.

There seem to be reasonable grounds for supposing that natural killer cells play a significant, if not a major, part in immune surveillance against tumours *in vivo*. Immune T cells, without doubt, are the most active agency. Although xenografts of tumours will grow successfully in athymic *nude* mice, these animals none the less possess significant antitumour activity. This has been attributed to increased levels of NK cell activity (Herberman and Oldham, 1980), but susceptibility to lysis by natural killer cells has not been positively correlated with lack of tumorigenicity in *nude* mice. It has been suggested that NK cells might provide a first line of defence against neoplastic cells (Herberman and Holden, 1978; Herberman and Holden, 1980).

Since it is believed that metastatic cells differ both immunologically and immunogenetically from cells of the primary tumour (*see* pp. 67-71), it would be relevant to ask whether NK cells may have a role also in the control of metastatic disease. An indication that they may indeed resist metastatic spread of tumours comes from work on tumour xenografts in *nude* mice. While a variety of tumours can grow as xenografts in *nude* mice, even the most malignant tumours only rarely show metastatic dissemination. Freedman *et al.* (1976) examined the behaviour of a number of established malignant cell lines implanted into *nude* mice. While they invariably produced tumours, none of the tumours was invasive or formed metastatic deposits.

A variety of human cancer lines and tumours have been shown to be highly transplantable in athymic *nude* mice. Schmidt and Good (1975) have successfully transplanted gastric, pancreatic and colonic carcinomas, and melanomas. Approximately 50% of lung carcinomas but only 1/13 carcinomas of the breast were successfully transplanted by Shimosato *et al.* (1976). Rae-Venter and Reid (1980) transplanted 32 human breast carcinomas. Of these, 7 survived but showed no metastatic spread. Giovanella *et al.* (1973, 1974) have reported the metastatic spread of some human melanomas. None the less, acceptance of xenograft and its metastatic dissemination can be improved by treating recipient animals with antilymphocyte serum (Klein *et al.*, 1978) or by anti-interferon antiserum

(Reid *et al.*, 1981). In these thymus-deficient animals, the effect presumably is due to destruction of NK cells by the antisera.

In contrast with *nude* mice with higher NK cell activity, another strain of mice, the *beige* (Chediak-Higashi) mouse, carrying the homozygous *beige* gene, are said to be selectively deficient in NK cells (Roder and Duwe, 1979). Human subjects carrying the analogous autosomal recessive Chediak-Higashi gene have also been found to be deficient in NK function (Roder *et al.*, 1980). *Beige* mice, which are more susceptible to transplantable syngeneic tumours, have also been described as allowing significantly greater metastatic spread of the Lewis lung tumour (Saloman *et al.*, 1980).

Therefore there may be sufficient justification in suggesting a role for NK cells in the secondary immune surveillance against circulating malignant cells.

Segal *et al.* (1980) have reported that metastatic cells of Lewis lung carcinoma are less susceptible to lysis by NK cells than cells of the primary tumour, and it has also been reported that the expression of an MHC determinant is associated with successful evasion of the immune surveillance by the metastatic cells (De Baetselier *et al.*, 1980). On the contrary, in an MCA-induced sarcoma maintained in syngeneic (DBA/2 × A) F-1 mice, Kerbel *et al.* (1978) had demonstrated that serial transplantation of the tumour resulted in the selection of an H-2^k negative variant with increased metastatic potential.

As described earlier, an increased expression of some determinant of the histocompatibility complex consequent upon interferon treatment has the effect of making the target tumour cells less susceptible to lysis by NK cells. In addition, it is believed that NK cell activity is not subject to MHC restriction as is cytotoxic T cell activity.

It would seem, therefore, that the role played by NK cells in immune surveillance and possibly metastatic dissemination is a complex one and as yet we have only a superficial understanding of it. Many questions need to be answered, e.g. about the activation of NK cells, their specificities, perhaps also their cell lineage, before their possible role in the control of tumour metastases can be elucidated.

Immunosuppressive proteins

Several investigators have reported the occurrence of proteins in sera and amniotic fluid which have immunosuppressive properties. An α-globulin fraction from mammalian serum has been found to produce immune suppression both *in vitro* and *in vivo* (Kamrin, 1958, 1959; Mowbray, 1963; Mowbray and Hargrave, 1966; Mannick and Schmid, 1967; Cooperband *et al.*, 1968; Glasgow *et al.*, 1971; Glaser *et al.*, 1972a, b; Glaser and Nelken,

1972; Nelken and Glaser, 1972; Nelken, 1973; Badger *et al.*, 1977). This fraction not only suppresses mitogen-induced lymphocyte transformation *in vitro*, but is also able to prolong allo- and xenograft survival.

Ovadia *et al.* (1975) showed that an immunosuppressive protein extracted from plasma promoted the "take" of MCA-induced tumours in C57BL mice. They found that the administration of this immunosuppressive protein 24 h before and again 24 h after inoculation of the animals with tumour cells promoted tumour growth. Secondly, they found that 25% animals inoculated with 10^3 tumour cells and all the animals inoculated with 10^4 cells developed tumours. Control animals, on the other hand, produced no tumours with 10^3 or 10^4 cells.

An increase in the serum or plasma levels of α-globulin in patients with neoplastic disease has been reported on several occasions (Petermann and Hogness, 1948; Seibert *et al.*, 1947; Hsu and Lo Gerfo, 1972; Ablin *et al.*, 1975). Hsu and Lo Gerfo (1972) have reported a correlation between the levels of α-globulin concentration in the sera of patients with cancer of the colon and the inhibitory effect of the plasma on PHA-induced lymphocyte activity. In advanced colonic cancer, patients not only show lower PHA response, but also high levels of the carcino-embryonic antigen (CEA). Ablin *et al.* (1975) also reported a clear relationship between the levels of α-2-globulin and the stage of carcinoma of the prostate. Patients with stage III carcinoma had twice the amount of α-2-globulin as stage I carcinoma patients. The levels in patients with stage II disease were intermediate. Besides, 3 out of 4 patients with stage I carcinoma possessed normal amounts of α-2-globulin. In contrast, only 2 out of 9 patients with stage III disease had normal amounts of the protein. Thus there appears to be some indication that the levels of α-globulins may be correlated with the state of progression of the neoplastic disease.

Alpha-fetoprotein (AFP) is also immunosuppressive (Murgita and Tomasi, 1975a, b; Aver and Kress, 1977), and AFP has been suggested as a component of the immunosuppressive α-globulin fraction. Contractor and Davies (1973) have observed inhibition of PHA-induced lymphocyte transformation by the glycoprotein hormone, human chorionic gonadotropin, and the peptide hormone human chorionic somatommamotropin. C-reactive protein is also known to possess similar suppressive action (Paik *et al.*, 1972).

Certain proteinase inhibitors such as α-2-macroglobulin (Chase, 1972) and α-1-antitrypsin (Arora *et al.*, 1978) also seem to possess immuno-suppressive ability. On this basis, it would be expected that the occurrence of these in serum would be conducive to tumour development and spread. Latner *et al.* (1976) found that levels of α-antitrypsin were higher in sera of patients with early (smear-positive) and late carcinoma of the cervix. The increased levels of this antiproteinase associated with increased malignant involvement is compatabile with an immunological inhibitory mode of action of α-antitrypsin.

PART II

The Epigenetics of Tumour Malignancy

Similarities between Embryonic and Neoplastic Systems

Introduction

Recently there has been an increasing awareness of the possibility that epigenetic mechanisms might operate in neoplastic systems (Sherbet, 1974a, b; Good, 1977). Epigenetic (developmental) systems share several features with neoplastic systems. These similarities were recognized by both pathologists and embryologists several decades ago.

Theories relating to the origin of neoplasia have been proposed in the past and have been based on embryological aspects. As early as 1829, the French investigators Lobstein and Recamier proposed that tumours originated from pockets of resting embryonic cells (*see* Gurchot, 1975). Cohnheim (1875) formulated a hypothesis which proposed that such cell nests were effectively sequestered from the host tissues, failed to mature and hence remained in an embryonic state. Cohnheim further suggested that a reactivation of these embryonic nests resulted in the formation of cancers. Over seventy years ago, the Scottish embryologist, John Beard, proposed the "trophoblast theory of cancer" (Beard, 1902). The general applicability of these theories to the pathogenesis of cancer is subject to considerable doubt and they have been refuted with sufficient justification. None the less, the pluripotency, i.e. the ability for diverse histological and morphogenetic differentiation of the stem cells of teratomas (Kleinsmith and Pierce, 1964; Finch and Ephrussi, 1967; Kahan and Ephrussi, 1970: M. Evans, 1972) and the detection of carcino-embryonic antigens in association with neoplasms, have given some credence to these theories and have defined a limited area of application, preventing them from lapsing into obscurity.

Neoplastic transformation represents a stable, heritable change suggesting that a genetic change, a mutation, may form the basic lesion of cancer. Paul (1978) has pointed out that the process of normal differentiation exhibits several characteristics of a mutation, but there is no demonstrable irreversible genetic alteration here. This is indicated by the process of regeneration (*see* reviews in Sherbet, 1974a) and by nuclear transplantation experiments. In the latter, it was shown that if nuclei derived from highly differentiated somatic cells were transplanted into enucleated *Xenopus* eggs, the new "differentiated' nuclei could organize the development of the eggs into mature adults, albeit only in a small proportion of cases (Gurdon, 1962; Gurdon and Laskey, 1970). On the other hand, mutagens may produce phenotypic changes analogous to those associated with differentiation (Siciliano *et al.*, 1978).

It has been suggested that neoplastic transformation might be a pathological counterpart of normal differentiation, an aberrant state of cell differentiation resulting from inappropriate and misprogrammed gene function (Markert, 1968; Sherbet, 1974b).

Waddington (1952) defined epigenetics as the science concerned with the causal analysis of development. This has, of late, been replaced by a more formal and precise definition. The epigenetic concept of cell differentiation, while retaining the essence of Waddington's definition, postulates that cell differentiation is an outcome of a concerted regulation of genetic activity (Sherbet, 1966). The concept has also been applied to neoplasia from time to time. The major criticism attracted by the epigenetic concept of neoplasia is that it is imprecise (for example, *see* Calman and Paul, 1978). While one might concur with this criticism, one can hardly agree with Calman and Paul that it is questionable whether epigenetic theories should be considered seriously at all. What is required unquestionably is a precise description of the epigenetic criteria. This has been attempted with some degree of success (*see* Anderson and Coggin, 1974; Uriel, 1979). Attempts have also been made to describe the epigenetic features of neoplasia and how epigenetic mechanisms might lead to the misprogramming of genetic activity, with the attendant aberrations in differentiation in and production of phenotypic products by neoplasms (Sherbet, 1974b). In this part of the book, epigenetic aspects are discussed in sufficient detail as to enable a cohesive picture to be drawn of the possible operation of epigenetic mechanisms in the expression of malignancy of tumours.

Growth

It is a common misconception that tumours ordinarily achieve very high rates of growth. High growth rates are not a characteristic feature of tumours. Tumours may grow as fast as embryos; there is hardly any noticeable difference in the rates of growth *in vivo* of normal fibroblasts of mouse embryos, such as 3T3 fibroblasts, and their malignant counterparts, the Simian virus-transformed SV-3T3 cells (Todaro *et al.*, 1964; Tobey and Campbell, 1965; Sheppard, 1972). Human astrocytoma cells in culture are known to grow faster than normal brain tissue (Chen and Mealey, 1972), but foetal brain cells appear to grow more than twice as fast as do Kernohan grade IV gliomas (glioblastoma multiforme) (Sherbet and Lakshmi, 1974a). Also, meningiomas, which are generally regarded as non-malignant tumours, have been reported to possess growth rates that are comparable with the highly malignant astrocytomas belonging to Kernohan grades III and IV (Sherbet and Lakshmi, 1974a) (histological grading of astrocytomas according to the system described by Kernohan *et al.*, 1949). It has been recognized, however, that by criteria of histology and behaviour some meningiomas can be considered as aggressive. Gibson and Halaka (1978) have reported that meningiomas may possess invasive properties. In these cases the histology provides little guidance as to the aggressiveness of the tumour or to prognosis. Bertalanffy (1969) had earlier examined the rates of proliferation of normal cell populations and compared them with those of normal tissue at certain cycles of physiological activity, and with the rates of growth of both malignant and non-malignant tumour cell populations. He found that rat mammary gland cells showed higher mitotic rates during pregnancy than the parenchymal cells of virgin rats, but they were comparable with mammary adenocarcinoma cells.

Another differentiating system which has yielded significant comparisons with neoplastic systems is regenerating tissues such as the regeneration blastema found in the regeneration of appendages in certain vertebrates (Carlson, 1974; Wolsky, 1974) or regenerating organs such as liver following partial hepatectomy. The dedifferentiating cells of the regeneration blastema show intense proliferation as compared with normal tissue (Carlson, 1974; Hay and Fischman, 1961; O'Steen and Walker, 1961). Bertalanffy (1969) reported that the mitotic rates of regenerating liver cells and hepatomas were roughly comparable. In some instances, regenerating liver showed greater mitotic activity than the hepatomas. (Authoritative accounts of the processes of growth and its regulation in neoplastic, embryonic and regenerating systems may be found in Sherbet, 1974a, 1981).

Proteolytic activity associated with neoplastic and embryonic cells

Normal cells cultivated *in vitro* on a finite substratum show contact-mediated inhibition of cellular movement (Abercrombie, 1961, 1970a, b) and a density-dependent inhibition of growth when a certain maximum cell density is achieved (Stoker and Rubin, 1967). This cell density is known as the saturation density. Such a density-dependent mechanism for the control of growth appears to be lacking in malignantly transformed cells, which often show considerable cell overlap and achieve high saturation densities.

Treatment with proteolytic enzyme has been shown to release normal cells transiently from density-dependent inhibition of growth (Burger, 1970; Sefton and Rubin, 1970). That proteolytic enzymes play an important part in the loss of contact inhibition by normal chick embryo cells transformed by avian RNA virus has been amply demonstrated (Unkeless *et al.*, 1973, 1974; Ossowski *et al.*, 1973a, b).

Schnebli and Burger (1972) showed that proteolytic enzymes are associated with 3T3 mouse fibroblasts transformed by polyoma virus and by Simian virus 40. Unkeless *et al.* (1973) also reported that fibroblasts transformed by RNA and DNA viruses exhibited greater fibrinolytic activity than normal cells. They appear to produce high levels of a serine protease which generates the active fibrinolytic protease, plasmin, by the hydrolysis of plasminogen (Ossowski *et al.*, 1973b; Rifkin *et al.*, 1974).

Plasminogen activator (PA) levels are negligibly low in normal hamster and guinea-pig embryonic cells, but those transformed by chemical carcinogens show high levels of this proteolytic enzyme. The close relationship between transformation and high enzyme levels is also suggested by the fact that in guinea-pig cells there is a prolonged lag period between exposure to carcinogens and actual cell transformation. This lag period is also seen in the appearance of increased amounts of PA. In other words, the phenotypic expression of the neoplastic state may be reflected in the ability of the cell to produce increased amounts of the enzyme.

Chick embryo fibroblasts which have been infected by non-transforming strains of avian leukosis virus or the temperature sensitive (*ts*) mutant of the Rous sarcoma virus (RSV) grown at non-permissive temperatures, show no fibronolytic activity. But cells infected with the wild-type RSV or the RSV *ts* mutant grown at permissive temperatures have shown distinct fibrinolytic activity. The plasminogen-activator activity appears to be associated with a specific membrane fraction isolated from the transformed cells (Quigley, 1976).

Mammary carcinomas of the rat induced by the administration of the carcinogen dimethyl benzanthracene (DMBA), are reported to be able to produce the plasminogen activator, while cells from lactating as well as from non-lactating mammary glands are unable to do so. The non-malignant breast tumour, the fibroadenoma, does not produce the activator, but malignant carcinomas do (Reich, 1974; Ossowski, 1979). Ossowski (1979) reported that the plasminogen activator content of two fibroadenomas was 140 and 28 Plong milliunits mg^{-1} protein. On the other hand, the plasminogen activator content of about 16 human breast carcinomas tested was in the range of 600-2200 milliunits mg^{-1} protein. This vast difference between malignant and non-malignant tumours was also noticeable when the tumours were tested in organ culture. The plasminogen activator content of extracts of prostatic cancers has been reported to be about 1·7 times higher, on average, than that of extracts of benign prostatic hyperplasia (Camiolo *et al.*, 1981). But in both neoplastic and benign groups the values were found to be distributed over wide ranges.

Studies on tumorigenic and non-tumorigenic clones of the B16 murine melanoma have tended to support these findings. The clone B_5-59 of the melanoma is a tumorigenic clone. If this is grown in the presence of 5-bromodeoxyuridine, the clone not only loses its tumorigenicity but also a greater proportion of its original fibrinolytic activity. When growth conditions are returned to normality, both tumorigenicity and fibrinolytic activity appear to return (Christman *et al.*, 1974). The teratocarcinoma cell line F9, which originated from a spontaneous testicular tumour of the strain 129 mouse and which is known to be non-invasive and to possess no metastatic ability, does not produce the plasminogen activator (Sherman *et al.*, 1976). Clifton and Grossi (1955) reported that plasminogen activator activity could be detected in association with breast carcinomas and adeno-carcinomas of the gastro-intestinal tract. In acute leukemia, a wide variation in fibrinolytic activity has been reported (Brackman *et al.*, 1970).

The proteolytic enzyme, plasmin, generated by the plasminogen activator cleaves fibrin into fibrin degradation products (FDP). It may be expected, therefore, that higher levels of FDP may be associated with malignant conditions.

Increased levels of fibrin degradation products have been found in non-cancerous conditions such as pulmonary embolism (Ruckley *et al.*, 1970), deep vein thrombosis and myocardial infarction (Cash *et al.*, 1969). Whur *et al.* (1978) found that in a series of bronchial carcinomas investigated, only 22% of the patients showed raised FDP levels in blood and/or urine. They concluded that elevated FDP levels may not be a feature of primary bronchial carcinoma. According to Gropp *et al.* (1980), FDP were detected in 40% of their patients with lung cancer. In patients with metastatic disease, 22 out of 26 had FDP in the serum. None of these patients had shown any signs of intravascular coagulation. In agreement with other investigators (Hedner and Nilsson, 1971; Carlsson, 1973), Gropp *et al.* (1980) suggest that the FDP may have been derived from the extravascular breakdown of fibrin by malignant cells.

It ought to be pointed out, however, that an association between malignancy and levels of plasminogen activator secretion must yet be considered uncertain. Wilson and Dowdle (1978) have recently examined 39 primary or early passages of human malignant neoplasms, 16 benign neoplasms and several normal tissues. Their general finding is that while normal cells secreted less plasminogen activator than malignant cells, high levels were also found in benign tumours and reactive tissue. Thus, reactive gliosis was found to secrete much higher quantities of plasminogen activator than did normal glial tissue, and the levels were comparable with those found in malignant melanoma. Primary cultures of the non-malignant meningiomas produced very low levels of the activator, but cells which had been passaged longer *in vitro* produced comparatively greater quantities. This could be a result of selection of cells which have greater plasminogen activator activity associated with them, although it is uncertain if such ability would confer any selective advantage on the cells. The overall impression one gains is that, more often than not, a higher level of plasmin-ogen activator activity may be found to be associated with the neoplastic state than the normal state, but quantitation of the plasminogen activator content for individual tumours may be of limited clinical value.

Proteolytic activity is undoubtedly associated with a wide variety of tumours (Ottoson and Sylvén, 1960; Taylor *et al.*, 1970; Yamanishi *et al.*, 1972; Dabbous *et al.*, 1977; *see also* review by Schnebli, 1974). Strauch (1971, 1972) reported an increase in collagenolytic activity in carcinomas of the breast. The levels of activity were considerably higher than non-malignant conditions of mastopathy and fibroadenoma. Such increases have also been observed in the squamous cell carcinoma of the head and neck (Abramson *et al.*, 1975).

Dresden *et al.* (1972) examined a variety of human tumours for their collagenolytic activity. Some tumours of epithelial origin such as basal cell and squamous cell carcinoma of the skin frequently possessed high collagenolytic activity. Adenocarcinomas of the colon also produced high amounts of collagenase, but chondrosarcomas and astrocytomas apparently possessed no enzyme activity. Hashimoto *et al.* (1973) have confirmed the association of high proteolytic activity with squamous cell carcinoma of the skin, while Yamanishi *et al.* (1973) found high collagenase activity in malignant melanoma. Koono *et al.* (1974) reported the occurrence of neutral proteases in rat ascites hepatomas. The surface proteolytic activity of transformed mouse epidermal cells has been reported to be 3-4 times higher than that of normal cells (Hatcher *et al.*, 1976).

Weiss and Holyoke (1969) reported increased pulmonary metastasis of a spontaneous mammary tumour of mice, which had been fed with excess vitamin A. This has been suggested to be due to a release of hydrolytic enzyme by the vitamin, which is known to activate lysosomal enzymes of many cells. Sylvén and Bois (1960) and Sylvén (1968) found marked increases in lysosomal hydrolases in the interstitial fluid from the periphery of tumours; and also in the interstices and soluble components of the cytoplasm.

Weiss (1977, 1978) noticed that the detachment of viable tumour cells from the Walker carcinoma 256 was facilitated if there were adjacent necrotic zones or if the tumours were exposed to extracts of necrotic tissues.

Using pure Walker carcinoma cells and necrotic extracts that were demonstrably rich in lysosomal enzymes, Weiss (1978) has shown that the necrotic extracts act directly upon the cells and facilitate their detachment. Robertson and Williams (1969) showed that an increased collagenase activity was detectable at the surface and beyond of an invading experimental breast tumour.

Tumours thus appear to make penetration space by means of hydrolytic enzymes. Invasion is also probably aided by peritumoral oedema. Burgess and Sylvén (1962) reported that the degree of oedema is related to the degree of malignancy and oedema is largely associated with the process of glycolysis occurring in tumours.

Since proteolytic activity in association with tumours may facilitate the detachment and release of tumour emboli (Weiss, 1977), and also the infiltration of tissue stroma of the host by enzymatic degradation, the postulate that these enzymes may be responsible for the invasive ability of tumours (Poole, 1973) has gained ground. Consistent with this view is the demonstration by Latner *et al.* (1973a) that the wide-spectrum antiproteinase, aprotinin (Trasylol®) inhibits the invasion of mouse kidney cortex in organ culture by malignantly transformed BHK cells. The growth of Ehrlich ascites tumour cells has been shown to be inhibited by soya-bean trypsin inhibitor (Verloes *et al.*, 1978). One could then envisage a situation where the proteolytic activity associated with a tumour which could facilitate its spread may be neutralized by the antiproteinases produced by the host. De Vore *et al.* (1980) found that the human small cell carcinoma was not invasive in athymic *nude* mice, although it possessed high collagenase activity. An investigation of the tumours after a few weeks following implantation revealed a thin fibrous capsule around the tumour implants. Homogenates of these capsular tissues were found to possess high anticollagenase activity. In contrast, the Lewis lung carcinoma, which also had associated collagenase activity, was only poorly encapsulated. When assayed, this capsular material was found to have much less collagenase-inhibiting activity than did the capsular tissue surrounding the small cell carcinoma.

The resistance of certain tissues to invasion by cancer cells has also been attributed to proteinase inhibitors occurring in such tissues. Hyaline cartilage, a tissue which is resistant to invasion (Eisenstein *et al.*, 1973), has been reported to contain antiproteinase (Sorgente *et al.*, 1975; Eisenstein *et al.*, 1975). None the less, it ought to be pointed out that certain strains of non-transformed fibroblast lines have been reported to show growth inhibition by proteinase inhibitors (McIlhenny and Hogan, 1974; Eisenstein *et al.*, 1975).

It would appear from the above discussion that the proteolytic activity may at least in part contribute to or aid the invasive behaviour of tumour cells. Its association with the metastatic process yet remains largely un-investigated. Thus, although plasminogen activator levels may be higher in some malignant cells, Nicolson *et al.* (1976a, c) found no differences in plas-minogen activator levels of B16 melanoma variant lines with different meta-static abilities. In any case, the advantages of possessing the ability to release the activator are not clearly understood. While, on the one hand this may enable the tumour cell to infiltrate surrounding tissue, the formation of fibrin deposit around tumour cell emboli may have a protective role and aid the metastatic behaviour (Hagmar, 1972a; *see also* pp. 24-29).

Giraldi *et al.* (1977a, b) have reported that the broad-spectrum anti-proteinase, aprotinin, which was earlier shown by Latner *et al.* (1973a) to inhibit invasion by tumour, also reduced metastasis in the lungs of the Lewis lung carcinoma. However, they also reported that Pepstatin and Leupeptin were ineffective both in the control of primary tumour growth and the formation of metastases. Giraldi *et al.* have therefore suggested that cathepsins B and D may not be involved in the formation of metastases. While the detachment of tumour fragments may be inhibited by anti-proteinases, how these enzymes could possibly reduce the incidence of metastases seems a complex question.

Although the work of Giraldi *et al.* shows that Leupeptin had no effect on spontaenous metastasis, Saito *et al.* (1980) have described Leupeptin suppression of the arrest and development into tumour nodules of a Yoshida ascites hepatoma injected intravenously.

It has been shown that treatment of tumour cells with aprotinin alters their surface properties (Latner and Sherbet, 1979), apparently by preventing the excision by the tumour-associated proteolytic enzymes of surface proteins of approximate molecular weight of 115K (Lakshmi *et al.*, 1982, *see* pp. 62-63). This presumably has the effect of making the aprotinin-treated cancer cells more antigenic. Whether Leupeptin and Pepstatin may act in a similar fashion is not known. Aprotinin has also been found to bind to sialyl residues of cell surface glycoproteins (Stoddart *et al.*, 1974; Thomson *et al.*, 1978). If such binding occurred on a large scale, on account of the basic nature (pI 10·5) of aprotinin, it is possible that the net surface charge density on the surface of the tumour cells may be reduced thereby creating an electrostatic environment that may be conducive to the adhesion of the aprotinin treated cells to the endothelial wall and subsequently to the parenchymal cells of the metastatic organ. It may be pointed out, neverthe-less, that it does not seem likely that aprotinin may bind the cell surface in large amounts, since Latner and Sherbet (1979) found that there was a dose-dependent increase in the surface charge density in cells treated with various concentrations of aprotinin.

Tumour cells are not unique in possessing the ability to invade neighbouring tissues. As discussed in later sections, embryonic cells are also known to be invasive. It seems, therefore, more than coincidental that high proteolytic activity should also be found in embryonic cells. It has been reported that sea-urchin eggs release proteolytic enzymes (inhibitable by soy-bean trypsin inhibitor) upon fertilization (Vacquier *et al.*, 1972, 1973). Slaughter and Triplett (1975a) found high proteolytic activity (and also proteinase inhibitors) in association with amphibian oocytes. The enzymes and the inhibitors also seemed to be closely linked with the process of differentiation of pigment cells, which is related to the metabolism of the amino acid, tyrosine (Slaughter and Triplett, 1975b).

Mouse embryos between the 7th and 10th day of development also secrete the plasminogen activator. A progressive appearance of plasminogen activator activity in different embryonic tissues has been described and it has been suggested that such activity may be associated with migratory ability and rapid growth of certain embryonic tissues (Bode and Dziadek, 1979). Thus the onset of secretion of the plasminogen activator on the 8th day is said to coincide with the formation of the primitive streak and the proliferation and migration of embryonic mesoderm. This is consistent with the suggestion of Adamson and Ayers (1979) that the migration of mesoderm between the ectodermal and endodermal cell layers may be aided by an enzyme-mediated degradation of the basement membrane present between these two tissues.

The invasive ability of trophoblast cells has often been attributed to associated proteolytic enzymes. Proteolytic activity has been demonstrated *in vitro* in guinea-pig, rat and mouse trophoblasts (Blandau, 1949; Owers, 1970; Owers and Blandau, 1971; Strickland *et al.*, 1976). Strickland *et al.* (1976) and Sherman *et al.* (1976) demonstrated the production of plasminogen activator by trophoblast cells when they invade the uterine desidua during implantation. They also suggested that the migration of parietal endodermal cells along the Reichert's membrane may be aided by the proteinase.

Plasminogen activator activity has also been implicated in the process involving tissue remodelling, such as the involution of the mammary gland in the post-lactation period (Ossowski, 1979).

Invasive and metastatic ability

Invasive ability is accepted as a characteristic feature of malignant tumours, but it is not an indicator of malignancy (Foulds, 1958). Tumour cells share this property with embryonic cells. The invasion of the endometrium by trophoblast cells of the developing embryo is an oft-cited example of invasive behaviour shown by embryonic cells. According to Glenister (1961), the initial phase of this process appears to depend upon direct interactions occurring between the embryonic cells and the endometrium, and the invasion is cellular and not syncytial in nature as once believed. Embryonic mesenchymal cells are one of the most invasive types of differentiated cells. Invasive ability may indeed be an intrinsic feature of differentiating cells. Sherbet (1970) stated that most embryonic cells appear to lose their motility in the course of embryonic development and that this is compatible with the acquisition of organization. Since neoplasia has been described as remarkable for the failure of normal regulation and organization (Foulds, 1963), it would be interesting if a correlation existed in neoplastic cells between this apparent loss of organization and the acquisition of invasive ability. It may not be out of place to point out here that leukocytes are also an invasive type of cell.

The distribution of argentiffin tissue in the primitive gut is another instance of invasiveness of embryonic cells. The argentiffin cells are derived from the neural ectoderm and have been found to invade and become distributed in the primitive gut and its derivatives, viz. the gastric glands and anterior pituitary.

Even more interesting is the migration of certain neural crest cells which somewhat characteristically show a cytoplasmic reaction with chromic acid and have been designated as chromaffin cells. Chromaffin cells may cluster in the proximity of the sympathetic ganglia to form para-ganglionic chromaffin bodies. Clusters of chromaffin cells are also associated with the mesoderm in the coelom. The largest clustering of these cells occurs in the adrenal gland to form the adrenal medulla. It is evident, therefore, that not only do the chromaffin cells invade other parts of the organism, but they also appear to become localized at certain sites, the process being akin to the process of the formation of secondary tumour foci in metastatic dissemination.

Embryonic induction and neoplasia

The interactions occurring between components of the embryonic system provide a basis for the operation of epigenetic mechanisms in cell differentiation and morphogenesis. Embryogenesis, which involves cell differentiation and morphogenesis, is the product of a complex but co-ordinated interplay of epigenetic processes. The most significant feature of gastrulation and post-gastrulation embryogenesis is the appearance of a series of inductive interactions. These interactions constitute a temporal hierarchy of interacting systems, with each interaction constituting a step in the process of differentiation. These have been classified as primary, secondary and tertiary interactions, according to the level at which they operate. Embryonic inductions are essentially interactions between component tissues of the embryo. As a result of these interactions, a selection appears to be made of a facultative genome in either or both of the reactant tissues and consequently the synthetic machinery of these cells is directed in such a way as to bring about their differentiation into specific cell types (Sherbet, 1966, 1974b). (*See* Toivonen *et al.*, (1976) for a review of the induction phenomenon which includes a discussion of the salient features of the historical development of the concept of embryonic induction.)

The process of embryonic induction which is divisible into evocation and individuation has superficial but important similarities with the process of induction and development of tumours. The initiation of the neural ectoderm into neural tissue is induced by embryonic mesoderm. Contact between the two cell types lasting no longer than 5 h (in the chick embryo system; Sherbet and Lakshmi, 1969) to 10 h (in the amphibian system; Toivonen and Wartiovaara, 1976) appears to be sufficient to induce the ectodermal cells to begin to differentiate into neural cells. If the inducer is removed from the ectoderm after the required duration of contact, the differentiation of the ectoderm into neural tissue will continue. Waddington (1941) therefore suggested that the process of differentiation be regarded as divisible into "evocation", which is the initiation of events leading to a state of differentiation, and "individuation", which is the morphogenesis of the induced structures. The latter is an autonomous process not dependent upon the presence of the agent that produces the "evocation".

The parallelism of the "evocation" and "individuation" concept with the concept of initiation and promotion of neoplasia proposed by Rous and Kidd (1941) and Berenblum and Shubik (1947a, b, 1949a, b), in their investigations on chemically induced neoplasia in the epidermis of rabbits and mice, is fairly obvious. Rous and Kidd (1941) found that application of tar to rabbit epidermis caused the appearance of warts, which regressed when the chemical stimulus was withdrawn. However, they reappeared quickly when the stimulus was applied again. Rous and Kidd (1941) argued that the first stimulus produced a sub-threshold neoplastic state, from which the epidermis did not revert to the normal state even after the stimulus was withdrawn. Berenblum and Shubik (1947a, b, 1949a, b) showed that when the sub-threshold state is reached, the second chemical stimulus need not necessarily be carcinogenic but could be a non-specific agent whose role is simply to promote the progression of the neoplastic change. Thus in embryonic induction and in the induction of neoplasia, the initial stimulus may be deemed to be responsible for the "determination" of the path of differentiation into neural tissue differentiation or into a sub-threshold neoplasia, respectively. The major point of difference, however, is the autonomous process of individuation which provides form and organization to the induced structures resulting as a consequence of an embryonic induction. This process of individuation may be lacking in the progression and development of the neoplasm. In other words, while the primary embryonic inductor is literally a primary "organizer", the neoplastic state is devoid of such organizational control. Needham (1950) has indeed suggested that the development of teratomas is an example of the failure of the individuation field in the process of neoplastic development.

Morphogenetic and neoplastic stimuli

No sooner was the phenomenon of embryonic induction discovered (Spemann and Mangold, 1924) than it was also discovered that the ability to provide a morphogenetic stimulus was not particularly a property of the living "organizer" but that killed tissues were also able successfully to produce embryonic inductions (Bautzmann *et al.*, 1932). Following this discovery, a large number of natural as well as unnatural substances have been tested and a variety of chemical substances (Needham, 1950), vitamins, plant auxins (Suomalainen and Toivonen, 1939), glycoprotein (Sherbet and Mulherkar, 1963, 1965; Sherbet and Lakshmi, 1967a, b, 1968a, c, 1969b, 1974b) and steroid hormones, and polycyclic hydrocarbons have been shown to be able to act as morphogenetic agents (Needham, 1950).

The most interesting feature of these investigations is the observation that several polycyclic hydrocarbons known to be potent carcinogens were also very active morphogenetic agents. Two important examples are 3,4-benzo(a)pyrene (BP), the isolation of which from coal tar by Kennaway and colleagues opened the doors to chemical carcinogenesis, and 3-methylcholanthrene (MCA), both of which are highly carcinogenic and both possess strong morphogenetic activity. On the other hand, non-carcinogenic hydrocarbons such as chrysene had no such ability.

Both carcinogenic and morphogenetic stimuli appear to produce their effects rapidly. Prostate cells in culture exposed to MCA for 24 h at a concentration of 1 μg ml^{-1} sufficed to produce a 100% malignant transformation (Mondal and Heidelberger, 1970). A 10% transformation of hamster cells was achieved by exposure to benzo(a)pyrene for 3 h (Berwald and Sachs, 1963, 1965; Huberman and Sachs, 1966). An even shorter exposure to nitrosomethylurea (NMU) (2 h) was required by pseudo-diploid Chinese hamster cells to obtain transformation (Sanders and Burford, 1967). The morphogenetic stimulus also takes effect over a comparable time course. In *Triturus* Brahma (1966) found ectoderm contact with inductor over a 6-h period was required for the inductive effect. In the chick embryo system, the minimum duration of contact was found to be 5 h (Sherbet and Lakshmi, 1969a). In these experiments, the inductor and the responding ectoderm were in direct contact with each other. In trans-filter inductions with filters of 0·2 μm pore size interposed between the interacting systems, the minimum time required for successful morphogenetic effect has been reported to be about 10 h (Toivonen and Wartiovaara, 1976).

The rapidity of both carcinogenic and morphogenetic transformation might indicate that both stimuli may interact with the genetic material and derepress sections of the genome which results in pleiotropic alterations of the reacting cells. The metabolic products of the carcinogens, which are probably the ultimate effectors of transformation, have been known to be strongly electrophilic, and as such would be expected to interact with electron-rich molecules of tissues such as the bases of nucleic acids (Sivak and Van Duuren, 1969; Miller and Miller, 1971). This can conceivably lead to a heritable change in the genome, and is seen as a variation in the normal genomic pattern of expression, as implied in the protovirus hypothesis of carcinogenesis (Temin, 1974). In other words, the evolution of "cancer genes" is seen in the phenotypic effects of this process of evolution. The process of differentiation is measured by the same yardstick, viz. the development of phenotypically distinct cell types. In order to induce the differentiation of the ectodermal cells into neural tissue, the morphogenetic stimulus imparted by the primary organizer must also achieve a "derepression" or activation of a certain section of the genome, and this effect could be described as heritable in *sensu stricto* as transformation of cells could be.

The argument that the morphogenetic stimulus of the primary organizer has a "genotropic" action (Waddington, 1962) is a sensible one. Trans-filter neural inductions (Toivonen *et al.*, 1976) can indeed be interpreted as demonstrating that the stimulus is macromolecular in nature. Its binding to the genetic material has not been demonstrated, but there is much circumstantial evidence that this may indeed be the case (Sherbet and Lakshmi, 1967a, 1968a, 1974a). In any event, there is little doubt that the inductive stimulus triggers the synthesis of rapidly labelled nuclear ribonucleic acids (RNA) which indicates that the inductive tissue interaction has either directly or indirectly derepressed genes which will, as judged by the subsequent phenotypic effect of the interaction, result in the differentiation of neural tissue. The synthesis of specific RNA has also been demonstrated in other induction systems, e.g. the induction of the lens by the optic vesicle (Scott and Bell, 1965; Yamada and Roesel, 1964; Yamada and Karasaki, 1963) and in the induction of differentiating pancreatic epithelium by mesenchymal cells (Rutter *et al.*, 1964; Wessels and Wilt, 1965).

Competence phenomenon in differentiation
and neoplasia

It was stated earlier that embryonic inductions are essentially interactions between component parts of the embryo. Every induction system, therefore, has at least two components. In primary embryonic induction, the "organizer" mesoderm and the presumptive neural ectoderm are the components which interact with each other, as a consequence of which the ectoderm is induced to differentiate into neural tissue. This neural tissue undergoes morphogenesis into the brain which, within a few hours of development, can be distinguished into the fore-, mid- and hind-brain. If we focus our attention on the forebrain, we will see it undergo further morphogenesis to give rise to the optic vesicles. These optic vesicles are then in contact with the presumptive neural ectoderm again, which induces the differentiation of lens tissue. This may be seen as a secondary interaction and described as a secondary induction. The most important feature, however, is that the presumptive neural ectoderm possesses two different modes of differentiation, i.e. it can produce to different types of tissue. Obviously, therefore, this could be due to one of two causes: (a) the different types of differentiation are due to qualitative differences in the inducing stimulus, or (b) the ectoderm may have undergone changes in the course of time which may have altered its state of responsiveness to the inducing stimulus.

Although it is now accepted that chemical mediators trigger genetic mechanisms in order to produce the differentiation of new tissues in embryonic induction systems, there are still considerable doubts as to the specificity of chemical mediators. There is much evidence in the literature that a variety of inductors derived from embryos or adult animals, inductors either in the living state or after a variety of chemical and heat treatments, can produce the same spectrum of cell differentiation (Saxén and Toivonen, 1962; Sherbet, 1962, 1963; Rostedt, 1968, 1971). Thus it appears that the inductive stimuli are non-specific in their action. It is inevitable, therefore, that mechanisms that confer the specificity, i.e. determine the nature of differentiation of the stimulated ectoderm, must reside in the responding tissue. In other words, there must be a built-in mechanism that allows the inductive stimulus selectively to activate the transcription of a particular section of the genome.

There is considerable evidence that the responsiveness of the embryonic ectoderm does indeed change in the course of time. It is well known, for example, that neuro-ectoderm isolated from early gastrula stage embryos and combined with an inductor, such as a neural plate, would differentiate into a neural plate. However, if the isolated ectoderm is left in saline to "age" and is then combined with the same inductor, a lens rather than neural tissue is formed from the ectoderm (Waddington, 1936, Holtfreter,

1934). Earlier, Waddington (1934) had introduced the concept of competence as an important factor in the determination of the path of differentiation being followed as a consequence of embryonic induction.

The competence of a tissue may be described as a state of being able to respond to an inductive stimulus. The differentiative competence may be said to arise in a temporal sequence. In the experiments described above, it may be said that the neuro-ectoderm had lost its "neural competence", i.e. the ability to be induced to differentiate into neural tissue, but had acquired "lens competence". Some states of competence are known to arise late in development, such as competence to be induced to differentiate into muscle, cartilage, cornea and other cell types (Waddington, 1962).

Although the concept was formulated over four decades ago, very little is known about the nature of changes that occur when certain states of competence are lost and others acquired. The changes obviously involve the genetic material, either its structure or function or both. Ultraviolet irradiation is known to depress neural competence. Actinomycin D is known to alter the state of competence (Lakshmi, 1970). Since actinomycin D reacts with the guanine bases of DNA and sterically prevents RNA polymerase activity, Sherbet (1974b) has suggested that altered competence may reflect changes in genetic function, such as alterations in the synthesis of specific proteins (repressor?) or other nuclear or cytoplasmic factors, changes in competence being associated with a gradual depletion of the factors with time.

Waddington (1966) proposed that a cell is switched to a certain developmental path when certain proteins are available in that cell that can become attached to and prime the genes which define the particular developmental pathway. Sherbet (1974b) suggested that these proteins could be viewed as analogous to a repressor that can exist in two forms at equilibrium with each other (Englesberg *et al.*, 1965, 1969). Sherbet (1974b) further suggested that competence may be thought of as a state of sub-threshold activation of the genes. In analogy with the L-arabinose operon, it was postulated that in the state of competence for a switch to differentiation into a given cell type, a regulator gene product, P, saturates the operator sites, with their true repressor form, P1, remaining in equilibirium with a P2 form. If the inductor molecules are transmitted into this competent cell, the repressor form P1 molecules are altered by a configurational change into the P2 form, which is the activator form. Such an alteration into the activator P2 form may not be possible, or be rendered difficult, by a dilution effect in the event of a late arrival of the inductive stimulus. The depression or alteration in neural competence described by Lakshmi (1970) may be due to an inhibition of the production of the repressor molecules (Fig. 5). However, hypothetical such a model might be, the simple message which emerges

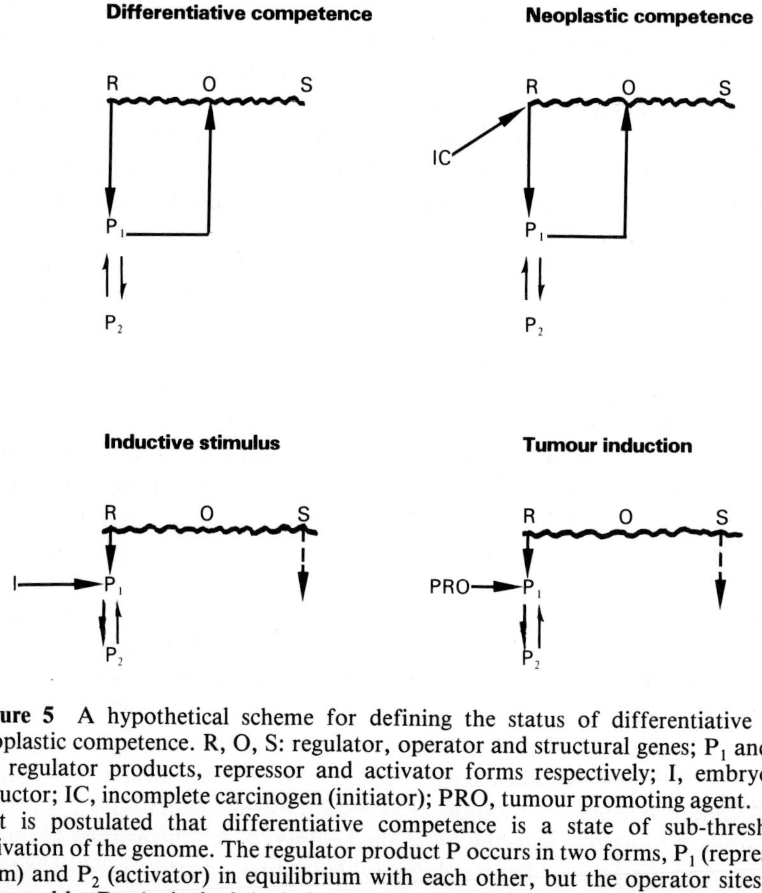

Figure 5 A hypothetical scheme for defining the status of differentiative and neoplastic competence. R, O, S: regulator, operator and structural genes; P_1 and P_2 are regulator products, repressor and activator forms respectively; I, embryonic inductor; IC, incomplete carcinogen (initiator); PRO, tumour promoting agent.

It is postulated that differentiative competence is a state of sub-threshold activation of the genome. The regulator product P occurs in two forms, P_1 (repressor form) and P_2 (activator) in equilibrium with each other, but the operator sites are saturated by P_1. Arrival of the inductive stimulus causes P_1 to alter in form to P_2, allowing an activation of the operon.

Neoplastic competence is postulated to be induced by a carcinogenic stimulus· which results also in the synthesis of the repressor form P_1. Neoplastic induction will result when P_1 is converted to the P_2 (activator form) by the tumour promoting agent. A complete carcinogen is postulated not only to induce synthesis of P_1, but also to convert it to the P_2 form.

from this discussion is that differentiating systems have intrinsic mechanisms which control their response to inducing morphogenetic stimuli. This is one major aspect in which the neoplastic system apparently differs from the epigenetic system.

It is commonly believed that application of an incomplete carcinogen to skin, for instance, initiates a sub-threshold neoplastic state or incipient neoplasia, in which the cells may remain for several weeks or remain permanently sensitized in this way. An application of a cocarcinogen or a promoting agent following the application of the carcinogenic stimulus results in the development of the tumour. This effect apparently is the result of the changes in gene expression caused by the agent. This is suggested by the ability of tumour promoters in general to mimic phenotypic expression of neoplastic transformation and to enhance such expression in cells which have undergone transformation. Tumour promoters also affect differentiation. Promoters such as phorbol esters, e.g. 12-O-tetra decanoyl-phorbol-13 acetate, are known to inhibit normal differentiation but induce differentiation in certain neoplastic systems (Weinstein *et al.*, 1979). A complete carcinogen possesses not only the ability to initiate but also to promote development of a tumour from the sensitized cells. However, the experiments of Bielschosky *et al.* (1968) on the carcinogenicity of urethane indicate that the promoting ability of urethane is genetically determined. From this, one may envisage a situation where in certain cases the promotion of the tumour from the subthreshold neoplastic state may be caused by some intracellular component whose availability may determine the requirement for an extraneous promoting agent. This is not incompatible with the analogous fact that although the embryonic organizer lays down the whole pattern of development, abilities comparable with the organizer can still be found in various organs of the adult animal.

It was suggested earlier in this section that the state of competence to differentiate could be viewed as a sub-threshold activation of the corresponding genes, with the actual progress of these cells in the path of differentiation being dependent upon the arrival of the inducing stimulus. One could postulate, in parallel with these thoughts on the differentiative competence of tissues, that the sub-threshold neoplastic state induced by the initiating carcinogenic stimulus may be analogous to the acquisition of a state of competence. It could be further postulated that when such a state of competence is achieved, provided that the promoting agents are available, the competent cells may be induced to develop into a neoplasm.

The acquisition of neoplastic competence may be due to an initiation of the repressor, which not only saturates the operator sites but is available in excess intracellularly. The promoter (non-carcinogen) may be the agent which would alter the P_1 repressor into the P_2 activator form. If the carcinogen is a complete carcinogen, one would expect that it will not only induce production of the repressor proteins by the regulator gene but will also bind the intracellular repressor.

Abell and Heidelberger (1962) identified a protein fraction in mouse skin cells to which carcinogenic hydrocarbons could bind but not the non-carcinogenic ones. This protein fraction was similar to the *h* protein of rat liver, which binds the carcinogenic azo dyes and 2-acetylaminofluorene. Not only did the mouse skin *h* protein bind carcinogenic hydrocarbons, but the ability of the hydrocarbons to bind the protein correlated closely with their carcinogenic activity (Abell and Heidelberger, 1962). Indeed, Pitot and Heidelberger (1963) suggested that this protein may be a repressor.

The neoplastic competence model may also be applied to viral carcinogenesis. The pathogenesis of paraneoplastic syndromes has similarly been attributed to the acquisition of new "neoplastic competence" (Sherbet, 1974b; see below).

Paraneoplastic Syndromes

Among the causes that lead to the death of cancer patients are the familiar syndromes of anorexia and cachexia (Theologides, 1974; Gold, 1974), recurrent fevers (Bodell, 1974) and several types of anaemia (Berlin, 1974). In addition to these generalized conditions, patients frequently suffer from metabolic disturbances caused by the production of specific hormones and peptides, etc. Hall (1974) has stated that about 20% of cancer patients will have such cancer-associated or paraneoplastic syndromes and that 75% of all patients will develop one in the course of time.

Brown (1928) first reported the occurrence of endocrine dysfunction in a case of oat-cell carcinoma of the bronchus. In 1932, Cushing described the syndrome bearing his name. Several syndromes of ectopic endocrinopathy have been described (*see* Haas, 1964; Lpsett *et al.*, 1964; Sachs, 1965; Bower and Gordon, 1965; Myers *et al.*, 1966; Fukase, 1978; Table 4). The possibility that detection of ectopic endocrinopathy with the sensitive biochemical and immunological aids currently available may result in early diagnosis of cancer, and also in assessing responsiveness to therapy, has generated intense interest in the study of paraneoplastic syndromes. Sachs (1965) opined that hypokalaemic alkalosis was so distinguishing a feature of the ectopic production of ACTH that, if discovered in a patient with Cushing's syndrome, one must suspect the presence of tumour. Ectopic endorinopathy has frequently been detected long before the detection of the neoplasm itself (Bower and Gordon, 1965).

The development of sensitive methods of assay of ectopic products may be of considerable use in assessing the efficacy of treatment (Bagshawe *et al.*, 1969); perhaps, as suggested by Dilman (1966), it may offer new modes of therapy. Equally important is the fundamental implication for understanding the mechanisms of neoplasia. The production of hormones or biologically active peptides by tissues which normally do not synthesize them is obviously concerned with the mechanisms of activation of certain sections of the genome which are normally inoperative, i.e. the tumours are acquiring new differentiated functions, and therefore this is a process akin to differentiation, which may be described in terms of sequential activation of the genetic material culminating in the production of a specific phenotypic product such as haemoglobin, myosin, crystallin, etc. This provides an obvious venue for exploration as to whether epigenetic models might be used for explaining the pathogenesis of paraneoplastic syndromes of ectopic endocrinopathy.

Ross (1972) pointed out that polypeptide hormones such as ADH, oxytocin, melatonin, etc. are produced in the hypothalamus in tissues which are embryologically ectodermal in origin, and in the pituitary gland, thyroid, parathyroid or parafollicular cells of the thyroid, which originate from the embryonic endoderm. Steroid hormones are produced by glands of mesodermal origin. A close examination of the neoplasms and their ectopic endocrine activities shows that polypeptide hormone activities are more often than not associated with neoplasms of organs that are endodermal in origin. Hall and Nathanson (1969) had suggested earlier that in certain syndromes the products ectopically synthesized corresponded with the normal synthetic activities of histogenetically related organs. Thus, ectopic ACTH syndrome was more frequently associated with thymic or bronchiogenic tumours. ACTH is normally produced by the anterior pituitary gland, which is derived, as also are the thymus and lung, from the same branchial embryological anlagen.

Sherbet (1974b) suggested a rational approach to the problem of paraneoplastic syndrome by classifying the neoplasms into epigenetic groups based on the embryological relationships pointed out by Hall and Nathanson (1969). Sherbet (1974b) further proposed the following genetic model for the pathogenesis of paraneoplastic syndrome.

1. All the cells in a differentiating system have the same genetic potentialities. Cell differentiation involves a progressive "determination" and restriction of "competences" and a sequential activation of the genome.

2. Neoplastic change, at least in part, constitutes a dedetermination and acquisition of an earlier state of competence. An abnormal genetic activation may be produced in the newly acquired competent state by chemical inducers already present in the cells or transmitted into

Table 4

Paraneoplastic syndromes[a]

Syndrome	Tumours involved	Ectopic hormone	References
Hyperadrenocorticism	Bronchogenic, thymic, pancreatic ca (infrequently tumours of the testis, thyroid, breast, ovary, kidney, etc.)	ACTH	Brown, 1928; Leyton *et al.*, 1931; Lipsett *et al.*, 1964; Bower and Gordon, 1965; Sachs, 1965; Hallwright *et al.*, 1964; Gordon, 1967; Brookes *et al.*, 1963; Liddle, 1960; Holub and Katz, 1961; Meador *et al.*, 1962; Azzopardi and Williams, 1968; Laurence and Neville, 1972; Omenn, 1970
Hypoglycaemia	Mesenchymal tumours, less frequently hepatic, adrenocortical carcinomas	Insulin (hypo-glycaemia-producing factor, HPF)	Nadler and Wolfer, 1929; McFadzean and Yeung, 1956; Lipsett *et al.*, 1964; Odell, *et al.*, 1963; Schonfeld *et al.*, 1961; Whitney and Massey, 1961; Barton and Labange, 1961; Omenn, 1970
Hypercalcaemia	Breast, renal and bronchogenic carcinomas	PTH	Thomas *et al.*, 1960; Bower and Gordon, 1965; Tashjian *et al.*, 1964; Munson *et al.*, 1965; Sherwood *et al.*, 1967; Berson and Yalow, 1966; Azzopardi and Whittaker, 1969; Mavligit *et al.*, 1971; Melick *et al.*, 1972

Erythrocythaemia	Erythropoietin	Renal carcinomas and benign lesions, cerebellar haemangioma, uterine myofibroma, rarely in adrenocortical carcinoma or carcinomas of the breast, lung, ovary, etc., hepatoma	Lipsett et al., 1964; Bower and Gordon, 1965; Fried et al., 1956; Rosse et al 1963a, b; Gurney, 1960; Hewlett et al., 1960; Korst et al., 1962; Murphy et al., 1967; Hammond and Winnick, 1974; Omenn, 1970
Hyponatraemia	ADH	Bronchogenic carcinoma	Schwartz et al., 1957; Amatruda et al., 1963; Bower and Mason, 1964; Bower et al., 1964; Lipscomb et al., 1968; Bartter and Schwartz, 1967; Imura, 1980
Hyperthyroidism	TSH	Chorio-carcinoma, tumours of the gastro-intestinal tract, bronchial tumours	Odell et al., 1963; Steigbeigel et al., 1964; Hennen, 1966, 1967; Omenn, 1970
Ectopic calcitonin production (no recognizable syndrome but elevated plasma levels)	Calcitonin	Tumours of the lung, oesophagus, pancreas, adrenal cortex, breast	Fukase, 1978; Coombes et al., 1974; Milhaud et al., 1974; Silva et al., 1974
Gynaecomastia	LH, FSH, HCG	Hepatoblastoma, bronchial carcinoma, adrenocortical tumours	Wyss, 1967; Hung et al., 1963; Omenn, 1970; Rudnick and Odell, 1971; Castleman et al., 1972

[a] *See also* Tables 5 and 6

the cells of the neoplasm from other tissues. The abnormal genetic activity so induced may be reflected in the synthesis of unusual products by a neoplasm, or in an altered level, heightened or reduced, of the usual cellular product (*see* Fig. 7, p. 129).

The concept that the ability of embryonic cells to respond to inductive stimuli varies with their state of competence and that the state of competence determines the specificity of differentiation was discussed earlier. Bonner's (1960) proposal that specificity of competence determines the specificity of differentiation was taken as a nucleus around which Sherbet (1966) formulated the sequential competence hypothesis, to which subsequently (Sherbet, 1974b) was added the idea that the determination of the competent state was a sub-threshold activation of specific sections of the genome, presumably by protein(s) analogous to "repressors". In the preceding pages it was also proposed that a state of neoplastic competence may be induced by incomplete carcinogens, with the associated synthesis of the repressor proteins. Anderson and Coggin (1974) argued that cellular proteins could be grouped into (a) phenotypic proteins, i.e. those which characterize the state of differentiation, and (b) transient gene products which are present in very small quantities and that these are concerned in the main with morphogenetic events. Although the presence of these can only be inferred at this stage, these could be the macromolecular "repressors" that define the state of competence of an embryonic tissue.

The histogenetic proximity of the neoplasm and the endocrine organ whose product the neoplasm is able to synthesize ectopically has suggested the classification of the neoplasms in terms of acquired states of competence (Sherbet, 1974b; Table 5) as reflected by the ectopic endocrine syndrome. The neoplasms and syndromes can be classified into 3 groups, I, II and III with the group I being subdivided into two further groups (IA and IB). Group I neoplasms may have acquired the preceding state of competence (IA) or one of the preceding competent states (IB). Bronchiogenic and thymic carcinomas with associated syndromes of hyper-adrenocorticism, hypercalcaemia and hyponatraemia are examples of group IA neoplasms. The hormone activities involved, viz. ACTH, PTH and ADH, are normal products of the anterior hypophysis and the parathyroid. Now the thymus and anterior hypophysis as well as the parathyroid are all derivatives of the branchial clefts which in turn are derived from the branchial endoderm.

Group IB neoplasms will produce hormones ectopically which are normally synthesized by endocrine organs derived from the same embryonic organ system, though not from the same anlagen as in group IA. Primary hepatomas and pancreatic tumours which show associated syndromes of hypercalcaemia, hyperadrenocorticism and gynaecomastia, which are

Table 5

Epigenetic group classification of neoplasms and paraneoplastic syndromes

Group	Neoplasm	Paraneoplastic syndrome
IA	Bronchial carcinoma	Hyperadrenocorticism, hypo-natraemia, gynaecomastia
	Thymic carcinoma	Hyperadrenocorticism
IB	Primary hepatoma	Hypercalcaemia, gynaecomastia,
	Pancreatic carcinoma	hyperadrenocorticism
II	Renal carcinoma	
	Benign renal lesions	Erythrocytosis
	Uterine fibroma	
	Cerebellar haemangioma	
III	Breast carcinoma	Hypercalcaemia
	Adrenocortical tumour	Hypoglycaemia, gynaecomastia
	Bronchiogenic carcinoma	Hyponatraemia
	Chorio-carcinoma	Hyperthyroidism

From Sherbet (1974b).

attributed to hormonal activities normally associated with parathyroid and anterior hypophysis, may be cited as examples of group IB. Group IB neoplasms produce ectopic hormonal activities farther removed embryologically than are IA neoplasms from their respective ectopic hormonal activities. In other words, a given neoplasm may have to undergo dedetermination to a greater degree in order to produce a group IB syndrome than a IA syndrome.

In group II are included tumours which have little in common with the paraneoplastic syndrome except that they originate from the same embryonic germ layer. In group III tumours, the ectopic activities are even further removed from the neoplasms than are group II. Indeed the dedetermination crosses the germ cell boundaries, and a neoplasm may acquire synthetic activity normally associated with an organ derived from a different germ layer than that from which the neoplasm itself originated.

This concept of acquisition of precedent competence in neoplasia would thus imply that the greater the degree of dedetermination required in order to produce a specific paraneoplastic syndrome, the lesser would be the frequency with which it would occur in association with a neoplasm. For example, hyperadrenocorticism is likely to be associated more frequently with a thymic carcinoma than with a hepatoma. Likewise, there is an even smaller chance of hypoglycaemia being associated with lymphomas than with a hepatic tumour.

The precedent competence concept also, therefore, provides a possible device for predicting the occurrence of paraneoplastic syndromes (Table 6). A retrospective study of neoplasms and associated syndromes has indeed confirmed this (Sherbet, 1974b). It ought to be pointed out, however, that in spite of the general validity of this hypothesis, some exceptions could be cited such as, for example, ectopic secretion of calcitonin (*see* Fukase, 1978).

It also follows from this hypothesis that since the ability to produce ectopically biologically active substances may be related to the degree of dedetermination, such ability may also reflect the degree of malignancy of a particular tumour (Sherbet, 1974b). Although no supporting clinical evidence is available, it may reasonably be suggested that an ovarian or a breast carcinoma that has associated ectopic ACTH syndrome would be more malignant than one that has not. In the same vein, a hepatic tumour which shows hypoglycaemic activity (IB) would be expected to be less malignant than the hepatoma with which erythrocytosis (Group III) is found to be associated.

This could indeed turn out to be a useful parameter in the clinical management of cancer patients. As mentioned before, about 20% of cancer patients will have one or more associated syndromes of endocrine dysfunction at a given time and up to 75% of all patients will develop one in the course of the disease. The epigenetic group classification might enable one not only to assess the status of malignancy of the tumour at the time of diagnosis, but it would appear possible that the course of progression taken by a particular tumour and its consequence to the patient in terms of prognosis can be assessed either independently of, or in conjunction with, conventional methods of histopathology and clinical staging, etc.

The precedent competence hypothesis also states that an abnormal genetic activation may be produced in the reacquired competent state by chemical inductors that are already present in the neoplasm or transmitted into the neoplasm from neighbouring tissues. Adult organs from a variety of species have been shown to be able to induce a wide spectrum of differentiation (Saxén and Toivonen, 1962) and indeed several substances possessing distinctive inductive properties have been isolated (Tiedemann, 1968). In interactions with host tissues it is possible also that neoplasms may exert various long range as well as close range effects on the tissue of the host. Ewing (1940) recognized this and pointed out that neoplasms can produce hyperplastic changes in neighbouring normal tissue. This was confirmed by Argyris and Argyris (1962) who transplanted a mouse tumour into the dermis of the host and noticed that the normal epithelium above the transplant became hyperplastic, although the epithelium itself was not in direct contact with the tumour. Presumably, this effect was produced by

Table 6

Epigenetic group and classification and incidence of paraneoplastic syndromes

Paraneoplastic syndrome and neoplasm	Incidence (%)	Group
Cushing's (ectopic ACTH) syndrome		
Bronchial carcinoma	50	IA
Thymic	25	IA
Pancreatic	25	IB
Phaechromocytoma, neuroblastoma, ganglioma	5	
Ovarian, testis, breast	Rare	III
Hypercalcaemia[a]		
Lung	29	IB
Kidney	29	
Ovary	10	III
Uterus	7	
Pancreas	7	
Liver	7	IB
Hyponatraemia		
Lung oat-cell carcinoma[b]	40	IB
Colonic carcinoma[c]	43	IB
Polycythemia (erythrocytosis)		
Renal carcinoma[d]	50	
Cerebellar haemangioblastoma	50	II
Uterine fibroma	20	
Hepatoma	8	
Phaeochromocytoma	2	III
Hypoglycaemia		
Hepatic tumour	75	IB
Adrenal carcinoma	25	
Lymphoma	5	III

From Sherbet (1974b).
[a]The correlation between epigentic group classification and frequency of occurrence of hypercalcaemia is not very consistent. This presumably is due to difficulties in establishing whether the syndrome was produced by ectopic PTH. It is known that other agents such as prostaglandin (PGE$_2$) (Tashjian *et al.*, 1972; Voelkel *et al.*, 1975; Seyberth *et al.*, 1975, 1978) and osteoclast stimulating factor, which has PTH activity (Horton *et al.*, 1972; Luben *et al.*, 1974; Mundy *et al.*, 1974) cause hypercalcaemia.
[b]Gilby *et al.* (1975).
[c]Odell *et al.* (1977).
[d]Hammond and Winnick (1974). However, the kidney is the major site of erythropoietin production (Fisher and Birdwell, 1961), hence its production by renal carcinoma may not be considered as ectopic.

some diffusible factor emanating from the tumour. Such interactions may be involved, for instance, in the occurrence of dermatological phenomena, such as the Bazex syndrome in association with bronchial carcinoma (Puissant and Benvenista, 1971; Logroscino *et al.*, 1967). The Bazex syndrome, which is also known as acromatic psoriasiform dermatosis and paraneoplastic acrokeratosis, was described by Bazex in 1965. The syndrome is indisputably associated with neoplasia of the upper respiratory tract, and often precedes any clinical sign of tumour (Puissant and Benveniste, 1971). Motlik *et al.* (1968) reported that excessive hyperplasia and extracapsular proliferation of the adrenal cortex occurs in association with malignant thymoma.

A histotopographic investigation by Ageeva (1969) has indicated the possibility that astrocytomas may induce neighbouring glial cells into pre-blastomatous hyperplasia and cause nodular proliferates to form tumours. Retrogressive changes, i.e. negative in character, may also be induced by tumours such as the involution of the thymus in rats by the Walker carcinoma (Ertl and Immich, 1968).

That such interactions occur has been demonstrated convincingly by Greene and Harvey (1968). They transplanted human glioblastoma multi-forme into guinea-pig brains and into subcutaneous spaces of hamsters and mice and found that the tumours induced the formation of endothelial sarcomas. Similar transplantation of a variety of animal as well as human tumours into embryos has demonstrable effects on the proliferation and differentiation of embryonic cells (Sherbet and Lakshmi, 1974c, d, 1978a; *see* pp. 178-183). The interaction between tumour and neighbouring cells, whether *in vivo* or *in vitro,* may involve transmission of chemical stimuli. Daniel (1970) showed that tumour cells may produce degeneration of embryonic epidermal cells if cultured with the basal layer of epidermis in contact with certain malignant fibroblasts of dermal origin. Daniel's experiments seemed to suggest that the malignant fibroblasts produce two substances, one of which is a toxic diffusible macromolecule and the other a low molecular weight substance which has a growth-promoting ability and which can cause premature keratinization of the epidermis.

The conclusion is inescapable, therefore, that not only are the genetic activity and *in vivo* behaviour of the tumour affected by the host tissues, but also the growth and behaviour of the latter are influenced to a consider-able degree as a consequence of the interactions of the cellular elements of the tumour with the host cell types.

The importance of such interaction in the natural history of tumours and the germs of the "precedent competence" hypothesis in relation to the interactions between the neoplasm and the host tissue have prompted several investigations by the author's laboratory into the interactions between embryonic and tumour cells. These studies will be discussed subsequently (*see* pp. 168-198). They have not only brought to light the fact that tumour cells can functionally resemble embryonic cells, but have also led to the use of embryonic systems as a means of determining the malignancy of tumours.

Paraneoplastic Markers for Malignancy

Ectopic hormones and peptides

Neoplastic cells produce an impressive array of phenotypic products which includes polypeptide and protein hormones as discussed before, and also a variety of other products, such as foetal antigens, enzymes and associated metabolic products, in the natural course of progression of neoplasms (Table 7). The presence of these products, which are demonstrably of tumour origin and tumour-specific, in the body fluids of patients has proved to be an invaluable aid in the detection of the neoplasm and in determining its rate of growth and therefore the tumour burden. They have also aided in determining the efficacy of treatment. Surgical removal of a tumour source may cause a fall in the circulating levels of the marker products and recurrence may be indicated by progressive increases in levels in the post-operative phase of management. The response of tumours to chemotherapy may also be assessed by regular monitoring of levels of the paraneoplastic products. The assessment of the extent of the disease and improvement of the accuracy of clinical staging will be dependent upon correlating the metastatic behaviour with the presence of tumour markers. It is proposed to review such a correlation here and the discussion is restricted, by design, to examining the expression of paraneoplastic markers as indicators of the degree of tumour malignancy.

The detection of ectopic products released by tumours has often been an aid in deducing the site of the primary tumour from the histogenetic relationship between the ectopic tumour product and the histogenesis of the organ which is the natural source of the product. Although there is a diversity of paraneoplastic products, several products often appear to be closely related in that they could be cleavage products of a larger precursor molecule. Tumours which produce ACTH ectopically (e.g. the oat-cell carcinoma of the bronchus) may be cited as an example of this. These tumours produce, in addition to ACTH, β-LPH (a protein molecule with 91 amino acid residues), α-MSH and CLIP (Hirata *et al.*, 1976; Tanaka *et al.*, 1978; Ratcliffe *et al.*, 1973; Imura *et al.*, 1978). γ-LPH and endorphins also may be found (Imura *et al.*, 1978). All these are known to be cleavage

Table 7

Paraneoplastic markers

Marker	Tumour type	Non-neoplastic condition
Foetal antigens		
Carcino-embryonic antigen	Carcinomas of the colon and rectum, pancreas, liver, bronchus, breast, uterus, ovary, prostate, kidney, leukemia and lymphoma, neuro-blastoma, testicular tumours (Gold and Freedman, 1965; Laurence et al., 1972; Neville and Cooper, 1976; Tormey et al., 1977; Wang, et al., 1975; Cove et al., 1979a; M.R.C. Tumour Products Committee Sub Group Report, 1980).	Colorectal polyps, pancreatitis, cirrhosis and alcoholic liver disease, chronic bronchitis and emphysema, tuberculosis, inflammatory bowel disease, ulcerative colitis and Crohn's disease, fibro-adenosis, prostatitis (?)
Alpha fetoprotein	Hepatoma, testicular tumours, ovarian pancreatic, colonic, bronchogenic carci-nomas (Abelev et al., 1967; Abelev, 1974; Hirai and Miyaji, 1973; Purves et al., 1973; Kohn et al., 1976)	Hepatitis, cirrhosis, pregnancy
Pancreatic oncofoetal antigen	Pancreatic carcinoma (Banwo et al., 1974; Gelder et al., 1978a, b; Wood and Moossa, 1977)	Possible raised levels also in pancreatitis, biliary stone and gastric ulcers
Enzymes		
Sialyl transferase	Metastatic breast cancer, rat mammary tumours, carcinomas of the lung, colon, prostate, lymphoma, melanoma (Bernacki and Kim, 1977; Bosmann and Hilf, 1974; Coombes et al., 1977; Dao et al., 1980)	Rheumatoid arthritis, chronic liver disease, drug-induced hepatotoxicity
Galactosyl transferase	Carcinomas of the breast, lung, oesophagus, pancreas, colon, ovary, acute lymphocytic leukemia (Podolsky and Weiser, 1978; Chatterjee et al., 1979; Bhattacharaya et al., 1976; Weiser et al., 1976)	Acute active liver disease, coeliac disease
Fucosyl transferase	Carcinoma of the breast, leukemia, carcinomas metastatic to the liver (Kessel et al., 1977; Chatterjee et al., 1979)	

Acid phosphatase	Carcinoma of the prostate with skeletal metastases, bronchial carcinoma (Coombes, 1978)	Gaucher's disease
Alkaline phosphatase	Osteogenic sarcoma, prostatic and breast carcinoma metastatic to the bone, multiple myeloma, Hodgkin's disease, leukemia, reticulum cell sarcoma (Schwartz, 1976)	Hepatitis, cirrhosis, tuberculosis, amyloidosis
Alkaline phosphatase (placental)	Ovarian and breast cancer	
Ribonuclease	Carcinoma of the pancreas (Reddi and Holland, 1976)	Patients with renal failure
Glycolytic enzymes	Cancers metastatic to the liver. LDH5 isoenzyme predominates in cancer tissues of breast, uterus, prostate, lung, kidney, stomach. LDH5/LDH1 ratio high in breast cancer as compared with fibro-adenoma tissue, also in prostatic carcinoma (Schwartz, 1976; Wood et al., 1973; Clark and Srinivasan, 1973; Bredni et al., 1973). LDH5 proportion high in cervical carcinoma tissue. Abnormal serum levels in patients with colorectal cancer	
Terminal deoxynucleotidyl transferase	Leukemias and lymphoma (Hutton et al., 1978)	
Plasminogen activator activity	Carcinoma of the breast, murine B16 melanomas, virally and chemically transformed cells (see pp. 86-88)	Benign tumours such as fibroadenomas, meningiomas, etc.
Proteins, carbohydrates Ferritin	Acute leukemia, Hodgkin's disease, locally recurrent or metastatic breast cancer (Jones et al., 1973; Worwood et al., 1974; Marcus and Zinberg, 1975)	Hepatitis, cirrhosis

Table 7 *(cont.)*

Marker	Tumour type	None-neoplastic condition
Acute phase reactants (proteins) (α_1-antitrypsin, α_1 acid glycoprotein, C-reactive protein, haptoglobin)	Cancers of the breast, bronchus, pancreas, prostate and colorectal (Hollinshead *et al.*, 1977; Ward *et al.*, 1977a, b; Neville and Cooper, 1976)	Trauma, inflammation
T23 protein	Hodgkins disease, non-Hodgkins lymphomas, also non-lymphoreticular tumours (Begent *et al.*, 1980)	
β_2-microglobulin	Increased levels in adenocarcinomas of the stomach and pancreas, chronic lymphocytic leukemia, Hodgkin's and non-Hodgkin's lymphomas (Rashid *et al.*, 1980; Späti *et al.*, 1980; Child *et al.*, 1980; Mavligit *et al.*, 1980)	
Immunoglobulins	Plasma cell tumours, lymphocytic tumours, e.g. Waldenstrom's macroglobulinaemia (Coombes, 1978)	
IgA/IgM ratio	In pancreatic duodenal fluid decrease in pancreatic cancer (Bramis *et al.*, 1978)	Increased ratio seen in pancreatitis
Serum bound fucose, sialic acid	Breast (Rosato and Seltzer, 1969; Evans *et al.*, 1974; Waalkes *et al.*, 1978)	
Ectopic hormones Common α-subunit of glyco-protein hormones	Lung, colorectal, breast cancers, pituitary adenomas, carcinoid, islet-cell tumour (Cove *et al.*, 1979b; Dosogne-Guérin *et al.*, 1978; Rosen and Weintraub, 1974; Blackman *et al.*, 1980; MacFarlane *et al.*, 1980)	Pregnancy, uremia, renal failure, hypoparathyroidism

HCG and HCG-α	Trophoblastic tumours and various non-trophoblastic tumours (references as above, esp. Blackman *et al.*, 1980)	
Metabolic and degradation products Hydroxyproline (HP) (collagen degradation product) measured as HP based on creatinine (c) (HP/c)	Tumours metastasizing to the bone. Variation in urinary levels in progression or regression of breast tumours (Powles *et al.*, 1975)	Hydroxyprolinaemia, inflammation
Fibrin degradation products (FDP)	Carcinoma of ovary, prostate, breast, adeno-carcinoma of the gastro-intestinal tract and cancers of the lung (*see* p. 87)	Endometriosis, uterine myoma, infection, renal disease
Putrescine, spermidine, spermine (and ornithine decarboxylase activity)	Rat hepatomas, murine leukemia, melanoma; certain human cancers such as Burkitt's lymphoma, breast cancer, brain tumours (Williams-Ashman, 1972; Russel and Levy, 1971; Russel, 1971; Russel and Russel, 1975; Takami and Nishioka, 1980; Nishioka *et al.*, 1977; Harik and Sutton, 1979)	

products of a pre-pro ACTH-LPH precursor molecule (Roberts *et al.*, 1978; Nakanishi *et al.*, 1978; Odagiri *et al.*, 1979). In other words, there seems to be a specific pattern in the production of phenotypic products by neoplastic cells.

On the other hand, even tumours of the same histogenetic origin may show a spectrum of aberrant genetic activity resulting in wide variations in the synthesis of a given family of phenotypic products. Thus islet cell tumours may be innocuous and discovered incidentally at necropsy or may actively synthesize insulin, causing the syndrome characterized by fasting hypoglycaemia (*see* Willis, 1967). Melanomas may range from amelanotic ones to those which are highly active producers of melanin. The functional activity is often independent of the size of the neoplasm. Clinically functional insulinomas may vary greatly in size, and tumours smaller than half a centimetre in diameter may be highly active producers of insulin and prove fatal (Willis, 1967; Bloom and Polak, 1980).

It would also appear that the ability for ectopic production of hormones could be related to the degree of anaplasia. Vorherr (1974) has argued that in bronchogenic carcinomas the more anaplastic the tumour the greater is its potential for the synthesis of ectopic products. Oat-cell carcinomas (lympocyte-like small cell carcinomas) which are highly anaplastic, invasive tumours, with much poorer prognosis than both adenocarcinoma and squamous cell carcinoma (Bondy, 1977), are most frequently involved in the production of single or multiple paraneoplastic syndromes. As we shall discuss in a following section (pp. 128-135), the degree of differentiation is held to be able to predict prognosis: the higher the degree of differentiation, the more favourable being the prognosis of the disease. The degree and extent of synthesis of paraneoplastic products may be related to the degree of malignancy of the tumour. Preliminary observations in the author's laboratory on murine B16 melanoma cell lines selected for increasing metastatic ability seem to show that increased ability to synthesize melanin may be accompanied by increased metastatic ability. The B16-BL6 variant cells, which produce metastases in 80% of animals within 4 weeks after injection of 25 000 cells (Liotta *et al.*, 1980), are intensely active in melanin production, which results in jet-black coloration of the primary tumour. In contrast, the B16-F10 cells, which are less metastatic (producing metastases in only 30% of animals) produce primary growths that are much paler with considerably reduced amounts of melanin in them. One might also cite oat-cell carcinomas, which are glaring examples of paraneoplastic function with the accompaniment of high metastatic ability. In this tumour, metastases are said to be present in 60-80% of patients at first presentation (Gilby, 1977; Smith, 1981). There is a substantial basis, therefore, for employing paraneoplastic products, the spectrum of their expression, or the variations in the expression of specified individual components as criteria for determining the degree of tumour malignancy.

Carcino-embryonic antigen (CEA)

The carcino-embryonic antigen is the most extensively investigated and arguably the most successful of biomarkers for human cancer. Gold and Freedman (1965) reported on its occurrence in colonic carcinoma and initially regarded it as a tumour-specific antigen associated with tumours of the gastro-intestinal tract. With the discovery that CEA was found also in association with cancer of the breast (Laurence *et al.*, 1972; Chu and Nemoto, 1973), lung (Laurence *et al.*, 1972; Vincent and Chu, 1973), pancreas (Holyoke *et al.*, 1972b) and urological tumours (Reynoso *et al.*, 1972), and in certain non neoplastic conditions (*see* Tables 7 and 8), CEA has lost the lustre of specificity, but still appears over the years to have retained its clinical usefulness.

Carcino-embryonic antigens (CEAs) form a well-characterized family of glycoproteins of molecular weight of approximately 200K ($K = 10^3$) daltons, containing 40-50% carbohydrate moiety. The CEA molecule has a single polypeptide chain (Slayter and Coligan, 1975) which contains antigenic determinants of the CEA molecule. Although CEA occurs in tumours of different histogenetic origin, these have not been shown to be chemically distinct species, but variations have been reported in the protein : carbohydrate ratio. The sialic acid content of CEA preparations from various sources appears to vary considerably. There may also be variation as regards the *N*-terminal end of the peptide chain (Shuster *et al.*, 1977). Preparations from different tumour sources may also vary antigenically. The antigenic as well as structural heterogeneity of CEA preparations would suggest that CEAs form a family of closely related species of antigens which share among themselves certain antigenic determinants. Some of the CEA antigenic determinants have also been detected in other normally excreted proteins, termed somewhat unhelpfully as the non-specific cross-reacting antigen (Burtin, 1978).

The discovery of CEA raised fervent hopes that it would help considerably in cancer management. Unfortunately, investigations over the past decade have not fulfilled these hopes. It has become apparent that, on account of its lack of specificity and high incidence in association with benign neoplasms and non-neoplastic conditions (Table 8), the use of CEA as a marker for the detection and/or diagnosis of neoplasms has met with little success. However, the hope that CEA could be used to determine the degree of spread has been sustained by a number of observations. The amount of CEA may be related to the total tumour burden, i.e. the primary tumour mass as well as metastatic deposits. One may also envisage a situation where the ability of the primary tumour cells and the secondary cells to synthesize CEA is a direct reflection of the malignancy of the tumour.

Table 8

Incidence of CEA

Neoplastic/non-neoplastic condition	Incidence of raised CEA in serum/plasma (%)
Carcinomas	
Pancreas	92
Colon and rectum	73
Bronchus	72
Liver	67
Gall bladder and biliary tract	66
Breast	52
Uterus	36
Ovary	36
Benign condition	
Fibro-adenosis	7
Non-neoplastic	
Emphysema	57
Alcoholics	65
Ulcerative colitis	31
Ileitis	40
Pancreatitis	53

From Neville and Cooper (1976), Holyoke *et al.* (1979), Al-Sarraf *et al.* (1979).

The relationship between tumour burden and levels of CEA in body fluids is easily understood. Ellison *et al.* (1977) found that in tissue culture conditions, the release of CEA by tumour cells was related to the number of cells present. Consistent with this is the observation in the clinical context that excision of the primary tumour results in a fall in CEA levels (Laurence *et al.*, 1972; Sharin *et al.*, 1974; Neville and Cooper, 1976; Cove *et al.*, 1979a).

The contribution of metastatic cells to circulating CEA levels is also quite convincing. Increase in CEA concurrent with the appearance of metastatic deposits has been reported (Neville and Cooper, 1976) in colorectal cancer. In cancer of the pancreas, the levels of circulating CEA are far higher in patients with metastatic disease. Kalser *et al.* (1978) described a five-fold increase in the mean CEA levels in more than 50% of a group of over 100 patients with advanced disease.

Loewenstein *et al.* (1981) have recently raised the possibility of identifying metastatic spread in patients from whom tumour effusions are available for investigation. They have described the CEA content of ascites fluid and plasma from 19 patients with various types of tumour. They found that patients who had higher CEA levels in ascites fluid (exudate) than in plasma invariably had peritoneal spread of the tumour. In patients with lower CEA levels in ascitic fluid (transudates) than in plasma, hepatic metastases were detected.

The correlation between high CEA levels and clinical progression of cancer has also been shown by several investigators for carcinoma of the breast. Steward *et al.* (1974) reported that whilst CEA levels were above 2·5 ng ml^{-1} in 6 out of 22 patients with primary cancer but without clinical evidence of metastases, 37 out of 47 patients with metastatic disease had CEA levels above 2·5 ng ml^{-1}. In post-operative patients, about 30-40% show raised CEA levels during the disease-free interval but more than about 70% of patients with metastatic disease will show raised levels of the antigen (MacSween *et al.*, 1972; Chu and Nemoto, 1973; Laurence *et al.*, 1972; Concannon *et al.*, 1973; Tormey *et al.*, 1975; Wang *et al.*, 1975). Cove *et al.* (1979a) used a high upper normal limit of 15 ng ml^{-1}, based on 269 control subjects with the criterion that more than 97·4% were below this limit. In local disease (stages I and II), only 13% of patients showed elevated CEA levels in plasma. On the other hand, in disseminated disease (stages III and IV), 65% of patients had elevated levels of plasma CEA. Earlier, Krebs *et al.* (1977) had shown a similar correlation of CEA levels with the clinical status of tumour progression in breast and bronchial carcinomas. Twenty-one percent of bronchial carcinoma and 11% of breast carcinoma patients with no nodal involvement nor metastasis ($N_0 M_0$) had >5 ng ml^{-1}CEA. The frequency of abnormality increased three-fold when there was lymph node involvement but no distant metastasis ($N_+ M_0$). There was an even greater frequency (95% and 65% respectively for bronchial carcinoma patients and breast carcinoma patients) when there was distant metastatic dissemination in addition to local lymph node involvement.

If the levels of CEA were not merely related in a stoichiometric way with tumour burden, but were also a reflection of the aberrant genetic activity coupled with the neoplastic change, one could expect that the degree of production and release of carcino-embryonic antigen, even at the early stages of development of the primary tumour, would be predictive of the metastatic potential of the tumour and hence of prognostic value.

Wang *et al.* (1975) found that elevated CEA levels (> 2·5 ng ml^{-1}) 10 days post-mastectomy were predictive of recurrence. The recurrence rates were signficantly higher for patients with >2·5 ng ml⁻¹ CEA than for patients with CEA below this level. In the 2-year post-mastectomy phase, 65% of patients with raised CEA levels showed recurrent disease, whilst only 20% of those with CEA levels below 2·5 ng ml⁻¹ did so. Cove *et al.* (1979a) have also subscribed to the view that raised post-operative levels of CEA may indicate early recurrent disease. This could be construed as evidence of residual tumour contributing to CEA levels in the post-operative phase. However, Wang *et al.* (1975) also found that the recurrence rates for women with low CEA levels *before* mastectomy were not significantly different from those for women with high pre-mastectomy levels of CEA. This could be interpreted as suggesting that the primary tumours are heterogeneous with regard to their ability to synthesize CEA, i.e. the low CEA values could only be indicating that a smaller proportion of tumour cells are actively engaged in CEA production in the low pre-mastectomy CEA group than in the second group with high CEA levels before mastectomy. In such a case, the size of the tumour alone will not dictate the circulating levels of CEA. Although the foregoing discussion has tended to suggest that there is a greater likelihood that CEA levels are dependent upon tumour burden, Krebs *et al.* (1977) have stated that tumour size bears no relationship to CEA in the blood.

It ought to be said, none the less, that a heterogeneity of tumours as regards CEA production has not been demonstrated. It would indeed be most interesting to examine this thesis of heterogeneity of neoplasms in relation to the metastatic potential of tumours. The notion that primary neoplasms are a heterogeneous mixture of cell types with different degrees of metastatic ability was mooted many years ago and in fact implied in Fould's concept of tumour progression. Linking this notion with the phenotypic ability to synthesize CEA may resolve the question of whether CEA can predict metastatic potential. The variability in the pattern of CEA production shown to occur in patients with colonic carcinoma (Mariani *et al.*, 1980) may, in fact, be attributed to the heterogeneity of the primary neoplasm with regard to the CEA-producing ability of the component cells. Mariani *et al.* (1980) found that a significant proportion of patients who had normal serum CEA levels before operation showed a steady rise in CEA titres post-operatively. Of these, the major proportion (9/11) showed local recurrence or metastasis of the tumour. It is possible that this could have been brought about by a change in the cell population composing the recurrent tumour. Whether similar changes occur in the pattern of CEA production in patients who have normal pre-operative CEA levels but who subsequently show metastatic dissemination is not known. An investigation of this may yield valuable results. However, the major problem is that when patients have normal CEA levels before operation is is often assumed to be unlikely that they will show increases in CEA post-operatively and in the follow-up CEA levels are not usually assayed.

It follows from the above thesis that a metastatic selection might occur of CEA producer cells. It is known that large quantities of the antigen may be prepared from metastatic deposits (Pritchard *et al.*, 1978), but no comparative figures for primary tumour and metastatic cells are available.

This inevitably leads one to a discussion of the possible relationship between the degree of differentiation and the CEA producing activity. Since the production of carcino-embryonic antigens or any other specific product may be considered as a differentiated function, anaplastic and active mitotic state will be incompatible with high CEA production. Consistent with this view was the observation of Denk *et al.* (1972) that the CEA content of tumours correlated with the degree of their cellular differentiation. In well-differentiated carcinomas of the colon, abundant CEA was detectable. CEA was absent in poorly differentiated or anaplastic tumours. However, it would be difficult to reconcile this with the widely accepted concept that the more anaplastic a tumour, the more malignant it is likely to be, without partially amending the stand that the expression of CEA is an intrinsic ability of certain neoplastic cells and that the degree of expression of this antigen reflects the degree of malignancy of the tumours.

Alpha fetoprotein (AFP)

Alpha fetoprotein is another oncofoetal antigen whose utility in cancer management has been examined extensively. AFP is a glycoprotein of molecular weight of approximately 70K, normally produced in the yolk sac and by liver cells in foetal life (Abelev, 1968, 1971), which appears in the blood (Ruoslahti *et al.*, 1974; Adinolfi *et al.*, 1975). It reaches a peak around early-mid gestation. The levels begin to fall rapidly as parturition approaches and in the following few months to those found in normal adults (Karlsson, 1970; Karlsson *et al.*, 1972; Sell *et al.*, 1974; Gitlin, 1975; Nayak and Mital, 1977). AFP appears to be associated with some stage in the differentiation of hepatocytes and the AFP-producing cells seem to switch over to the production of albumin (Carlsson and Ingvarsson, 1979). It has been suggested that the fall in AFP is due to the synthesis of a repressor in later embryonic life (Grabar, 1968).

The elevation of levels of AFP has been described mainly in hepatocellular carcinomas and testicular tumours (Abelev, 1974; Hirai and Miyaji, 1973; Newlands *et al.*, 1976; Javadpour, 1979). As with CEA, excision of the AFP-producing tumour causes a fall in the circulating levels of the antigen. Subsequent increases often indicate recurrence of the tumour.

Cancers of the gastro-intestinal tract and the pancreas (10-35%) are also known to have an associated increase in AFP levels, although it appears possible that this increase is due to the occurrence of hepatic metastases. The metastatic process could produce liver damage, and presumably stimulate a compensatory regenerative response. One could envisage a situation where, in the process of regeneration, the hepatocytes produce the antigen at a specific stage of differentiation. This suggestion is consistent with the reported appearance of AFP with the processes of liver regeneration (Ruoslahti *et al.*, 1974).

The specificity of AFP as a paraneoplastic product is impressive. As far as it has been reported, this antigen appears to be associated with tumours which are histogenetically endodermal in origin (Table 9). Many of these tumours may also produce HCG. But is has been shown by Kurman *et al.* (1977) that different cellular elements of germ cell tumours are responsible for the production of AFP and HCG. In choriocarcinomas and embryonal carcinomas, syncitiotrophoblastic cells show localization of HCG. AFP, on the other hand, is apparently a product of mononuclear embryonal cells of embryonal carcinoma and endodermal sinus tumours. Although about 10% of hepatocellular carcinomas may have no associated AFP, the apparent histogenetic specifity of AFP lends considerable credence to the concept of epigenetic control of the synthesis of paraneoplastic products.

Table 9

Frequency of paraneoplastic incidence of AFP

Neoplasm	Incidence %	Reference
Hepatocellular carcinoma Teratocarcinoma containing yolk-sac elements	approx. 80	Abelev, 1968, 1974; Adinolfi *et al.*, 1975; Wepsic and Sell, 1974; Sell and Wepsic, 1975
Pancreatic and gastric tumours	approx. 10-35	Wood and Moossa, 1977
Lung adenocarcinoma	lower	McIntire *et al.*, 1972, 1975
Non-endodermal tumours	very rare	Mihalev *et al.*, 1976

Cell surface markers for malignancy

There is considerable evidence that neoplastic transformation is accompanied by a variety of alterations at the cell surface (*see* Hynes, 1979; Sherbet, 1978). The putative markers for malignancy listed in Table 7 have a diversity of postulated sites of origin located in the cancer cell itself or in cells and body fluids of the host. Markers such as the carcino-embryonic antigen, sialyl transferase, etc. are postulated to be of glycocaleal or membrane origin, while others might be of cytoplasmic or intranuclear origin.

The goal of establishing surface markers for malignancy has been pursued with great zeal, in the hope that discovery of such markers might lead to the development of specific antibodies directed against the tumour for achieving a selective destruction of tumour cells and, if common antigens occurred on the surfaces of the cells of the primary tumour and its metastases, also for the eradication of the metastatic tumour. In addition, there is also the attractive possibility that chemotherapeutic agents could be tagged on to specific antibodies so that the latter might home in on the specific target. This has been attempted, albeit with limited success, with antitumour agents such as daunomycin, adriamycin and methotrexate tagged to antibodies raised against tumour-associated surface antigens (Levy *et al.*, 1975; Ghose and Blair, 1978). A more recent development is the linking of toxins such as abrin (*Abrus precatorius* toxin) and ricin (*Ricinus communis* lectin) to monoclonal antibodies raised against cell surface antigens (Youle and Neville, 1980; Blythman *et al.*, 1981).

The essential criteria to be met are obviously that the markers be specific and closely linked with malignancy. A close link with malignancy does not imply that it is required that the markers necessarily participate in the process of malignancy. In other words, the expression of malignancy and the expression of the markers need not be subject to the same control mechanism. It is essential, however, that the markers appear invariably in the neoplastic state at least as a cognate event.

Two possibilities have been examined. One of these is that there could be a common marker for malignancy. Price and Stoddart (1976) have identified a glycoprotein of pI 4·0 in neutral detergent extracts of the cell membrane of a variety of tumours of the rat, e.g. the D23 hepatoma, mammary carcinomas, epitheliomas and fibrosarcomas. This glyco-protein(s) was also found in homogenates of certain human tumours, a lymphosarcoma of the pig, murine leukemias and a chondrosarcoma of the rat. In contrast, a range of normal adult tissues of the rat showed no trace of this component.

Bowen and Kulatilake (1979) have provided supporting evidence for the occurrence of the pI 4·0 glycoprotein. They detected the glycoprotein in ten specimens of prostatic adenocarcinoma. It was not detectable in 10/13 benign prostatic hypertrophy cases. Three cases of this benign condition did, however, reveal the presence of small quantities of the pI 4·0 glyco-protein.

The close association of the pI 4·0 glycoprotein had been described earlier by Bramwell and Harris (1978a), who described it as a glycoprotein of molecular weight 100K. It bound the lectins Con. A and WGA. They also reported that the 100K protein bound more Con. A and less WGA in malignant cells than in normal cells since Con. A binds to mannose and glucose residues, while WGA binds N-acetyl glucosamine; this indicated an abnormality in the glycosylation of the 100K component. It has been suggested that the 100K protein may be a major component involved in the transport of glucose across the cell membrane. Bramwell and Harris (1978b) have also indicated that it could have specific binding sites for insulin.

Genetic evidence for linkage of the 100K marker with malignancy has also been most elegantly demonstrated by Bramwell and Harris (1978a) using the celebrated cell hybridization technique. Harris and his co-workers had shown earlier that if malignant cells are fused with non-malignant diploid cells, the phenotypic features of malignancy are suppressed. However, continued cultivation of the hybrid cells gradually results in the segregation of the genetic elements of the malignant and non-malignant component cells, accompanied also by the reappearance of the malignant phenotype (Harris, 1971; Wiener *et al.*, 1974a, b; Jonasson *et al.*, 1977).

In hybrid cells with suppressed malignancy, the amount of Con. A bound to the 100K protein was much lower than in the malignant parent line. In the malignant segregant clones, on the other hand, the Con. A binding showed a substantial increase. The binding of WGA showed a reverse situation. McCormick *et al.* (1979) and Shiu *et al.* (1977) have described an underglycosylated form of a glycoprotein of approximately 97K in transformed cells.

Although the occurrence of the 100K protein may not be deemed as fully established, the concept of a single protein or even a family of closely related proteins unifying the diversity of neoplasia is certainly a most attractive one and deserves the devoted attention of the doyen of cancer research.

In spite of its demonstrated genetic linkage, the 100K protein is not a convincing indicator of malignancy. Albeit in the form of a mere statement not supported by properly documented data, Price and Stoddart (1976) have claimed that the concentration of the protein showed no relationship to the degree of lymphocytic infiltration of the tumours, their antigenicity, mitotic index or their metastatic ability, all essential features of malignancy. These authors seem to believe, therefore, that the 100K protein could be a characteristic feature of neoplasia, not necessarily associated with the expression of malignancy. But the alterations undergone by this marker in hybrids of normal and malignant cells with suppressed malignant state, and the inability of Bowen and Kulatilake (1979) to detect its presence in 10/13 benign prostatic hyperplasias would suggest that the protein may indeed be involved in the expression of malignancy.

The occurrence of a protein of mol. wt 97K has been reported on certain human tumours (Woodbury *et al.*, 1980, 1981; Brown *et al.*, 1981). The tumours that were assayed by immunoprecipitation with monoclonal IgGs against this protein have included melanomas (5/9 positive) and carcinomas (one each) of the breast, thyroid and lung. The 97K protein was not detectable in a variety of normal human tissues, but tissues of foetal colon and umbilical cord had detectable amounts of the protein. Only two benign tumours have so far been investigated.

As discussed in previous sections (*see* pp. 38-42; 60-63), the differences in the metastatic ability of tumours have been shown to be accompanied by changes in surface components (*see* Yogeeswaran *et al.*, 1978; Brunson *et al.*, 1978; Turner *et al.*, 1980b). The establishment of a marker associated with the malignant behaviour of tumours, i.e. their ability to invade and form distant metastases, would be of importance not only in the understanding of the biology of the tumour but, as stated earlier, in the clinical management of patients.

We have therefore recently examined the surface proteins expressed on a series of breast tumours, benign as well as malignant, and have discovered differences in the expression of certain species of protein/glycoprotein by benign tumours and carcinomas (Wildridge and Sherbet, 1981).

In this investigation, breast tumours were grown in culture and their surface proteins labelled by radioiodine and separated by electrophoresis on polyacrylamide gels (Fig. 6). The expression of two components with molecular weights of 265K and 233K showed marked differences. The 265K protein occurred in cystic hyperplasias (2) and 4/5 fibroadenomas. The 233K component occurred as a defined peak in 3/5 carcinomas (Table 10), but there was no statistically significant difference between the fibroadenomas and the carcinomas as regards incorporation of radioiodine. On the other hand, the ratio of 265K/233K was higher in the fibroadenoma group than in the carcinoma group (Table 11). In other words, the 265K peak was less in the carcinomas than in the fibro-adenomas. A second feature of difference between the fibro-adenomas and the carcinomas related to a 63K component(s) which was detected in greater quantities in the carcinomas than in the fibroadenomas.

Although this investigation concerns only a small number of mammary tumours, a correlation between the expression of the 265K and 233K proteins and the malignancy of the tumours has already become apparent. It may be seen from Table 12, that for fibroadenomas the ratio of 265K : 233K is between 3 and 6. The ratio for carcinomas varied from 1·3 to 3·0. There seems to be an overlap in the middle, where there were two cases: a fibroadenoma which recurred after two years and a carcinoma which showed metastasis to the pelvis after 3 years. With these exceptions in mind,

Table 10

Cell surface proteins of fibrocystic hyperplasias, fibroadenomas
and carcinomas of the breast

Tumour identification	Histology	Major components (approx. mol. wt)			
		265K	233K	145K	63K
EBA	Fibrocystic	$+^a$		+	+
VHG	hyperplasia	+		+	
MAT	Fibroadenoma	?		+	
AFH		+		+	+
JFE		+		+	
MEA		+		+	
WRA		+		?	
MCP	Carcinoma		?	+	+
HOR			+	+	+
AME			+	+	+
BAS			?	+	+
MCF			+	?	?

a + indicates the presence of a well-defined peak of incorporation of radioiodine.
From Wildridge and Sherbet (1981).

it could be suggested that the lower this 265K : 233K ratio, the greater was the metastatic ability of the carcinoma. It is needless to emphasize that this apparent relationship needs to be established in a large number of cases before the 265K : 233K ratio can be suggested as a possible marker for malignancy.

Histological and Epigenetic Correlates of Malignancy

Introduction

One of the most difficult conceptual problems which has attracted a great deal of attention is the state of differentiation of tumours. Tumours are known to show a varying degree of histotypic differentiation. More often than not they are anaplastic. Indeed, the degree of anaplasia of a tumour has been used as a criterion in the determination of the malignancy of the tumour, and has provided the basis for the histological grading of tumours (*see* pp. 128-135). Anaplasia has often been described as a state of dedifferentiation, perhaps with an implied reversion of the cells to an embryonic

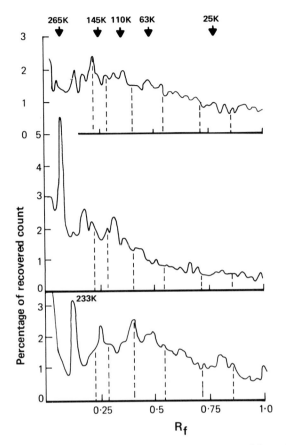

Figure 6 Patterns of radioiodinated surface proteins separated by polyacrylamide gel electrophoresis of a fibrocystic hyperplasia (top), fibroadenoma (middle) and a carcinoma of the breast (bottom). From Wildridge and Sherbet (1981).

state. In embryological parlance, a dedifferentiated tissue is one which has available to it a wider choice of pathways of differentiation as a consequence of the processes of dedifferentiation than before. In essence, this is a reversal of the processes of differentiation, where a progressive restriction occurs of the options available for differentiation. On the other hand, the neoplastic state has also been described as a state of aberrant differentiation. Thus Markert (1968) suggested that neoplastic transformation might be a pathological counterpart of normal differentiation.

Table 11

Distribution of radioactivity associated with cell surface components of fibroadenomas and carcinomas of the breast

Tumour identification	Tumour type	Mean total counts recovered per gel × 10⁻³	265K	233K	265K/233K	145K	63K
			% radioactivity			% radioactivity	
MAT	Fibro-adenoma	26·3	5·6 ± 0·9	2·8 ± 0·8	2·0	6·57 ± 1·3	17·76 ± 0·7
MEA		27·5	10·07 ± 0·5	1·74 ± 0·8	5·79	5·56 ± 0·5	16·26 ± 0·4
JFE		47·5	11·92 ± 1·8	2·38 ± 0·09	5·01	6·67 ± 0·4	12·70 ± 1·5
WRA		34·9	6·77 ± 1·4	2·22 ± 0·9	3·05	6·21 ± 0·8	16·92 ± 4·0
AFH		17·0	11·97 ± 1·5	2·27 ± 0·9	5·27	5·79 ± 0·8	12·62 ± 0·6
MCP	Carcinoma	52·6	3·83 ± 0·7	1·50 ± 0·5	2·55	6·93 ± 0·4	21·21 ± 0·9
AME		121·3	4·47 ± 0·3	3·27 ± 0·7	1·37	6·58 ± 0·8	18·36 ± 0·5
BAS		23·5	3·72 ± 0·2	1·29 ± 0·2	2·88	5·82 ± 0·8	18·67 ± 0·9
HOR		84·1	9·27 ± 2·8	5·79 ± 2·0	1·60	7·51 ± 0·4	15·09 ± 0·7
MCF		28·3	4·07 ± 0·5	2· ± 0·2	1·67	6·41 ± 0·3	18·25 ± 0·8
Probability values in Mann-Whitney test			0·016	N.S.ᵃ	0·016	N.S.	0·028

ᵃN.S.: not significant
From Wildridge and Sherbet (1981).

Table 12

Possible correlation between expression of 265K/233K proteins and histology/follow-up

Patient identification	$\dfrac{265K}{233K}$	Histology/follow-up
BAI	5·99	Cystic hyperplasia
MEA	5·79	Fibroadenoma
AFH	5·27	Fibroadenoma
JFE	5·01	Fibroadenoma
WRA	3·05	Fibroadenoma
MAT	2·0	Fibroadenoma—further tumour removed 2 years later
BAS	2·88	Carcinoma 3 years, pelvic metasases
MCP	2·55	Carcinoma No metastases 7 years
MCF	1·67	Carcinoma. No metastases 4 years
HOR	1·6	Carcinoma. 3½ years, metastases (bone and liver), deceased
AME	1·37	Carcinoma. 3½ years, pulmonary metastases, deceased

Based on Wildridge and Sherbet (1981) and Sherbet and Lakshmi (1981b)

The opposite view, crystallized in the rules of tumour progression proposed by Foulds (1954), includes the argument that neoplastic development is an extension of the process of differentiation rather than a retracing of the steps of differentiation. The concept of tumour progression may therefore be seen as a rejection of the notion that anaplasia reflects a dedifferentiated and totipotent stage.

This conceptual impasse has been opened up somewhat by the precedent competence hypothesis of neoplasia, which covers the middle ground. The proponents of the "totipotent differentiation" and the extended differentiation hypotheses appear to be taking extreme positions. It is neither necessary to invoke a state of "totipotency" nor to propose progressive differentiation into the neoplastic state in order to explain several or even a few features of neoplastic development. The definition of anaplasia as dedifferentiation in the sense of a return to a state of totipotency is in fact erroneous and indeed unwarranted, as the subsequent discussion here will show. It will be equally inadequate to argue that neoplasia is a state of terminal differentiation extending a stage or more beyond the normal bounds of differentiation, in so far as this argument fails to explain the progressive anaplastic alterations tumours generally tend to show and the acquisition of embryonic features, such as the expression of carcino-embryonic antigens or of abilities to induce differentiation of tissues which are normally an essential attribute of embryonic tissues.

According to the precedent competence hypothesis, neoplasms may acquire one of several preceding states of competence, and respond to inducers present intracellularly or to those transmitted from neighbouring tissues by synthesizing biologically active products which characterize related differentiated cells. This may be described as aberrant differentiation (Fig. 7). Could such acquisition of a precedent competent state be demonstrated experimentally? Would neoplasms in their newly acquired competent state be amenable to influences of embryonic inductors and could such interactions be used to induce normal differentiation of neoplasms? Although some of these questions have been received with levity, it is proposed here to discuss the experimental work which has attempted to answer these questions with the seriousness which they rightly deserve.

An examination of the literature reveals two ways by which this problem has been approached, which have one thing in common and that is their reliance on the interactions between tumour and embryonic cells. One approach is to see if embryonic tissues influence the phenotypic differentiation and probably also the functional differentiation of tumours. The second approach, while not totally ignoring the influence on tumour cells, has tended to emphasize the importance of possible alterations in the state of differentiation of embryonic cells consequent upon interaction with tumour cells in their precedent competent states. This latter approach has in fact resulted in the establishment of embryonic systems as a means not only for distinguishing between normal and neoplastic cells, but also of determining the degree of malignancy of tumours. The rest of this section will be devoted to a discussion of histological correlates of malignancy and the most salient features of the interactions between embryonic and tumour cells that could serve as a means for assaying the malignant behaviour of tumours.

Histological correlates of malignancy

Histological grading of tumours

Hausemann (1892) may be considered to have introduced the concept of histological grading of tumours with his contribution on the anaplasia of, and mitosis in, breast tumours, thus providing a basis for the now oft-quoted principle that the malignancy of a tumour is reflected in the degree of its cellular differentiation. One may state in general terms that the more anaplastic a tumour, the more malignant it is likely to be. This approach to the assessment of malignancy has stood the test of time, for the basic principle, in spite of contraindications, has proved to be sound and it has provided adequate guidelines for determining the degree of, and the potential for, malignancy, i.e. to invade and form metastatic deposits, possessed by a tumour.

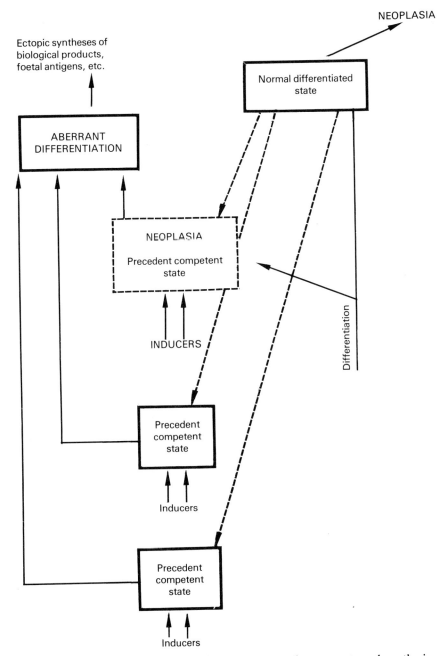

Figure 7 A diagrammatic representation of the precedent competence hypothesis
(*see also* pp. 96-109).

The histological assessment of malignancy hinges mainly on the tissue and cellular architecture of, and the intensity of mitotic activity in, the tumour tissues. Broders (1920) recognized the need to classify tumours with regard to the degree of malignancy. Using the state of differentiation and the degree of mitosis, he graded over five-hundred cases of squamous cell carcinoma of the lip. If three-fourths of the tumour was differentiated, it was considered as grade 1 and where approximately half of the tumour was differentiated, grade 2. When only a quarter of the tumour presented differentiated structures, it was termed grade 3. Grade 4 comprised tumours in which no differentiation was seen. Since the degree of differentiation is reflected also in the state of mitosis, the mitotic index was included as a second criterion. The classification of the squamous cell epitheliomas of the lip showed not only that the lower grade tumours had better prognosis, but also a clear correlation was apparent between the tumour grade and the incidence of metastasis. Of patients without metastasis, 92% had grades 1 and 2 tumours. In contrast, 60% of patients with metastatic disease had grade 3, 3% had grade 4 tumours and 37% of the patients had grade 2 tumours.

Histological grading has been used for breast cancer with much success. Patey and Scarff (1928, 1929) introduced a complex system of grading for these tumours, based on the histological criteria proposed by Greenough (1925). These were the extent of tissue organization as indicated by the degree of tubule formation and nuclear pleomorphism, hyperchromatism and mitotic index. Patey and Scarff (1929) reported on the histological grades of 163 breast carcinomas. The tumours were subdivided into three histological grades (low, moderate and high). The correlation between the latter and the incidence of metastasis in these patients was impressive. Ninety per cent of patients with high histological grade tumours had disseminated disease while only 44% of low grade and 68% of moderate grade tumours showed metastasis.

Bloom applied histological grading techniques to a large series of breast cancer patients and has demonstrated that histology can provide an accurate guide to prognosis (Bloom, 1950, 1956; Bloom and Richardson, 1957; Bloom, 1965). For assessing a possible relationship between histological deviation of the tumour from normality and prognosis, Bloom and Richardson (1957) evolved a method of numerical scoring of histological features in order to arrive at a composite histological grading for the tumours.

The criteria used by Bloom and Richardson (1957) were as follows. (a) The state of differentiation of the tumour. A well-marked tubular organization or acinar arrangement of cells in a regular manner around a central space was considered to be a feature of a high degree of differentiation and indicative of good prognosis. If a greater part of a section of the tumour showed good differentiation, the tumour was assigned 1 point, if there was only a moderate amount of differentiation, 2 points, if none, 3 points. (b) Nuclear morphology was assessed as a second criterion of deviation from normality. If nuclei were of regular shape, size and staining, the tumour was given one point, tumours with moderate variation, 2 points, tumours with marked pleomorphism, 3 points. (c) The third feature assessed was hyperchromatic and mitotic nuclei. If these occurred occasionally, the tumour was assigned 1 point, if with more moderate frequency, 2 points, but if their incidence was markedly frequent, 3 points. The sum of the scores provided the basis of grading: tumours with scores of 3, 4 and 5 being considered as grade I (low), those with scores of 6 and 7 as being grade II, and tumours with scores of 8-9 as constituting grade III.

The results of Bloom and Richardson (1957) and Bloom (1965), based on the follow up of over 1400 patients over a fifteen-year period after treatment, are given in Table 13. These clearly establish the close link

Table 13

Histological grade and prognosis in breast carcinoma

Histological grade	7-year results		10-year results		15-year results	
	No. of cases	% survival	No. of cases	% survival	No. of cases	% survival
1	362	75	215	53	96	31
11	640	47	349	27	162	18
III	407	32	250	19	101	10

From Bloom (1965); Bloom and Richardson (1957).

between low histological grade and good prognosis, confirmed subsequently by Tough *et al.* (1969) and Champion and Wallace (1971), though these investigators have reported somewhat higher survival rates. Bloom and Field (1971) included 20-year survival rates which were as follows: grade I 41%, grade II 26% and grade III 21%. A recent large series of breast tumours investigated has been described by Freedman *et al.* (1979), which also supports Bloom's method of histological grading as a valid prognostic indicator. They reported that the distribution of deaths over a 10-year period after treatment varied according to histological grade (Fig. 8). It may be seen from the figure that patients with grade III tumours show a risk peak between 1 and 2 years after treatment, much earlier than those with grade II and I tumours.

A histological classification has been introduced, albeit with less success, for astrocytomas. Kernohan (1949) and Svien *et al.* (1949) employed the

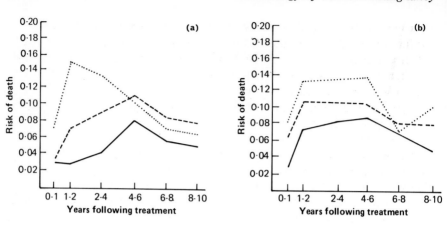

Figure 8 (a) Risk of death for carcinoma of the breast grade I (___); grade II (- - - -); Grade III (......). (b) Risk of death for clinical stage 1 (___); stage 2 (- - - -); stage 3 (......). From Freedman *et al.* (1979).

now well-established criteria of anaplasia, nuclear pleomorphism, hyperchromatism and mitotic activity for grading these tumours of the glial series. For astrocytoma patients in grade I-IV the average post-operative survival times were 74, 24, 12 and 7 months respectively (Svien *et al.*, 1949). The difference in average survival times for grades I and II is very large and not compatible with the only slight differences in the histological features of these low-grade tumours. The grade I tumours are described as being composed of apparently normal astrocytes, with no detectable anaplasia. In grade II, the majority of the cells are said to be normal, but a small number show nuclear pleomorphism and hyperchromatism. Both grade I and II show no mitotic activity. The distinctions between grades III and IV and I and II are much clearer, as far as the anaplasia and mitotic activity are concerned. Although Kernohan grading is widely used, there are no detailed reports on the correlation between histology and prognosis. In a short series of patients investigated by us from the point of view of establishing a correlation between epigenetic grade (*see* pp. 185-188) and prognosis, one patient with Kernohan grade I tumour showed a post-operative survival of longer than 16 months; two with grade II tumours showed a survival of 9 months. On the other hand, patients with grade III (7 patients) and grade IV (10 patients) tumours on average survived for a period of 6 months. Thus with the exception of grade IV, these survival figures were markedly different from those provided by Svien *et al.* (1949). None the less, there is a general trend towards better prognoses for the lower grade well-differentiated tumours. Tumours of the astrocytic series are known to show a spectrum of differentiation, but even more disconcerting is the observation that even well-differentiated tumours may infiltrate into neighbouring areas of the brain (Willis, 1967). Also, well-differentiated low-grade gliomas not infrequently progress into more malignant tumours as indicated by serial biopsy (Richmond, 1959). These factors will undoubtedly influence patient survival and could contribute to the less impressive correlation between histological grade and survival in the astrocytoma series than that in the breast tumour series.

These studies leave little doubt in one's mind about the clinical value of histological grading. Although clinical aggressiveness of a tumour is reflected in patient survival, it is still unclear if histological grade can unequivocally reflect the metastatic potential of the tumour. The early reports of Broders (1920) on squamous cell carcinoma of the lip and of Patey and Scarff (1920) on a series of breast carcinomas did show that metastatic dissemination was generally associated with high grade tumours and a small proportion (<10%) of patients who showed no metastatic dissemination had high grade tumours (Table 14). However, the results published by Bloom and Richardson do not show as remarkable a difference in distribution as that seen in the Patey and Scarff series. In the Bloom and Richardson series, approximately 20% of the patients with metastases had grade I tumours, about 45%, grade II and about 34% had grade III tumours. The distribution was slightly different in the patients who showed no invasion and axillary node involvement. Approximately 35% of the patients had grade I carcinoma, about 46% had grade II and about 20% had grade III tumour. This gives a distribution ratio between the 3 grades of 1:2·5:1·7 for patients with invasion and axillary node involvement and 1:1·3:0·6 for patients without invasion and axillary node involvement. The corresponding ratios for the Patey and Scarff series were 1:1·6:2·0 and 1:0·6:0·2.

From the more recent series reported by Bunting *et al.* (1976), the correlation existing between histological grade and metastatic distribution is fairly obvious (Table 15). The differences in the distribution of metastatic deposits in the lungs and the liver is even more striking than that in the bone.

Although the formation of metastatic deposits is also influenced by the immunological response of the host, one may conclude with sufficient justification that histological grading indeed reflects in some measure the metastatic potential of a given tumour. None the less, there are two important points which should be stressed. Firstly, patients with grade II carcinoma of the breast are just as likely to develop metastases as not, for the extent of distribution of this grade is almost identical between patients with metastatic disease and those without. Secondly, about half of breast cancers at presentation are grade II tumours (Table 16). It is imperative,

Table 14

Histological grade and metastatic behaviour of tumours

	Histological grade			References
	I	II	III	
% Patients with metastases	—	37	60 (3% grade IV)	Broders (1920)[a]
	6	30	52	Taylor and Nathanson (1939)[a]
% Patients without metastases	20	72	8	
% Patients with metastases	44	68	90	Patey and Scarff (1929)[b]
%Patients without metastases	56	32	10	
%Patients with invasion and axillary node involvement	21[c] 20[d] 20[e]	46 45 46	33 35 34	Bloom and Richardson (1957)[b]
% Patients without invasion and axillary node involvement	33[c] 36[d] 33[e]	47 42 49	20 22 18	
% Patients with lymph node metastasis	2	49	49	Hultborn and Törnberg (1960)[b]
%Patients with no lymph node metastasis	23	55	22	

[a]Squamous cell carcinoma of the lip; [b] breast tumours.
[c]% of patients followed up for 5 years.
[d]% of patients followed up for 10 years.
[e]% of patients followed up for 15 years.

therefore, that additional criteria be evolved to complement and improve the histological criteria for assessing tumour malignancy for use as an aid in the primary treatment of cancer.

Clinical staging of neoplasms has been used by some investigators to improve and refine prognostic predictions made using histological grading.

Table 15

Metastatic distribution of breast carcinomas in relation
to histological grade

Site of metastasis	Per cent distribution		
	Grade I	II	III
Bone	23	31	37
Lungs	3	14	15
Liver	7	21	20

From Bunting *et al.* (1976).

Before discussing these investigations and the possible advantages of combining clinical staging and histological grading for the assessment of patients, it might be worthwhile to digress briefly to describe the widely adopted technique of clinical staging according to the TNM system.

Clinical staging of tumours

The TNM classification   The widely accepted TNM staging of tumours was developed under the auspices of the International Union Against Cancer (UICC) and has been described extensively in a handbook published by the UICC in 1974.

The TNM classification of tumours arose from the need to rationalize the selection of patients for radical primary treatment by grouping patients with

Table 16

Distribution of histological grades of breast tumours

No. of patients	Tumour grade			Reference
	I	II	III	
	(% distribution)			
1409	29	45	26	Bloom and Richardson (1957); Bloom (1965)
525	11	52	37	Hultborn and Törnberg (1960)
687	11	52	37	Tough *et al.* (1969)
496	23	52	25	Champion and Wallace (1971)
1759	21	36	43	Freedman *et al.* (1979)
1000	3	27	70	E. R. Fisher *et al.* (1975)
524	24	44	32	Bunting *et al.* (1976)

Table 17

TNM Classification (AJC-UICC)—1977

Primary tumour (T)

T_x	Tumour cannot be assessed	T_1	Tumour of greatest dimension <2 cm
T_0	No evidence of tumour	T_2	Tumour >2 cm but <5 cm
T_{is}	Carcinoma *in situ*	T_3	Tumour >5 cm
		T_4	Tumour >5 cm in its greatest dimension

Note: Depending upon the site of the tumour, additional attributes which could add to the precision of describing the anatomical extent may be considered in determining the parameter T. Thus, for instance, in breast cancer, the T categories may be subdivided depending on the involvement of skin and the underlying pectoral fascia and/or muscle thus:

T_{1a} No fixation to pectoral fascia or muscle
T_{1b} Fixation to pectoral fascia and/or muscle present
Similarly T_{2a}, T_{2b}, T_{3a}, T_{3b}, etc.

Regional lymph nodes (N)

N_x State of regional lymph nodes cannot be assessed
N_0 No palpable lymph nodes
N_1 Movable homolateral lymph nodes
        N_{1a} Nodes not considered to contain growth
        N_{1b} Nodes considered to contain growth
N_2 Movable contralateral or bilateral lymph nodes
N_3 Fixed lymph nodes

Distant metastases (M)

M_x Not assessed
M_0 No (known) metastases
M_1 Distant metastases present
        To be specified as to site of metastasis

After assigning the T, N and M categories, tumours may be grouped into 4 stages.

Stage grouping

Stage I	$T_{1a} N_0/N_{1a}$	M_0
	$T_{1b} N_0/N_{1a}$	M_0
Stage II	$T_0 N_{1b}$	M_0
	$T_{2a} N_0/N_{1a}/N_{1b}$	M_0
	$T_{2b} N_0/N_{1a}/N_{1b}$	M_0
Stage III	Any $T_3 N_1$ or N_2	M_0
Stage IV	T_4 Any N	Any M
	Any T_3	Any M
	Any T Any N	M_1

From American Joint Committee for Cancer Staging and End Result Reporting. Manual for Staging Cancer (1977), pp. 101-114: UICC; TNM Classification of Malignant Tumours (1974).

confirmed neoplasms who could be predicted to have higher recovery rates and those with different degrees of tumour dissemination. It may be stated in general terms that this system of staging is related to the progression and extent of the disease, being essentially a representation of the topographical extent of the tumour (T), the status of the regional lymph nodes (N) and the presence of metastases (M). The exact clinical stage of the disease is simply described by taking into consideration the size of the primary tumour, the degree of involvement of regional lymph nodes and the degree of metastasis (Table 17).

The Manchester classification of breast tumours   In the past few years, several systems of clinical staging have been described especially to aid in the management of breast cancer. Some of these systems have been reviewed by Mansfield (1976). The effects of combining histological grading and clinical staging have been examined, mainly using the Manchester classification, by Bloom (1965), Bunting *et al.* (1976) and Freedman *et al.* (1979). Hence this system of classification will be summarized here before discussing the advantages of combining histological grading and clinical staging (Table 18A). A third most widely used system is the Columbia classification (Haagensen, 1974). This is given in Table 18B.

Table 18A

The Manchester classification of breast tumours (Paterson, 1948)

Stage I   Growth confined to the breast
1. An area of adherence to skin smaller than the periphery of the tumour does not affect staging, even ulceration of the skin in the area does not alter it.

Stage II
2. Same as Stage I, but there are affected mobile lymph nodes in the axilla.

Stage III
1. Skin involvement larger than tumour and/or:
2. Lymph nodes fixed and/or:
3. Tumour fixed to pectoral muscle and/or:
4. Affected lymph nodes in supraclavicular fossa

Stage IV
The same as stage III plus distant metastases either blood or lymph-borne; this includes metastases to opposite breast, axilla, supraclavicular fossa or satellite skin nodules

---

From Mansfield (1976).

Table 18B

Columbia clinical staging for breast cancer

Stage	Clinical criteria
A	No skin oedema, ulceration, nor tumour solidly fixed to chest wall, axillary nodes not involved
B	As in A, but clinically involved axillary nodes <2·5 cm in transverse diam., not fixed to skin or deeper structures of the axilla
C	Any one of five grave signs of advanced carcinoma present: 1. Oedema of skin (involves <$\frac{1}{3}$ of breast surface) 2. Skin ulceration 3. Tumour fixed to the chest wall 4. Massive axillary node involvement (>2·5 cm transverse diameter) 5. Fixed axillary nodes
D	All more advanced carcinomas including: 1. Any two or more of grave signs given under stage C 2. Extensive oedema of the skin (>$\frac{1}{3}$ breast surface) 3. Satellite skin nodules 4. Inflammatory carcinoma 5. Clinically involved supraclavicular lymph nodes 6. Parasternal tumour indicating mammary metastases 7. Oedema of the arm 8. Distant metastases

From Haagensen (1974).

Combination of histological grading and clinical staging

Bloom presented a scheme for linking histological grading with clinical staging in order to obtain a more accurate guide to prognosis (Bloom, 1950, 1956). In a large series of breast tumours, Bloom (1965) found that histological grading and clinical staging by the Manchester classification (Paterson, 1948) provided comparable results. But combining the two appeared to produce interesting results. The 5-year, 10-year and 15-year results for a series of 1391 treated cases of breast cancer, classified by histological grade and clinical stage published by Bloom (1965), are reproduced in Table 19. It may be seen from these data that in each clinical stage, the percentage of survivals has been subdivided according to histological grade. In all the stages, patients with grade I tumours show higher survival rates than those with grade III tumours. Such reductions in survival rate with increasing histological grade are seen for all three follow-up periods, viz. 5, 10 and 15 years. Thus, there could be a refinement of the prediction of prognosis if such a combined classification is employed. The data could

Table 19

Stage, grade and prognosis of carcinoma of the breast

Stage	Grade	Five-year results Cases 1936-49	Survivals %	Ten-year results Cases 1936-45	Survivals %	Fifteen-year results Cases 1936-40	Survivals %
1	I	162	86	98	55	45	40
	II	212	70	109	49	50	34
	III	93	70	58	48	22	27
2	I	120	71	66	58	21	19
	II	247	42	131	22	50	16
	III	181	25	103	12	38	10
3	I	63	67	45	42	28	28
	II	130	30	76	13	41	7
	III	97	19	64	9	26	0
4	I	11	36	2	50	—	—
	II	42	5	28	4	19	5
	III	33	3	24	4	15	0
	Total	1391	50	804	31	355	17

From Bloom (1965).

also indicate greater accuracy of prediction; for instance, patients with stage 3 disease but grade I tumour could have better prognosis than patients with stage 2 grade III tumour.

If one examined the distribution of survivals in relation to histological grade and clinical stage, however, the effects of combining the two systems are not as convincing as the data presented in Table 19 would seem. We have re-analysed the data to see if the proportions of survival bore any relationship to histological grade and/or clinical stage. The reworked data are presented in Table 20.

The major conclusions one may draw are as follows: as far as 5-year survival is concerned, prognosis for patients with grade I and II is similar, irrespective of the clinical stage. The chances of survival at 5 years are considerably lower for patients who have histological grade III tumours, notwithstanding the clinical stage.

Combining histological grading with clinical stage appears to make some difference in the 10-year survival group. The distribution of 10-year survival is similar for patients with grade I and II tumours of clinical stage 1 or 2. But patients with stage 3 disease appeared to have a better chance of 10-year survival if the tumours were histologically grade I. Again, patients with grade III tumours showed lower survival rates, irrespective of the clinical

Table 20

Survival distribution in relation to histological grade and clinical stage

Survival group	Clinical stage	Total no. of patients surviving	Grade I %	Grade II %	Grade III %
5-year	1	343	38	43	19
	2	233	36	44	19
	3	99	42	39	18
	4	7	57	29	14
10-year	1	135	40	39	21
	2	79	48	37	15
	3	35	54	29	17
	4	3	33	33	33
15-year	1	41	44	41	15
	2	16	25	50	25
	3	4	72	28	—
	4	1	—	—	—

Based on data of Bloom (1965).

stage of the disease. As far as 15-year survival is concerned, the distribution is similar for patients with grades I and II/clinical stage 1 tumours, but much lower for grade III tumours of the same clinical stage.

As a general rule, a more favourable prognosis could be predicted for patients with grades I and II tumours, even if they happen to belong to higher clinical stages. In other words, histological grading may be more valuable a guide for predicting prognosis than is clinical staging. Perhaps combination of clinical staging and histological grading could contribute to greater accuracy in predicting prognosis over 10-15 year periods.

Freedman *et al.* (1979) disagree with Bloom (1965) and Bunting *et al.* (1976) that histological and clinical staging stratification of survival gives comparable results. They believe that histological grading is more important than clinical staging. For they found that the distribution of deaths of treated patients over a 10-year period varied according to the histological grade of the tumour rather than the clinical stage of the disease. Also, as shown in Fig. 8 (p. 132), the high risk peak for patients with grade III tumours occurs between 1 and 2 years after treatment. This peak occurs much later at about 6 to 7 years after treatment, for those with histological grades II and I tumours. In contrast, no such difference is seen in patients with tumours of different clinical stages.

The attempts at discriminating between clinical staging and histological grading on the basis of the possible advantages which each has over the other are wholly laudable but inconsequential. The technique of clinical staging describes the extent of the disease as it appears in physical examination, radioisotopic scans, etc. There seems to be little rationale for suggesting that either method should be used to the exclusion of the other.

Clinical staging describes the status quo of the disease and allows one to evaluate prognosis of the disease on the basis of its apparent extent. But it cannot determine the malignancy potential of a tumour, nor predict the course of tumour progression. On the other hand, as discussed earlier, histological grading does in some measure determine the potential for malignancy possessed by a tumour. A combination of the two systems can do nothing but enhance the value of either method. The importance of the contribution made by histological grading to cancer management has been recognized, and the 1977 TNM classification incorporates the degree of differentiation of the tumour.

The method of histological grading has been criticized on several counts, the most important one being reproducibility. The subjective nature of the assessment of some of the parameters may cause some variation in the grading of the same tumour by different observers and even by the same observer on different occasions (Foote, 1959). Even the least subjective feature, viz. the mitotic count, could be a cause of disagreement between observers (Champion and Wallace, 1971). The variation in grading is obvious from the distribution of breast tumours over the three grades reported in a number of investigations (Table 16). The ratios of distribution are widely different. With the exception of Fisher *et al.* (1975) and Freedman *et al.* (1979), the investigators graded about 50% of all breast tumours as grade II. Three of the six series published classed between 20 and 30% to be grade I tumours. Two series showed 11% of tumours as being grade I. Fisher *et al.* (1975) claimed only 2·5% low grade tumours, while they found 70% of the tumours to be grade III. Also, Freedman *et al.* (1979) have stated that in their series (1961-68) the distribution ratio at the end of the series was different from that at the beginning and that the variations in the ratios which were more pronounced at the early stages of series could have coincided with the period in which "the pathologist was gaining experience in this grading method".

Another factor which adds to these difficulties is the possible variation in differentiation in different parts of the tumour. Foulds (1954) has argued most cogently that different parts of a tumour may undergo progression to different degrees, and even more disconcertingly, along different paths. It would be impracticable to examine an entire tumour in histology. Grading more often than not depends upon an examination of one section, except where the growth is large. Where there is considerable variation in the histological grade of different parts of a tumour, the highest grade is taken into account.

The numerical element in the scoring and the final histological grading has also attracted much comment. Bloom (1965) has stated in unambiguous terms that the histological grades are not defined entities but merely "represent arbitrary subdivisions of a continuous malignancy scale". None the less, not infrequently pathologists have opined that numerical histological grading may be no more reliable than simple histological descriptions of the tumour, from which the clinician may draw his own conclusions as to the degree of its malignancy.

Combination of histological features and
stromal responses

These criticisms concern the application of histological grading technique and do not call into question its intrinsic merit. Therefore, in spite of the unremarkable attempts at combining clinical staging with histological grading, it would be worthwhile examining if features such as the nature and extent of cellular contribution from outside the tumour itself could complement the grading system. The infiltration of tumours by host cells has been known for a long time, and has often been referred to as "stromal reaction", a term coined by Russel (1908). Grading systems including stromal features have been described in the past (Sistrunk and MacCarty, 1922; Smith and Bartlett, 1929; Haagensen, 1933) but without much success. With the realization that host-cell infiltration represents an immunological response to the presence of the aberrant cells, much effort has been invested in uncovering the possible role played by these cells in the growth and dissemination of the tumour. Sistrunk and MacCarty (1922) recognized the significance of stromal response in determining the prognosis of carcinoma of the breast. They reported that the post-operative survival life-span was about 42% shorter for patients with tumours showing no lymphocytic infiltration and hyalinization than the average survival span of patients with tumours that did contain lymphocytic infiltration and hyalinization. Also the occurrence of fibrosis appeared to be associated with a favourable prognosis. At present, there is much additional evidence which links the nature and degree of host cell infiltration with favourable prognosis for the patients. Some of this evidence has been reviewed earlier (*see* pp. 48-56).

Recently Pagnini *et al.* (1980) have advocated the inclusion in histological examination not only of the stromal response but also of other features such as vascular invasion, depth of invasion and mode of invasion. They reported on a series of 125 patients with squamous cell carcinoma of the uterine cervix and examined histological grading in relation to prognosis. They make the interesting claim that 5-year survival within the group clinical stages I and II correlated favourably with histological grading, with 87% of patients with low histological grade carcinomas surviving the 5-year period but only 54% surviving in the group with high histological grade carcinomas. This correlation was found also in stages III and IV carcinomas (Table 21). Unfortunately, the value of this analysis is diminished greatly because Pagnini *et al.* did not break down the histological grades into the usual subdivisions and separate the four clinical stages. This is presumably because, if this had been attempted, the numbers of cases in each group would have been too small for statistical analysis.

Table 21

Histological grading and 5-year survival of infiltrating
squamous cell carcinoma of the uterine cervix

Histological grade	Stages I-II		Stages III-IV	
	No. of cases	% 5-year survivals	No. of cases	% 5-year survivals
Low	77	87	9	44
High	28	54	11	9

From Pagnini *et al.* (1980).

It would seem from the study of Pagnini *et al.* that histological typing of squamous cell carcinoma into keratinizing, large cell and small cell carcinomas alone may not suffice in evaluating prognosis for patients who have been treated surgically. Combining histological typing with clinical staging seems to hold no obvious advantages. But combining histological classification with the degree and depth of stromal invasion into the tumour could, it would appear from the manner in which the data are presented, have considerable predictive value.

It is reasonable to conclude from the preceding discussion that certain "extraneous" factors such as stromal response and clinical staging can usefully complement histological grading in predicting the course of neoplasia. It would be of more than academic interest, therefore, to inquire if histological grading can be aided by other systems, such as those incorporating epigenetic criteria, which might refine the technique of assessing differentiation which forms an integral part of histological grading, and make determination of the degree of differentiation with greater reliability than could be associated with morphological descriptions.

Epigenetic correlates of malignancy

*Effects of individuation fields on tumour
differentiation*

In embryonic development, the initiation of cellular differentiation by
morphogenetic stimuli, i.e. the process of evocation, is followed by an autonomous process of "individuation", which involves the regional
organization and pattern formation of the induced structures (Needham *et
al.*, 1933, 1934). Individuation has been considered to be a field phenomenon, this notion being implicit in the work of Waddington and Schmidt
(1933). The most important feature of the forces operating in the
individuation field is their ability to influence all tissue in that field to
organize and build up into the whole embryo or to be fashioned into a
specific organ, depending upon which part of the individuation field the
tissue happens to be in. Although the nature of the forces acting in the field
is not understood, the actual process of individuation has been adequately
demonstrated.

One of the outstanding examples of the operation of the individuation
process is the regeneration of limbs in, for instance, the adult newt. In this
animal, the stump area left after amputation of the leg is so strong a
regenerating zone that it moulds any component tissue grafted on to it into
a limb. It was inevitable, therefore, that attempts would be made to test the
possible effects of any individuation field such as that occurring in
regeneration upon tissues which are grafted onto it.

Since the ability to regenerate lost limbs is not possessed by all animals, it
has been argued that the possession of such an ability may be an indication
of the persistence of the individuation field in adult life (Needham, 1942).
Needham extended this argument to explain the origins of neoplasia. He
suggested that neoplastic development may be the result of a failure of the
individuation field. If this should be the case, persistence of the individuation field should bear some relationship to the incidence of neoplasia.
Some support for this view had in fact been adduced by Needham. For a
search of the literature on the incidence of cancers in amphibia indicated
that the occurrence of neoplasms is far higher in anurans than in the
urodeles. Such retrospective studies are, as often as not, inadequate. As
Needham himself has pointed out, the reported occurrence of neoplasms
tends to concern species which are being investigated and therefore does not
provide an accurate reflection of natural incidence but exaggerates the
incidence in certain species which are suitable for laboratory experiments.

An examination of the list of accessions to the Registry of Tumours in
Lower Animals, National Museum of Natural History of the Smithsonian
Institution (Harshbarger, 1965-78) has revealed much useful information

regarding the incidence of neoplasia in amphibians. The accessions included 32 neoplasms from anurans, of which 84% were malignant tumours. On the other hand, only 61% of the 85 neoplasms of urodeles were malignant tumours. Thus, although the incidence of neoplasms may not be higher in anurans than in urodeles, the incidence of malignant tumours is far higher in the former than the latter. The data in Table 22 includes only spon-

Table 22

Incidence of malignant neoplasms in anurans and urodeles

Order	No. of neoplasms	Malignant	Non-malignant
Anura	32	27 (84%)	5 (16%)
Urodeles	85	52 (61%)	33 (39%)

Data from Harshbarger (1965-78). A statistical analysis by X^2 distribution using 2×2 contingency tables (Fisher and Yates, 1974) shows that the difference between the two orders in the incidence of malignant neoplasms is significant ($X^2 = 5.9$; P<0.02).

taneous tumours, but not *en masse* contributions to the Registry. Admittedly, the numbers of tumours involved are small. None the less, the difference in the incidence of malignant tumours in the two orders is significant enough to provide support to the lobby which is inclined to attribute a possible role to the controlling influences of the individuation field. It ought to be pointed out that Balls (1962) assembled data on the reported incidence of neoplasia in the amphibia which showed no significant differences in the frequency of the incidence of malignant and non-malignant tumours in the two amphibian orders. Thus, of 68 reported neoplasms of anurans, 44% were malignant and 56% non-malignant, while of 40 tumours of urodeles, 38% were malignant and 62% non-malignant. The two sets of data, viz. that taken from Harshbarger (1965-78) and Balls (1962), are widely divergent. Since it is based on the accessions to the Registry of Tumours in Lower Animals, the pattern of incidence of malignant and non-malignant tumours based on the data of Harshbarger may reflect the true situation more accurately. The data of Balls (1962), on the other hand, is based on published work up to 1962 and this may contribute to a distortion of the true picture, the distorting factor being the selection by the investigators of certain suitable tumour and animal systems. The reported incidence of tumours should also be treated with great caution because the susceptibility to develop tumours appears to be dependent upon several factors. Thus, Camerini and Zavanella (1968) and Seilern-Aspang and Kratochwil (1963a) noticed that the susceptibility of urodeles to chemical carcinogens is dependent upon seasonal factors. The spontaneous incidence of neoplasms is also reported to be related to unknown geographical factors (Camerini and Zavanella, 1968).

To take an overview of the situation, there is as yet little firm evidence that neoplastic change is due to a failure of the individuation field, but the data available to date do not warrant a total rejection of the view that the expression of malignant behaviour could conceivably be influenced by the individuation field.

Some experimental evidence is available which appears to support the view that regenerating field forces may influence and possibly control the growth and differentiation of tumours. Seilern-Aspang and Kratochwil (1962, 1965) examined the behaviour of chemically induced epithelial tumours of *Triturus cristatus* placed in the regenerating tail region of the animal. These authors claimed that the tumour differentiated into normal epidermal tissue. Rose and Wallingford (1948) had earlier reported that tissue of the Lucké renal adenocarcinoma of *Rana pipiens* differentiated into normal muscle, cartilage and connective tissue when tumour fragments were implanted into the limb and the limb was subsequently amputated. Apparently, therefore, the regeneration field induced the adenocarcinoma to differentiate.

Mizell (1960, 1961) implanted the Lucké renal carcinoma into the tail fin of *Rana pipiens* tadpoles and amputated the tail after the tumours had taken and had begun to grow. It seemed that the portion of the tumour in the regeneration field broke down, but the portion of the implant proximal to the area of regeneration retained the tubular characteristics. The cells were intact and mitosing.

Subsequently, Mizell (1965) labelled tumour cells with tritium before implanting them and claimed its recovery in normal tissue. Unfortunately, the detection of the radioactive label in normal cells does not constitute incontrovertible evidence that the cells carrying the label were derived from the original tumour now differentiated into a normal state. Even in heterologous systems, such induced differentiation of tumours has been reported. Thus, Seilern-Aspang and Kratochwil (1963b) described the differentiation of a chemically induced tumour of the planarian *Dendrocoelum lacteum* placed in the regeneration field following amputation of the limb in an amphibian.

There is, however, considerable evidence which totally refutes such claims. As early as 1955, Rubens reported that Lucké carcinoma implants were unaffected by various stages of regeneration. Neither were chemically induced lymphosarcomas of *Xenopus laevis* affected in any way on implantation into regenerating forelimbs of post-metamorphic *Xenopus laevis* (Rubens and Balls, 1964a). Sheremetieva (1965) found that spontaneous melanomas grew without any subversive effects of the regeneration field in regenerating tails of *Axolotl*. Consistent with such a lack of effect is the observation that regeneration field forces in no way impede the induction of tumours by chemical carcinogens. Breedis (1951) could induce sarcomas to develop in regenerating salamander limb; while Rose and Rose (1952) reported the induction of chondrosarcoma in adult limb cartilage. Rubens and Balls (1964b) implanted methylcholanthrene crystals on regenerating limbs and abdomen of immature *Xenopus laevis*, and noticed that the carcinogen induced lymphosarcoma irrespective of whether the carcinogen was placed in the regenerating limb of abdomen. Leone (1953) reported that the experimental induction of cancers in urodeles which have considerable regenerative capacity is in fact far more successful than in anurans. There is little basis for believing that factors other than pure experimental conditions might have dictated such differences. Recently, Khudoley and Picard (1980) showed about 54% incidence of tumours in *Xenopus* following induction by *N*-nitrosodimethylamine. These investigations seem to suggest that the processes of neoplastic transformation and development of tumours are not impeded or interfered with by the regeneration field, and also that the state of differentiation of the tumours placed in such a field is not altered in any way.

Effects of embryonic tissues on tumour differentiation

The association of embryonic cells and tumour cells as a means of harnessing the morphogenetic stimuli emanating from the embryonic cells to influence the state of differentiation of tumours has attracted considerable attention, although in hindsight this approach has been as unfruitful as that which employed regeneration field forces as a means to achieve the same ends.

Some of the earliest work in this type of investigation was published by De Lustig and De Matrajt (1961). De Lustig and Lustig (1964) and De Lustig (1968) examined the effects of the chick embryo organiser, viz. pieces of the anterior part of the primitive-streak embryo, on mouse sarcoma 180. They reported that, after culture with the embryonic tissue, the tumour showed a tendency towards tubular organization and slower growth on reimplantation into host animals. These tumours also appeared to be less invasive. They reported further that when a mouse osteogenic sarcoma was co-cultivated with 3-day-old chick chorda and neural tube, the sarcoma showed differentiation into osseous trabeculae and a reduction in the number of giant cells (De Lustig and Lustig, 1964). In order to ensure that the differentiated components were not of the chick origin, these authors separated the embryonic and tumour components by vitelline membrane of the egg.

Seilern-Aspang *et al.* (1963a, b) and Seilern-Aspang and Kratochwil (1963c) obtained the differentiation of cartilage in human and mouse sarcomas combined *in vitro* with 5-day chick embryo notochord. Pretreatment of the notochord with x-rays at 500 rads in order to limit the proliferation of the embryonic cells resulted in the formation of reduced amounts of cartilage, suggesting a major contribution of differentiated tissue from the embryonic component.

Ellison *et al.* (1969) performed similar experiments and cultured mouse sarcoma 180 in combination with notochord and/or spinal cord of 3- to 5-day-old chick embryos. Differentiation of cartilage seemed to occur in the tumour tissue, but this was found to be of chick origin. This appeared to be due to the fact that precartilaginous condensations could not be completely removed from the 5-day chick notochord. This was confirmed by the observation that no cartilage differentiation was seen in tumour explants combined with notochord from younger embryos, where a complete isolation of notochordal tissues was possible. Besides, interposition of Millipore filters of 25 μm thickness and 0·8 μm pore size completely prevented the formation of cartilage in explants grown in association even with 5-day chick embryo notochord. Ellison *et al.* (1969) also tested a homologous combination, viz. rat renal tumour and dorsal spinal cord of mouse and rat embryos, which is considered to be an inductor of kidney tubules (Grobstein, 1977; Moscona, 1957; Lash, 1963). Of a total of 28 trans-filter combinations, one explant showed a clear differentiation of tubules. These authors also found that some control explants of tumour, i.e. not combined with embryonic tissues, also showed tubule differentiation in a small number of cases. Unfortunately these experiments do not exclude the involvement of embryonic factors in the differentiation of the tumour explants, since the growth medium used in these experiments contained embryo extracts prepared from 9- to 11-day-old chick embryos. Embryo extracts do indeed exert differentiative influences as shown by Seilern-Aspang and Weissberg (1963). They have reported several instances of redifferentiation in chicken sarcomas injected with extracts of 2- to 4-day-old chick embryos.

Crocker and Vernier (1972) examined the differentiative ability of a congenital nephroma which frequently occurs in children. This tumour, which is regarded as a variant of Wilm's tumour, is composed predominantly of sheets of spindle-shaped mesenchymal derivative cells, and differs from Wilm's tumour in that it does not possess renal structures. Crocker and Vernier (1972) grew pieces of this tumour in organ culture along with pieces of dorsal spinal cord of foetal mouse. The latter is known to act as an inductor of kidney tubules (Grobstein, 1975; Moscona, 1957; Lash, 1963). Within 48 h of co-cultivation with the inductor, the nephroma tissue adjacent to the inductor was found to differentiate into kidney tubules which included recognizable Bowman's capsule, glomeruli and proximal tubules.

The most convincing piece of work which describes the induction of differentiation of tumour was published by De Cosse *et al.* (1973). These authors used a mammary adenocarcinoma BW10232 of C57BL/6J mice and the homologous embryonic inductor, viz. mammary mesenchyme derived from CF 1 Swiss white embryos of 12-day's gestation. The tumour and the embryonic inductor were combined with or without the interposition of Millipore filters of 1 μm thickness and of 0·45 μm pore size. A histological examination showed that tumour pieces exposed to mammary mesenchyme showed changes in the tumour morphology in 33% of cases. The morphological changes included the appearance of tubules, changes in nuclear and cytoplasmic morphology and also reduction in mitoses and DNA synthesis. Interposition of Millipore filter made no difference in the frequency of differentiation. However, if tumour pieces were exposed to embryonic brain tissue instead of the homologous inductor, no differentiation occurred.

De Cosse *et al.* (1973) also demonstrated that there may have been some functional differentiation as well in the tumour exposed to the embryonic inductor. Since acid mucopolysaccharides have been associated with the epithelial-mesenchymal interface in induction (Pessac and Defendi, 1972), De Cosse *et al.* (1973) stained their preparation with Alcian blue for acid mucopolysaccharides. While control cultures failed to stain, Alcian blue-positive material was detected between epithelial areas where tubule formation had occurred.

The investigations of both Ellison *et al.* (1969) and De Cosse *et al.* (1973) tend to underline the importance of employing homologous inductors. None the less, it ought to be pointed out that embryo extracts had been used in the culture medium in both investigations. That factors present in the embryo extract may be involved in the differentiation obtained in the control cultures of Ellison *et al.* (1969) appears to be confirmed by the experiments of De Cosse *et al.* (1973). These latter authors found that when the embryo extract concentration was raised, the incidence of differentiation in the tumour tissue exposed to the embryonic inductor increased by a factor of 2 or 3. Increase of the embryo extract concentration also produced some differentiation in tumours exposed to the heterologous inductor, suggesting the possibility that some factor present in the embryo extract may act as a co-factor or promoter of differentiation.

Another interesting series of experiments aimed at establishing comparability in the differentiative status of embryonic cells and tumour cells has resulted in the demonstration that teratoma cells can produce perfect chimeras with embryonic cells. Chimeric mice have been successfully produced by the injection of teratocarcinoma cells into the blastocyst of mice (Gardner, 1968; Brinster, 1974; Mintz and Illmensee, 1975; Illmensee and Mintz, 1976). The contribution of, and the complete participation by the teratocarcinoma cells in the formation of the chimeras has been adequately demonstrated by the use of specific genetic markers associated with the teratocarcinoma cells (Mintz and Illmensee, 1975; Illmensee and Mintz, 1976; Dewey and Mintz, 1978; Mintz and Cronmiller, 1978). The degree of such participation or the degree of chimerism could vary considerably, but this ability of teratocarcinoma cells to participate in the orderly and sequential processes of differentiation and embryogenesis indicates not only the parity of pluripotency, but also the possibility that the embryonal carcinoma cells are in a state of competence at which they can impart as well as respond to morphogenetic stimuli.

Growth and Maintenance of Tumours

In the evaluation of the progression of a neoplasm and prognosis of the disease, it would be essential to have sufficient knowledge of the biological attributes of the neoplasm. Since the behaviour of the tumour *in vivo* is affected, modified and controlled, though often unsuccessfully, by host factors, a determination of the intrinsic abilities of a tumour would be of considerable assistance in extrapolating or predicting its possible behaviour *in vivo*. Several tests have been described for assessing the invasive ability of the tumours and their growth characteristics. The other distinguishing property of tumours, i.e. their ability to form metastases, however, is neither a function nor a reflection of the invasive ability. None the less, the tests could be used to examine preferential arrest and lodgement of tumour cells and emboli at distant sites. Among other objectives pursued by the designers of these tests were their application to the screening of suspected carcinogenic substances and possibly also examining the effects on tumour cells of potential therapeutic agents.

The investigations which have led to the development of such tests may be discussed in two broad groups, viz. transplantation in embryo and transplantation in association with organ culture of mainly embryonic tissues or organs.

The history of transplantation and maintenance of tumours goes back several years, but the techniques available are still limited in number. The transplantation of tumours into immunologically privileged sites such as the anterior chamber of the eye (Eichwald and Chang, 1951; Greene, 1952) and the cheek pouch of the hamster (Handler, 1956) and in immuno-suppressed animals (Toolan, 1954) is not simple enough in practice to commend itself to general and widespread use. Hence simpler systems such as the chick embryo or the chorio-allantoic membrane (CAM) have been tested for their ability to support the growth of human tumours as well as those of other mammals. As Leighton (1970) has stressed, it is essential that the technique is conducive to the maintenance of the original histological characteristics in the tumour before it can be accepted for assaying the biological features of the tumour.

Leighton (1963, 1967) demonstrated that a variety of tumours may be grown successfully in chick embryos or on the CAM system, and also provided examples where tumours had retained their characteristic histo-logical appearance. Co-cultivation of tumour tissue with embryonic tissues appears to be conducive to the growth of tumours, whether the latter are maintained *in vitro* (Wolff and Schneider, 1957; Wolff and Sigot, 1961a, b; Wolff *et al.*, 1964) or on the CAM (Leighton *et al.*, 1972). Thus, the mouse mammary carcinoma T2633 and the rat ascites hepatoma not only grew successfully in association with mesonephros of 8- to 9-day-old chick embryos, but also showed no variation in histological appearance from the original tumour (Wolff and Sigot, 1961a, b). Embryonic liver was also found to be most conducive to the maintenance of the HZ hepatoma (Wolff *et al.*, 1964). Leighton *et al.* (1972) reported that, when inoculated on the CAM, Wilm's tumour formed small nodules which appeared irregularly, but when embryonic mesonephros, liver or heart tissue was included in the inoculum with the tumour tissue, the tumour grew in abundance, with the original histology being retained. Embryonic liver was found to be most suitable.

In spite of the striking success of Leighton and colleagues with the chick embryo or CAM system, serial transplantation of tumours from egg to egg has invariably failed. Easty *et al.* (1969) attempted an investigation of the factors contributing to the success or failure to maintain tumours in the embryo system. After investigating the behaviour of a variety of tumours, they came to the conclusion that tumours which had lost their strain specificity for the original species grew vigorously in embryos and the CAM. Those tumours which had retained their original species speci-ficity could be grown less successfully. According to Easty *et al.* (1969), immunological responses of the host are not a factor in determining the success rate. Easty *et al.* have used 11- to 14-day-old embryos for tumour implantation, the embryos being maintained for several days following inoculation. Solomon (1964) has stated that chick embryos become immunologically competent after 15 days of growth. Hence immunological interference with the growth of the tumours cannot be excluded. This is, in fact, compounded by the observations of Easty *et al.* (1969), that the use of 7- to 8-day-old embryos remarkably improved the growth of all tumours.

Röller *et al.* (1966) described an organ culture system for the growth of human tumours. This consisted of steel, 40 mesh grids placed in 35 × 10 mm sterile disposable plastic Petri dishes. Tissue culture medium is added to the Petri dish until the grid surface is just wet. On these grids are placed Millipore filters (0·45 μm pore size), to which the tumour pieces for culture are transferred. Röller *et al.* (1966) cultured about ninety human tumours and claimed that the organ cultures had retained the original histology.

Yarnell *et al.* (1964) used siliconized lens paper in which 1 mm diam. holes were cut. These siliconized papers were floated on tissue culture medium in a small, sterile, disposable plastic Petri dish. A small square of unsiliconized paper was placed on the hole, to which tumour pieces of 1-2 ml volume were transferred for cultivation.

Hodges (1981) has written an authoritative review on organotypic cultures of neoplasms. She has pointed out that the survival of neoplasms *in vitro* greatly depends upon their degree of differentiation. Thus well-differentiated malignant tumours can be maintained in culture with greater success than less well-differentiated or more anaplastic tumours.

Tests for Invasiveness

Conventional tissue culture methods

The invasive ability of tumour cells may be attributed not only to intrinsic features of the tumour cell, but also determined to a large extent by the interactions of the tumour cells with host tissues. Among other factors postulated to contribute to invasion by tumours are the intratumoral pressure presumably occasioned by rapid cellular multiplication (Willis, 1973; Eaves, 1973), and release of toxins and proteolytic enzymes (*see* pp. 85-90) by the tumour. However, using the CAM system, Nicolson *et al.* (1977) demonstrated that invasion by malignant cells could take place even under conditions where such mechanical pressure did not appear to exist.

Actively growing tumours may induce inflammatory response and cause accumulation of neutrophils, lympocytes and macrophages. Leukocytes contain a variety of proteolytic enzymes and these may be released upon breakdown of the cells and thus help invasion by tumour cells of surrounding host tissues (Fidler *et al.*, 1978). Susceptibility to invasion also depends upon the structure of the organ. Tissues rich in elastic and collagen fibres may successfully ward off invasion (Easty and Easty, 1973). The biochemical, physiological and also the immunological status of the host could be of significance in determining the degree of invasion achieved by a tumour. To this extent, invasive ability, which could be regarded as an attribute of the cell surface, cannot be assessed objectively in isolation. Therefore, tests for invasiveness have suffered from the drawback that even the vaguest approximation of the natural conditions cannot be reproduced *in vitro*. None the less, investigations into interactions between tumour and normal tissue *in vitro* would provide useful background data which could be of considerable assistance in understanding the biological behaviour of tumours *in vivo*.

Three-dimensional sponge matrix culture

The conventional tissue culture methods have some application in the study of invasiveness. Some underlying cell interactions such as the contact inhibition of cell movement (Abercrombie, 1970a, b), the density-dependent inhibition of growth (Stoker and Rubin, 1967) and the phenomenon of contact guidance (Weiss, 1934) are amenable to investigation by the conventional methods.

The early attempts at determining tumour invasiveness in two-dimensional *in vitro* systems have been described by Abercrombie *et al.* (1957). They argued that since normal fibroblasts *in vitro* showed contact-mediated inhibition of movement, this phenomenon might be absent in cultures in which the tumour cells are confronted with normal fibroblasts, which Abercrombie and his colleagues had indeed demonstrated previously (Abercrombie and Heaysman, 1954; Abercrombie and Ambrose, 1958; Abercrombie, 1970b). When two colonies of fibroblasts were initiated, cellular outgrowths ("outwanderings") appeared to proceed symmetrically until the populations met. At this point, the cellular movement was inhibited and over a few days, if the cells of the two populations could be distinguished, the colonies were found to invade each other slightly.

Abercrombie *et al.* (1957) investigated the social behaviour of cellular outgrowths from explants of two mouse sarcomas (S37 and Crocker) and mouse muscle and chick heart, and reported that normal fibroblast movements were obstructed by sarcoma outgrowths. No such inhibition was noticed in the movement of the sarcoma cells. Subsequently, Abercrombie and Heaysman (1976) and Abercrombie (1979) published a quantitative study of the invasive behaviour of five transplantable mouse sarcomas and a melanoma and of neonatal mouse fibroblasts in confronted cultures. The explants were placed 1 cm apart, and the cultures incubated for between 1 and 3 days, fixed, stained and mounted. They essentially confirmed the previous finding that, after between 12 and 24 h incubation, mutual invasion was much greater in sarcoma vs. fibroblast cultures than in fibroblast vs. fibroblast cultures. When normal mouse muscle fibroblasts were confronted with standard chick heart fibroblasts, a high degree of obstruction was seen. This was indicated by the occurrence of a narrow (approximately 20 μm) invasion zone which is defined as the zone occupied by cells from both explants. When one of the tumours was confronted with the standard fibroblast explant, the breadth of the invasion zone was found to vary between 130 and 290 μm. Three of the tumours were still obstructed by the normal fibroblasts. Abercrombie (1979) demonstrated this by measuring the mean distance migrated from each explant medially and the free sides. The ratio between the distances will be less than unity if movement is obstructed, but if the invasion is unobstructed, the ratio remains at unity.

Barski and Belehradek (1965) performed similar experiments and found that malignant cells tended to infiltrate colonies of normal cells. However, the infiltration was found to occur where intercellular gaps occurred, and no invasion was seen when the tumour cells were confronted by coherent sheets of normal cells. Thus, not only does there appear to be basic disagreement about the nature of invasiveness, but as Leighton *et al.* (1968) have pointed out, a severe limitation is that these studies are based on observations on two-dimensional interactions, while *in vivo* the situation is three-dimensional.

Abercrombie (1979) was indeed aware of the difficulties in relating the invasive behaviour *in vitro* to that occurring in vivo, and stated that while quantitation of invasiveness in explant culture is easy, ascertaining its relevance *in vivo* is complicated by the fact that no quantitation of invasion *in vivo* can be made, which is at best inferred from histology.

Leighton (1951) brought the tissue culture situation closer to the *in vivo* one by introducing the three-dimensional sponge matrix system. He employed a cellulose sponge matrix impregnated with plasma clot. Since the plasma-clot sponge matrix was unsuitable for tissues which are highly lytic for plasma clot, as were many carcinomas, Leighton *et al.* (1967) modified the method and used collagen-coated cellulose sponge. In these early experiments, they demonstrated satisfactorily the growth of the Walker carcinoma. Subsequently, Leighton *et al.* (1968) extended the study to several other tumours, such as mouse mammary carcinomas, ascites rat hepatoma (No. 7974) and also embryonic tissues. They reported that the growth characteristics of all the tumour and embryonic tissues were superior in collagen-coated cellulose sponge matrix culture to culture in either cellulose sponge or collagen sponge alone.

The application of this technology to the study of the invasive behaviour of tumours was described by Leighton *et al.* (1957). The method adopted by these authors was to establish host cultures of chick embryonic tissue, or foetal human liver, adrenal gland, lung, etc. by cementing the tissues to rectangular slices (12 × 6 × 1·0-0·5 mm) of cellulose sponge. Inoculation of these cellulose sponge host cultures is achieved by implanting pieces of gelfoam containing the tumour cells. Leighton *et al.* (1957) grew HeLa cells in suspension culture in gelfoam and used fragments of the gelfoam for inoculating the host cultures. These thick cellulose sponge cultures need to be examined histologically for possible interactions between host cells and tumour cells. Hence they also used 100-μm thick cellulose sponges. Host explants of connective tissue could be established easily by cementing the explants to the sponge surface by plasma clot. When the host cultures are established, the tumour explants could be applied wherever desired. In this system, HeLa cells have been shown to infiltrate and replace normal tissue. Leighton *et al.* (1956) used this *in vitro* system also to demonstrate differences between various tissues as regards the resistance offered to invading tumour cells. HeLa cells could invade embryonic mesenchyme and heart tissue extensively, but embryonic brain and liver tissues appeared to resist invasion.

Leighton *et al.* (1957) also claim that the combination of tumour and normal tissue in cellulose sponge matrix provides a histological picture comparable with the *in vivo* situation. Based on these observations, these authors have suggested the possible use of this system in testing chemotherapeutic agents on tumour invasiveness and on tumour-host tissue interactions.

Kaluš and colleagues (Kaluš and Klement, 1966; Kaluš and O'Neal, 1968) employed human fibrin foam for growing animal as well as human tissues. This spongy foam matrix prepared from human fibronogen was found to be suitable without further preparation for the culture of tissue. Kaluš *et al.* (1968) studied about 160 explants of human tumours, benign as well as malignant, for between 3 and 21 days in culture. Fifty-five benign tumours showed no proliferation into the matrix. In contradistinction, over one-hundred malignant tumours which were investigated showed invasion of the matrix to various degrees. It is of considerable interest to note that examination of a group of 72 adenocarcinomas of the gastro-intestinal tract revealed that tumour cell infiltration into the matrix correlated with the degree of differentiation seen in the biopsy; the greater the differentiation, the lower was the degree of infiltration into the matrix.

Organ culture systems

The invasive ability of tumours has also been monitored using many variations of the organ culture system. Two of them used fairly extensively have been described by Wolff and Haffen (1952) and Wolff and Wolff (1961). Wolff and Haffen used 1% agar impregnated with plasma clot and made up in tyrode solution. The tumour and embryonic explants are cultured side by side on the semi-solid agar. Wolff and Wolff (1961) subsequently modified this technique for the culture of human neoplasms. The tumour and embryonic tissues were wrapped in vitelline membrane of the hen's egg. The tumour and embryonic tissues could also be separated from one another by merely interposing the vitelline membrane. Wolff and Schneider (1956, 1957) demonstrated the invasion by sarcoma 180 of various embryonic tissues such as intestinal muscles, mesonephros, etc. and Sigot-Luizard (1974) the invasion of embryonic mesonephros by T2633 mammary carcinoma.

Tickle *et al.* (1978) used wing buds of chick embryos at stage 20-21, obtained after approximately 3 days' incubation. The wing bud, which is approximately $1 \cdot 5 \times 1$ mm, consists of loose mesenchyme covered by ectoderm. A square hole is cut into the bud using tungsten needles, the tissues to be tested being implanted into the cut hole. One to two days after implantation, the wing buds are examined in histology for the behaviour of the implanted cells. Tickle *et al.* (1978) have investigated the behaviour in this system of a variety of normal and malignant cells. Three types of carcinoma, viz. a mouse lung tumour, rat bladder tumour and human breast tumour, showed no invasion at all. On the other hand, sarcoma 180 and neuroblastomas did. Of a series of hamster fibroblast lines, normal as well as virus-transformed, the normal BHK cells, polyoma virus-transformed BHK cells, Nil 8 cells and their transformed counterparts were all found to be invasive.

In a subsequent paper, Tickle *et al.* (1979) claimed a distinct difference in the ability of the wing bud to support growth of normal and malignant cells. Cell lines derived from normal rat brain were unable to survive longer than one day, but malignant glioma cell lines could grow and invade unimpeded. Tumour cells showed first signs of degeneration after 7 days following grafting. It would seem, therefore, that these investigations have not revealed a consistent pattern of behaviour of heterotypic cells implanted into the wing bud.

Since the carcinomas, which are epithelial in origin, failed to invade the wing bud, Tickle *et al.* (1978) have suggested that these tumours may invade by mechanisms other than cellular motility. An epithelial invasion by sheets of cells or tongues of cells has been considered as a possiblity. Sträuli and Weiss (1977) earlier alluded to this possibility and suggested also that movement at the edge of such tongues or protrusions could be achieved by locomotion of the cells. It has been suggested that the invasive drive arises possibly by exertion of a mechanical force accruing from cellular division (Eaves, 1973; Willis, 1973), but Sträuli and Weiss (1977) consider that cell proliferation *per se* may not be a mobilizing mechanism. Tickle *et al.* (1978)

cite the work of Ambrose and Easty (1976a) in confirmation of their observation of non-invasiveness of carcinomas. While Ambrose and Easty (1976a) did state that fibroblasts growing out of human breast carcinoma cultures were non-invasive in the CAM system, they made no such claims for the epithelial cells growing from these explants. On the contrary, three established cell lines provided for their investigation by Professor Lasfargues did invade the CAM, but Ambrose and Easty (1976a) add a rider that the characterization of two of the three lines was uncertain.

One must agree with the statement of Tickle *et al.* (1978) that the limb bud system may not provide an ideal site for assaying invasiveness, since the embryonic tissues themselves are growing and differentiating. None the less, their work has been described clearly enough to enable the reader to evaluate the behaviour of the various implanted tissues.

Lohmann-Matthes *et al.* (1980) have recently used organ culture for examining differences between metastasizing and non-metastasizing tumours. The method adopted by these authors is very simple. They maintain pieces of syngeneic lung tissue in culture in rotating flasks, to which the test cells are added 48 h later and then left in organ culture for 6 days with a change of medium every 48 h. At the end of the 6-day period, the organ cultures are fixed and examined histologically. According to Lohmann-Matthes *et al.*, the metastasizing tumours adhered to and invaded the lung tissue while no such invasion was shown by non-metastasizing tumours.

Latner *et al.* (1971) developed a technique for studying invasiveness using a modified Trowell organ culture flask. The apparatus consists of an open-necked vessel with a ground glass flange containing a filter well. The latter is made by attaching a 25 mm diameter cellulose acetate Millipore filter to the base of a Pyrex glass ring. The well is supported by three legs so that the membrane is in contact with 5 ml of culture medium added to the flask. Latner *et al.* produced cell cultures in the filter wells. In order to test invasion, they used 1-2 mm^2 pieces of adult mouse kidney cortex. The culture is then incubated for 7 days and the kidney tissue is examined histologically for possible invasion by the cultured cells. Using this system, Latner *et al.* (1971) showed that while BHK-21 fibroblasts were not invasive, their malignant counterparts which had been transformed by polyoma virus showed extensive invasion into the kidney tissue.

While these observations relating to differences in invasion by various tumour cells of organ cultures may be accepted without question, their relevance to the intricate and complex processes of the metastatic cascade is open to question. Although processes of adhesion and invasion are involved in the development of metastasis, the organ culture system as employed in these studies is highly artificial.

Chorio-allantoic membrane (CAM) system

Organ cultures maintained on CAM have also been used for the assay of invasiveness. Leighton (1963, 1967) showed that by using double implants, i.e. normal and neoplastic tissue, invasion of the former by neoplastic cells could be demonstrated.

Subsequently the CAM has been used in a variety of ways and for varying purposes. The invasion of the CAM tissue itself has been used as a parameter of neoplastic behaviour. Easty and Easty (1973) used a modification of Trowell's (1954) grid technique and the CAM mounted on expanded metal grids previously coated with a film of agar gel. The grids are immersed in culture medium. Appropriate numbers of tumour cells are dispersed over the surface of the CAM. The whole system is incubated. At suitable intervals, the CAM is fixed and examined histologically for cellular infiltration. Normal hamster fibroblasts BHK-21 were unable to invade the exposed ectodermal layer of the CAM, even when a dense suspension of cells had been applied. On the other hand, polyoma virus-transformed BHK cells penetrated the ectodermal layers and invaded the underlying mesodermal layer of the CAM within 24 h, while by 48 h they had infiltrated deep into the CAM mesoderm. BHK cells transformed by SV-40 virus similarly showed invasion of the CAM.

It would appear, therefore, that normal and virus-transformed cells show differential invasive behaviour in the CAM system. However, it is doubtful how truly the simian virus transformation of cells may be deemed to be representative of malignant transformation. These cells are derived from an established line and very little is known about their invasive ability. Virus-transformed cells do form tumours in compatible hosts, but the natural history of these tumours has hardly been a subject of serious study. Apart from their tumorigenicity, normal and SV-40 transformed BHK cells are known to show certain differences in their social behaviour in tissue culture.

Recently, however, the CAM system has been able to highlight the differences between the B16 melanoma variants with high and low metastatic ability. The B16-F10 variant cells are known to be highly invasive *in vivo* (Fidler, 1975). Nicolson *et al.* (1977) found that when applied to the CAM, the F10 variants invaded the membrane within 12 h, but the F1 line was unable to do so. The invasion by the F10 variants was accompanied also by the destruction of the CAM, although these cells are not known to possess greater proteolytic activity.

Subsequently, Easty and Easty (1974) have attempted to quantify the invasion of the CAM system. They measured the depth of invasion into the CAM by untransformed BHK cells and SV-BHK and PyBHK cells. Their observations indicated that while BHK cells infiltrated into the CAM up to

30-40 μm, SV-BHK cells invaded to a depth of up to 160 μm. Also, up to approximately 1% of total BHK cells invaded the CAM to 40 μm, but about 80% of total SV-BHK cells penetrated the CAM to 40 μm; approximately 2% to 70 μm and about 1% of total cells invaded to depths between 90 and 160 μm. Similar differences in the degree of invasion were also demonstrated by Easty and Easty (1974) for the lowly tumorigenic P4 cells and the highly tumorigenic line P4T.

A quantitation of the invasion of CAM by cancer cells has also been attempted by Hart and Fidler (1978). Their method involves the preparation of an invasion chamber consisting of a latex rubber cylinder with a CAM tied to seal one end; the endodermal side of the CAM faces the lumen. This is then placed inside a glass vial on a piece of photographic sponge. Hart and Fidler (1978) employ cells which are labelled with ^{125}I-iododeoxyuridine. These are added inside the latex rubber cylinder. At various times after addition, the numbers of cells which have passed through the membrane are estimated. Unlike the study of Easty and Easty, here the cells are introduced on the endodermal surface. While the method is much simpler than that described by the Eastys, the integrity of the CAM is an important factor. Obviously, for general application, the test would have to be standardized.

There seems to be little doubt about the ability of tranformed cells, but not normal ones, to invade CAM. Scher *et al.* (1976) showed by scanning electron microscopy that the process of invasion is much more rapid than described previously. They demonstrated the penetration of the CAM ectoderm by single Kirsten sarcoma virus transformed 3T3 cells within 6 h, but viable untransformed cells did not penetrate the ectoderm in 24 h. Scher *et al.* also observed the penetration of the transformed cells into the mesoderm where the cells produced proliferating tumours. When 5×10^5 cells had been applied, up to 43% of CAMs showed the development of tumours in the mesoderm within 5 days, while no tumours were detected even when up to 5×10^6 normal 3T3 cells had been applied to the CAM surface.

Very little is known about the mechanism of invasion into the CAM system. Ambrose and Easty (1976a) have shown that the invading zone of the tumour cell shows extensive pseudopodial activity. This is consistent with the observation of Easty and Easty (1973) that the invasive behaviour of a highly invasive melanoma cell, which seems to invade by extension of long pseudopodia, could be inhibited by treatment with colcemid, which is known to inhibit pseudopodial activity. They point out, none the less, that mouse peritoneal macrophages, in spite of adhering to the ectoderm of the CAM and being capable of forming pseudopodia, were unable to invade. Also, colcemid had little effect on the invasion of the CAM by virus transformed BHK cells (Easty and Easty, 1974). Colcemid appears to be able to achieve either enhancement or inhibition in different systems, presumably because it can produce multiple effects, such as the loss of directional mobility (Vasiliev *et al.*, 1970) and conversion to amoeboid form of movement and enhanced membrane activity (Bhisey and Freed, 1971).

The invasion by individual cells by means of pseudopodial or cytoplasmic extensions has been described by several other authors (Dingemans, 1974; Ambrose and Easty, 1976b; Campbell, 1977; Roos *et al.*, 1977). The invasion by tumours can also occur, in addition to single tumour cell locomotion, through extension in the form of tongues or cords of cells infiltrating into normal parenchyma. A similar conclusion was also drawn by Tickle *et al.* (1978) from their investigation of the invasion of chick wing-buds by carcinomas. Invasion could also occur by migration of cell aggregates (Easty and Easty, 1973; D. M. Easty and Easty, 1974; Sträuli and Weiss, 1977).

In a review article, Poste (1977) has briefly mentioned his observation that the ability of cells to invade the CAM is closely correlated with tumorigenicity in nude mice. Apart from showing that he was using tumour cells, this statement adds little to the CAM story, for the objective is to assay the invasive behaviour of cells which are tumorigenic with a view to predicting *in vivo* behaviour. It would be worthwhile to examine tumour cell lines spanning a spectrum of invasive and metastatic abilities.

Recently Tchao *et al.* (1980) have described an *in vitro* model on much the same pattern as the CAM system but which uses amnion epithelium in place of the chorio-allantoic membrane. The advantages of this system over CAM are hardly apparent, unless it could be shown that the modes of invasion of the CAM and amnion (of human origin) were markedly different for tumour cells of human and non-human origin.

Much in the same way as CAM is employed for testing the invasiveness and tumorigenicity of cells, Petricciani (1977) has used embryonic skin in organ culture. Skin from 9-day chick embryos is cultured on a nutrient agar base. The cells being tested are applied to the skin surface. After incubation, the cultures are examined histologically for tumour formation. Using this system, Petricciani (1977) reported that up to 89% of embryonic skins inoculated with HeLa cells, all cultures inoculated with a human adenocarcinoma of the colon (WIDR) cells, and 86% of skins to which SV-40 transformed human embryonic lung cells had been applied, produced tumours. No tumour formation was noticed in skin cultures inoculated either with normal Muntjak or normal human embryonic lung fibroblasts. Unfortunately, the paper does not contain sufficient experimental detail to assess the results.

Cell aggregation assays

Schleich (1967, 1973) employed the technique of Moscona (1961) of cellular reaggregation in order to study the invasive ability of HeLa cells. The procedure adopted in these investigations is to rotate the cell types under investigation in tissue culture medium in a gyratory shaker. When normal human fibroblasts and HeLa cells were incubated in the gyratory shaker, initially the fibroblasts alone reaggregated; invasion by HeLa cells appeared to be prevented by the cellular capsule around the aggregate. However, in the same system when pieces of embryonic liver or kidney were included, invasion was apparent within a few hours after the normal tissue was confronted with HeLa cells. Although these experiments on the reaggregation behaviour of confronted normal and tumour cells may be of interest in regard to surface affinities between the component cell systems, one can hardly envisage meaningful estimates being made of the amount of invasion. The processes involved in histotypic reaggregation of cells are poorly understood owing to the complexity of the interactions. There are several views regarding the mechanisms involved in histotypic reaggregation of cells which have been reviewed by Sherbet (1978). The hypotheses most relevant to the experiments described by Schleich are those propounded by Steinberg (1978) and by P. Weiss (1947, 1961). Steinberg showed that the configuration adopted in a reaggregated mass of cells was the most stable or an equilibrium configuration, the assembly behaviour being dependent upon the strengths of adhesion between the component cell types. Thus, in a mixed population, cells would tend to rearrange themselves spontaneously until an equilibrium configuration is achieved where the interfacial free energy of the system is minimized. In the non-equilibrium state, the system may therefore be producing mobile cells which interact with one another and the extracellular milieu to specify the configuration.

In the experiments described by Schleich (1973), normal human fibroblasts formed aggregates initially and only after several hours did the HeLa cells adhere to the normal cell aggregate. From the author's description there does not seem to have been infiltration into the interior of the cell aggregate. It is possible that HeLa cells are less cohesive than the fibroblasts, as Steinberg's differential adhesion hypothesis requires. This conclusion would seem to be confirmed by the fact that no tumour cells were seen in the interior of the cell aggregate. Invasion of endometrial cell aggregates can occur if the surface of the aggregate is punctured or wounded.

The results are therefore inconclusive. The failure may be due to the choice of cell types. Such reaggregation experiments may be more informative if two cell types, one of them malignant, are chosen which do show co-aggregation, so that the formation of increasingly stable configurations could be correlated with malignancy.

This may not work out in practice, however, since Maslow and Mayhew (1975) and Maslow *et al.* (1976) found that Ehrlich ascites tumour cells inhibited the aggregation of neural retinal cells. Maslow and Weiss (1978) found that this was due to a decrease in the initial adhesion of neural retinal cells, apparently brought about by the malignant cells. For they found that the adhesion of neural retinal cells to microtest plates was significantly reduced, not only by Ehrlich ascites cells but also by cell-free medium conditioned by growing the malignant cells. In a recent paper, Maslow and Weiss (1979) demonstrated that human colonic carcinoma cells inhibited the aggregation of neural retina cells. Such inhibition is also produced by mouse Ehrlich ascites cells and rat Walker carcinoma cells. Macrophages also cause an inhibition of aggregation of neural retina cells and this was neither additive nor synergistic with that of the tumour cells. Macrophages are commonly present in solid as well as ascites tumours (Alexander, 1976; Evans, 1973). Macrophages are known to secrete lysozyme continuously, and also lysosomal acid hydrolases and neutral proteolytic enzymes (Davies and Allison, 1976). Therefore, tumour macrophages may be involved in the interaction between malignant and normal cells and consequently could modify reaggregation patterns.

Minor complications involve the need to use trypsin or other proteolytic enzymes or chelating agents to produce unicellular suspensions. There is considerable recent evidence which shows that these treatments bring about a loss of surface components and/or produce changes in the organization of the surface components (Sherbet, 1978; Sherbet and Lakshmi, 1974a, 1978b; Huggins *et al.*, 1976; Latner and Turner, 1978). Such changes will no doubt affect the aggregability and locomotive properties of the cells used in the tests (Sherbet, 1978). Besides, the work of Dorsey and Roth (1973) on the aggregability of normal 3T3 fibroblasts, spontaneously transformed 3T12 cells and SV-40 transformed 3T3 cells has shown that the capture of cells by aggregates of both normal or transformed cells depends upon the state of confluency of the cell cultures and the method used for harvesting the cells for the purposes of the assay.

An altered version of the aggregation technique has been described briefly by Schleich (1976). Instead of using dissociated normal cells, Schleich has used 1 mm^2 pieces of human decidua graviditatis. These pieces were maintained in culture medium for 48 h before HeLa cells were added to the culture. HeLa cells showed aggregation soon after addition (the exact time was not mentioned); the aggregates remained floating for a while and then adhered to the decidua pieces. This was followed by invasion of the decidua by HeLa cells. Invasion in this system is also shown by a fibro-sarcoma strain AF$_1$.

This method does appear to be more flexible than the dual aggregation technique. In addition, as the author has claimed, it can be used to test invasiveness of cells before and after modification of the tumour cells. Nevertheless, in common with other procedures for the assay of invasiveness, it would be difficult to assess the amount of invasion. Since the degree of invasiveness will obviously depend upon the type of tissue used as a "target" for the invading cells, no one assay system can be applicable in all cases.

The major hurdle in the way of acceptance of *in vitro* systems for assaying tumours for their invasiveness is determining the relationship between invasiveness in *in vitro* systems and the behaviour of the tumour *in vivo*. No such comparative studies appear to have been done. To demonstrate differential invasive behaviour in an *in vitro* system and ask whether those cells which invade the CAM, for instance, can produce tumours would be to put the cart before the horse. The question surely is, are malignant tumours only able to invade the CAM? Unhappily there appears to be a tendency in the literature to use the word tumorigenicity as synonymous with malignancy. The only correct approach has been made by Kaluš *et al.* (1968), who showed that invasiveness in their fibrin sponge matrix system is related to the degree of differentiation of the tumours examined.

Testing of Antitumour Agents and Suspected Carcinogens

Apart from investigating the growth characteristics and invasive abilities of tumours, the organ culture method may be employed for studying the response of tumours to potential antitumour agents, hormones, antisera, etc. (Yarnell *et al.*, 1964). The use of *in vitro* systems for assessing the effects of chemical agents on invasion holds much promise. Leighton *et al.* (1957) used the cellulose sponge matrix culture method for testing the inhibitory effects of acetylpodophyllotoxine-W-pyridinium chloride (NCI3022) on HeLa cells, while Simpson (1969) used Wolff's technique of combining human tumour with $8\frac{1}{2}$-day chick mesonephros separated by vitelline membrane to demonstrate the antitumour effects of the alkylating agent Melphalan. Yarnell *et al.* (1964) employed their method of organ culture on siliconized lens papers to demonstrate the inhibitory effects of methotrexate and Melphalan.

The organ culture systems, especially the CAM system, lend themselves to the testing of suspected carcinogens. Alteration in behaviour in the CAM system, such as acquired invasiveness or tumorigenicity, may be an adequate preliminary indication of cellular transformation. Needless to say, extrapolation from any such changes in behaviour to possible carcinogenicity *in vivo* may be difficult, since these assays do not take into account several host factors which determine the behaviour of tumours *in vivo*. Even more basic is the objection that we know little about the extent to which invasiveness and locomotion of cells is related to *in vivo* tumour penetration and formation of metastases.

Experiments on Mechanisms of Invasion

One of the properties of the tumour cell from which the invasive ability of the cell is postulated to flow is reduced cell-cell adhesiveness of malignant cells. Easty (1974) has discussed in detail the structural and chemical bases of reduced adhesiveness of malignant cells. Cell locomotion involves the formation of transient adhesive bonds with the substratum, directional response being produced either by haptotaxis, i.e. by the occurrence of a continuous gradient of adhesiveness to the substratum (Carter, 1967) or by contact guidance given by the form of the substratum. The formation and the strength of adhesive bonds depend upon a balance of electrostatic forces of repulsion and Van der Waal's forces of attraction in relation to Brownian and other movements (Weiss, 1968; Sträuli and Weiss, 1977). If the surface charge on the cells is altered experimentally, this should also result in an alteration in the invasive behaviour.

Yarnell and Ambrose (1969a) tested this proposition by treating tumour cells with polycationic substances and examining the invasive behaviour of the cells in organ culture. They inoculated explants of foetal mouse heart muscle with BHK-21, Py-BHK cells and Py-BHK cells which were pretreated with poly-L-lysine. Pretreatment of Py-BHK cells with 75 μg ml^{-1} of poly-L-lysine appeared to reduce the invasive behaviour. Yarnell and Ambrose (1969a) attribute this effect to the adsorption of the polylysine molecules to the tumour cell surface and a consequent decrease in their cellular motility, although they made no measurements of the surface charge densities before and after treatment with the polycationic compound. However, they have cited the work of Nevo *et al.* (1955) which described such effects on mammalian cells. Latner *et al.* (1971), on the contrary, noticed an increased ability of BHK cells treated with histones, which are also polycationic in nature and known also to adsorb to the cell surface, to invade mouse kidney cortex in organ culture. In fairness to Yarnell and Ambrose, it ought to be stated that Latner and Turner (1974) failed to detect by cell electrophoresis any alterations in the surface charge of BHK cells treated with histone, although it is difficult to see how basic proteins such as histone can fail to adsorb to the cell surface, which is negatively charged.

Yarnell and Ambrose (1969b) adduced further support for the involvement of surface charge in invasion by demonstrating that enzymatic removal of sialic acids also resulted in a reduced invasive ability. Again, the authors have made no attempt to measure the liberated sialic acids, nor determine the alteration in surface charge consequent upon treatment with neuraminidase. The latter determination is important, since the removal of surface sialic acid moieties is known to alter the deformability of the membrane and produce changes in the configuration of surface components. For sialic acids are known to confer structural rigidity to membrane glycoproteins (Gottschalk, 1960), and probably thereby contribute to the rigidity of the cell membrane (Weiss, 1963; Ray and Chatterjee, 1975; Bretscher, 1973).

It appears unlikely that any relationship exists between the degree of adhesiveness and surface negative charge densities. Thus, Dorsey and Roth (1973) found that the adhesiveness of SV-3T3 was no greater than that of the untransformed cells, even though the surface negative charge density of SV-3T3 cells is less than that on the untransformed cells.

The implication of cell surface components, if not the negative charge densities, is still credible, since the removal of surface components appears to affect the migration of cells *in vitro*. Varani *et al.* (1979) examined the migration of a mouse fibrosarcoma cells on an agarose substrate in the presence of medium containing either foetal calf serum or human serum. While the cells migrated actively in medium containing foetal calf serum, migration was greatly inhibited in the presence of human serum. The authors attributed this difference to the higher proteinase inhibitory activity of the calf serum than that of the human serum. When antiproteinases were included with human serum, the migration was comparable with that in the presence of foetal calf serum. This work suggests the possibility that some components which are associated with the migratory ability are being excised by proteinases. The higher antiproteinase activity presumably prevents the loss of these components. Latner and Sherbet (1979) in fact reported that treatment of malignant cells with the antiproteinase, aprotinin, induced surface changes. These changes included increase in surface negative charge density, a reduced agglutinability and reduced adhesiveness to Concanavalin A-linked plates. Recent (Lakshmi *et al.*, 1982) work in the author's laboratory indicates that there is an increased expression of certain components of molecular weight of approximately 115 000 and 50 000 on the surface following treatment of the cells with the antiproteinase. Such changes could bring about alterations in the adhesiveness of the cells. Recent work has also shown that adhesive functions are subserved not only by the high molecular weight glycoprotein components collectively known as fibronectins, but that considerably smaller macromolecules apparently mediate adhesive interactions (Pagano and Takeichi, 1977; Wildridge and Sherbet, 1982).

The status of adhesiveness of tumour cells and possibly the tissues which are invaded *in vivo* by the tumour can also be inferred from the reaggregation-type experiments described by Schleich (1967, 1973). The formation and size of cellular aggregates in Moscona's (1961) method is a reflection of the collision efficiency (Curtis, 1969), which is determined by the degree of inter-cellular adhesion; the higher the adhesion between colliding cells, the greater being the likelihood of adhesive bonds being formed between the colliding cells. The size of the aggregates depends also on the rate of separation of adherent cells (Weiss, 1976). As pointed out already, Dorsey and Roth (1973) demonstrated that there was no reduction in adhesiveness between normal and virus-transformed cells by using the technique of reaggregation. It would be interesting to see if the pattern of reaggregation of tumour cells and cells of the host's stroma correlated with the local invasiveness of the tumour *in vivo*.

Whur and Koppel (1975) examined the kinetics of aggregation of normal BHK and transformed BHK cells and concluded that the adhesive-ness of malignant cells was only 2% of the corresponding normal cells. It would be surprising if the differences in adhesiveness turned out to be as great as these authors claim. More recently, Edward *et al.* (1979) have claimed that the BHK-21 cells transformed by polyoma virus or RSV show reduced ability to aggregate compared to normal cells, i.e. the transformed cells show less intercellular adhesiveness. Unless adhesiveness as demonstrated in these experiments has no relationship to invasiveness, it would be difficult to reconcile these results with the invasion studies of Yarnell and Ambrose (1969a, b), who found both normal, as well as transformed, BHK cells invasive in foetal mouse organ cultures. Latner *et al.* (1973b) found that the "normal" BHK cells produced tumours in 80-90% of Wright's hamsters, although the tumours were neither locally invasive nor were they able to metastasize. Sherbet and Lakshmi (unpublished observations) tested the malignancy of BHK-21 cells (passage no. 62) by epigenetic grading tests and found that they were only slightly less malignant than a hamster fibrosarcoma cell line (TRES) transformed by means of histone treatment (Latner *et al.*, 1973b). The BHK cells have in fact been considered as premalignant cells by Defendi *et al.* (1963). In spite of all this evidence, it ought to be pointed out that BHK cells passaged less than 70 times have been found to be noninvasive in the CAM system (Easty and Easty, 1974).

Multicellular Spheroids as a Tumour Model

Several years ago it was shown that certain cell types, normal as well as neoplastic, could be grown in suspension as multicellular spheroids (Sutherland *et al.*, 1970, 1971, 1976). Histologically, these spheroids have been claimed to possess morphological and organizational similarities with certain carcinomas *in vivo*, thus commending them for possible use as an *in vitro* model. Since the introduction of the multicellular spheroid, several papers have appeared in which this model has been used in comparative studies of the kinetics of growth of tumours *in vivo* and as multicellular spheroids (Inch *et al.*, 1970; Durand, 1976a, Yuhas *et al.*, 1977), in the testing of anti-tumour agents (Durand, 1975a, 1976b; Sutherland *et al.*, 1979) and in the study of radiosensitizers. In the multicellular spheroid, the hypoxic core cells may simulate a situation obtaining in solid tumours and therefore the spheroid has been suggested as a model for testing compounds for radio-sensitizing ability (Sutherland and Durand, 1972, 1973; Hetzel *et al.*, 1973).

The multicellular spheroid tumour model has also been used for testing the tumour cell sensitivity to hyperthermia (Durand, 1975b) and in the assessment of the effects of combining radiation treatment or cytotoxic drugs with hyperthermia (Durand, 1975b; Lucke-Huhle and Dertinger, 1977; Morgan and Bleehen, 1981). Jones (1981) has advocated the use of multicellular spheroid models in the assessment of sensitivity of human tumours to toxic drugs. In a preliminary investigation, Jones has shown that the sensitivity of certain human multicellular tumour spheroids to cytotoxic drugs was comparable with the sensitivity of the tumour as xenografts and in the response observed clinically. Much work would be required, however, before an *in vitro* system can be proposed as a reliable model in assessing the sensitivity *in vivo* of human tumours.

A more recent development involves the use of the multicellular spheroid in assessing the interactions between tumour cells and the host cells. Lord *et al.* (1979) produced spheroids (700-900 μm diam.) of EM6 mammary sarcoma cells and implanted them into the peritoneal cavity of non-sensitized as well as sensitized hosts. These were subsequently recovered to check for host cell infiltration. Lord *et al.* found that spheroids recovered 24-48 h after intro-duction into sensitized allogeneic mice were heavily infiltrated by lympho-cytes and macrophages. A similar infiltration of the spheroids by host cells also occurs in non-sensitized animals, but the process of tumour cell destruction takes 6-8 days as compared with 1-2 days required for maximal cell destruction in the sensitized hosts. Sutherland *et al.* (1977) had indeed proposed earlier that the kinetics of tumour cell destruction by sensitized host lymphocytes could be investigated using the spheroid as a model. Also, the spheroid model could be profitably employed to test the relationship between the extent of host cell infiltration and the degree of malignancy of the primary tumour. The invasive ability and possibly also the organ specificity of invasion could also be assessed using the multicellular spheroid model.

There are, however, two major drawbacks in the model which may distort the picture of host cell infiltration into a spheroid of tumour cells or the invasion of spheroids of normal cells by malignant cells. One is the absence of the stroma or the structural elements normally found in solid tumours growing *in vivo*. Of no less significance is the degree of cohesive forces holding the spheroid together will be dependent upon how the component cells were grown and harvested before aggregation into a multicellular spheroid. The aggregability of trypsinized cells is known to differ markedly from those subjected to the action of chelating agents (Steinberg *et al.*, 1973). Both proteolytic enzymes and chelating agents have been shown to strip the surface coat material from tissue culture cells (Burger, 1970; Hynes, 1973; Sefton and Rubin, 1970; Kemp *et al.*, 1967; Neville, 1968; Allen and Snow, 1970). There is little doubt that these surface alterations will affect the degree of cohesion of the multicellular spheroid. In addition, the cells may be at different stages of the cell cycle and may possess different surface properties. Such a heterogeneity of surface properties will be reflected in their topographical distribution. In other words, the cohesive forces operating between component cells of a spheroid will vary at different depths of the spheroid (*see* Steinberg, 1970; Steinberg *et al.*, 1973). All these physical features are bound to determine the extent to which cells can invade the multicellular spheroid.

The Epigenetic Basis of Tumour Grading

Introduction

The biological characteristics of a tumour most likely to reflect the degree of its malignancy are the state of its differentiation, rate of growth, the extent of deviation of its karyotype from normality, and its invasive potential. As discussed earlier, neoplastic tissues share these features, possibly with the exception of karyotype deviation, with embryonic systems. In embryonic systems, the processes of differentiation, morphogensis and growth are under epigenetic control. Foulds (1958, 1975) has argued that neoplastic development follows a course similar to that followed by a developing embryo. Willis (1967) believes that the "programme of development" of teratomas can be compared with embryonic development itself, for teratomas show the whole spectrum of differentiation as does the developing embryo. In embryonic development there is a restriction of the available developmental pathways. This is achieved by a progressive determination and restriction of "competences" and by a sequential activation of genes mediated by the operation of a temporal hierarchy of inductive interactions (Sherbet, 1974b). Sherbet (1974b) also proposed an epigenetic basis for the pathogenesis of cancer. This epigenetic model is based not only on principles of developmental biology but also on the occurrence of paraneoplastic syndromes in association with certain forms of cancer. These syndromes are predominantly a consequence of "inappropriate" or ectopic production of certain hormones by the neoplastic tissue not produced by that tissue in its normal state.

According to the epigenetic model of Sherbet, neoplastic change constitutes a de-determination and acquisition of a preceding state of competence. In this newly sensitized genetic state, the tissue may be re-subjected to inductive cellular interactions resulting in an abnormal genetic activation that is characterized by the various differentiative and growth processes, and by the synthesis of inappropriate cell products and embryonic antigens by the neoplasm (*see also* pp. 96-109 and 129).

Tumours often show a loss of histotypic differentiation. Not infrequently, neoplastic tissues retain to a large extent not only their original histotypic features but also some functional characteristics. The loss of differentiation or the anaplastic state has often been erroneously described as a state of dedifferentiation. In embryological parlance, the term dedifferentiation implies a reversion to a state where the tissue has acquired the potential to differentiate in response to an appropriate stimulus into a definable, structurally and functionally, new tissue.

The question we asked ourselves as early as in 1964, at the suggestion of the late Sir Alexander Haddow was: can interactions between embryonic and tumour cells be used as a means for determining the state of differentiation of a tumour? Indeed, the homology between epigenetic (developmental) and neoplastic systems strengthened our view of the possibility of interpreting the interactions between embryonic cells and tumour cells using epigenetic criteria as a means of determining the degree of malignancy of tumours. It has been known for over 25 years that cancerous tissues induce specific changes in embyronic cells when they are brought together under experimental conditions (*see* Lakshmi and Sherbet, 1974). Our early experiments with HeLa (human carcinoma of the cervix) cells and animal tumour lines, such as Yoshida ascites sarcoma and Ehrlich ascites cells, indicated that embryonic cells may provide a valuable means of distinguishing between normal and tumour cells (Sherbet and Lakshmi, 1968b). Our research work in subsequent years has resulted in the development of an *in vitro* system for assaying the degree of malignancy of neoplasms. The assay system has been variously called the "embryonic system" or "embryological system", and the numerical grades of malignancy termed "embryonic malignancy grade", "embryological grade" or "tumour grade in embryos", in our publications to date. This uncertainty in nomenclature has arisen mainly because the word "embryonic" connotes "an under-developed" or "rudimentary" stage, while "embryological" is equally unacceptable because the assay is not concerned with the developing embryo. We therefore propose to use the terms "epigenetic grade (EGG) of malignancy" and "EGG test" for the assay. The latter is probably appropriate since the starting material for the assay is fertilized hens' eggs.

The epigenetic grading (EGG) test for malignancy

Principle of the EGG test

The assay involves bringing together embryonic and tumour cells under experimental conditions *in vitro*. The embryonic cells are obtained in the form of a blastoderm from fertilized hens' eggs incubated for about 18 h. The cells of the blastoderm respond to the presence of the tumour (or test) cells in the form of specific cellular responses which are described below. These responses depend upon the normality or degree of deviation from normality of the test cells. A numerical grading is given to the cells, and this is based on the nature, frequency and the intensity of the responses made by the embryonic cells.

Techniques

The two principle techniques involved in the assay are the *in vitro* culturing of 18-h-old chicken blastoderm and the implantation of the test cells into the blastoderm. The *in vitro* explantation and culturing of the blastoderms has been described by New (1955). In this method, the blastoderm disc is removed with the vitelline membrane from the egg yolk into a watch-glass. A glass ring is placed over the membrane. The edges of the membrane are folded over the glass ring and it is stretched to provide adequate tension to the blastodisc. The assembly is placed in a moist chamber constructed from Petri dishes.

The 18-h-old embryonic disc is composed of two cellular layers, viz. the ectodermal and the endodermal layers with the mesodermal layer in the process of being formed. The two cellular layers can be separated locally using fine tungsten needles in areas where there is no intervening mesoderm, and the test cells implanted between the two layers. This technique of implantation represents a modified version (Waddington, 1932) of the well-known *einsteckung* method devised by Hans Spemann, with which he demonstrated the presence of the organization centre in the amphibian embryo (Spemann, 1938). The blastodisc with the implanted test cells is supplied with adequate nutrients and culture media and incubated for a further 16-18 h, after which the cultures are fixed and serially sectioned for assessing the embryonic cellular responses.

The cellular responses

The cellular response may be discussed in three sections, viz. the host mesodermal response, the histogenetic response and morphogenetic displacement. Each of these parameters of embryonic response is related to particular tumour attributes.

The host mesodermal response (HMR)   As the name implies, the host mesodermal response is produced by the embryonic mesenchymal cells. When a normal adult heterologous tissue is implanted into the blastodisc, the highly mobile mesenchymal cells migrate towards the implant, cover it and virtually isolate its (Figs 9-11). This response is greatly reduced or absent when tumour cells are implanted into the blastodisc. Adult mouse liver and pituitary tissue of goat induced 70-100% HMR, but HeLa cells and Landschütz ascites tumour induced the response only in 3 and 27% of the implants respectively. Yoshida ascites sarcoma cells and a rat tumour induced by the administration of benzpyrene elicited no mesodermal

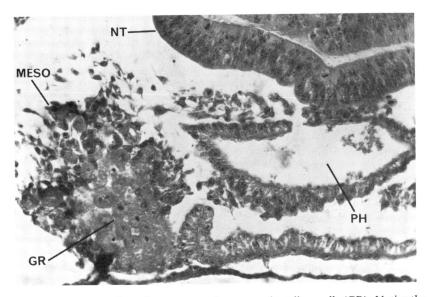

Figure 9   Host mesodermal response against normal rat liver cells (GR). Notice the mesenchymal cells covering the implant. × 330 (approx.) From Sherbet *et al.* (1970).

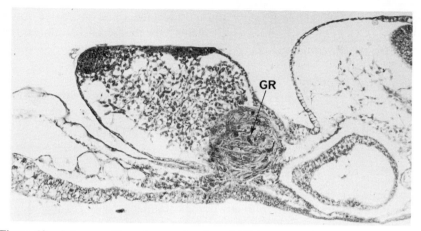

Figure 10   A human fibroadenoma implant (GR) in an ectodermal vesicle replete with mesenchyme. × 84 (approx).

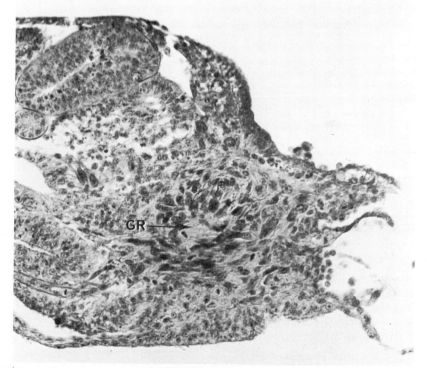

Figure 11   A benzo(a)pyrene-induced sarcoma graft (GR) in the chick embryo. Notice the invasive nature of the cells. × 250 (approx.)

response at all (Sherbet and Lakshmi, 1970; Table 23). HeLa cells are derived from a malignant carcinoma of the human cervix, and the ascites tumours are known to be one of the most malignant forms of cancer maintained in laboratory animals.

Table 23

Host mesodermal response induced by normal liver and some tumour cell lines

Tumour	No. of implants	Frequency of HMR (%)
Rat liver	32	100
Goat pituitary	24	70
HeLa cells	17	3
Landschütz ascites carcinoma	11	27
Yoshida ascites sarcoma	23	0
Benzpyrene-induced sarcoma	6	0

From Sherbet and Lakshmi (1970).

Less malignant and more differentiated tumours induced HMR to a greater degree. We examined a series of hepatomas induced by the administration of N-2-fluorenyldiacetamide and N-(2-fluorenyl)phthalamic acid which show a spectrum of growth rate and differentiation (Morris and Wagner, 1968). Many of these tumours have even retained their functional characteristics (Morris and Wagner, 1968; Miyaji *et al.*, 1968). These tumours have been classified as minimum deviation tumours (Potter, 1961; Potter and Watanabe, 1968) on the postulate that they may not have undergone extensive changes over and above those essential for neoplastic transformation. Their highly differentiated state and the minimal deviation from normality appear to be reflected accurately in the degree of HMR elicited by these hepatomas. While normal liver induced the reponse in all the grafts, the HMR induced by the minimum deviation hepatomas ranged from 71-92% (Sherbet *et al.*, 1970; Table 24). In addition, a clear correlation emerged between the extent of deviation of the karyotype of the tumour and the freqency of induction of HMR (Table 24).

The occurrence of the HMR has been confirmed by the work of Palayoor and Batra (1971) and Camon (1976). Palayoor and Batra (1971), who used the experimental techniques as employed in our laboratory, found that while xenografts of C_3H/J mouse normal kidney were encapsulated by embryonic mesoderm, no such encapsulation was encountered in the case of the C_3H/J mammary adenocarcinoma. It is now fairly well estab-

Table 24

Relationship between HMR, EPR, and Karyotype deviation
of some Morris minimum-deviation hepatomas

Tumour	Karyotype[a] score	HMR (%)	EPR (%)
Normal liver	0	100	20
9633	0	89	27
7794A	0·5	85	58
9618B	1·0	83	61
7793	4·0	80	67
7787	5·0	71	77
5123C	11·0	92	52

[a]The greater the abnormality of, and deviation from normality of, the karyotype, the higher is the karyotype score. The karyotype scoring system is described in Sherbet *et al.* (1970).
From Sherbet *et al.* (1970).

lished that the karyotype continually alters with the development and progression of tumours (*see* Lakshmi and Sherbet, 1974). Although the correlation between HMR and karyotype deviation may be described as unequivocal, we have not devoted much attention to the mechanisms underlying the induction of this response because our efforts have been directed towards developing the EGG test for clinical use. None the less, preliminary experiments indicate that the surface charge may be involved in the interaction. Sherbet *et al.* (1970) showed that the frequency of the mesodermal response could be altered by changing the net negative surface charge of the cells before implantation into the embryonic discs.

Morphogenetic displacement (MD) of implants The embryonic discs used in the assay consist of two germ layers, viz. the epiblast (ectoderm) and the hypoblast (endoderm). In the epiblast, streaming cellular movements occur which are related to the morphogenesis of the "primitive-streak" and its future development into the embryo. The primitive streak is in the middle of the blastodisc. The morphogenetic movement of cells of the epiblast takes place inwards towards the "primitive streak". The cells then invaginate at the primitive streak and form the primitive mesenchyme (Fig. 12a). When heterografts are placed between the germ layers, they may be carried along with the morphogenetic current (Sherbet and Lakshmi, 1968b; Sherbet *et al.*, 1970) (Figs 12b and 13). Similar graft movements have been described by Mareel *et al.* (1968) and also by Palayoor and Batra (1971). We describe this movement of the grafts as "morphogenetic displacement" (MD).

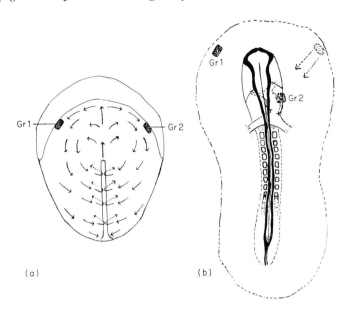

Figure 12 (a) Position of implants at the beginning of the experiment. The arrows show the morphogenetic current of cellular movement in the epiblast. The grafts are often carried along these currents towards the developing embryo. (b) GR2 has moved into the heart. From Sherbet *et al.* (1970).

In the minimum deviation hepatomas, the frequency with which the implants showed morphogenetic displacement was clearly related to the growth rate of the hepatomas. The higher the growth rate, the greater was the frequency of morphogenetic displacement (Table 25). There is considerable evidence in the literature which indicates an unequivocal correspondence between growth rates and surface negative charge density in embryonic, neoplastic and in regenerating tissue systems. In general, the faster the growth, the greater is the surface charge density (Sherbet, 1978). A high surface charge may indeed be involved in the regulation of growth. This is indicated by the high sialic acid content reported for fucosylsialoglycoproteins of, and the high sialyltransferase activity associated with, the mitotic cell membrane (Buck *et al.*, 1971; Warren *et al.*, 1972a, b; Van Beek *et al.*, 1973).

Therefore, we examined the surface charge status of implanted cells in relation to the morphogenetic displacement. HeLa cells showed morphogenetic displacement in 58% of the grafts. If their surface charge was increased experimentally, the frequency of MD increased to 82%. Yoshida

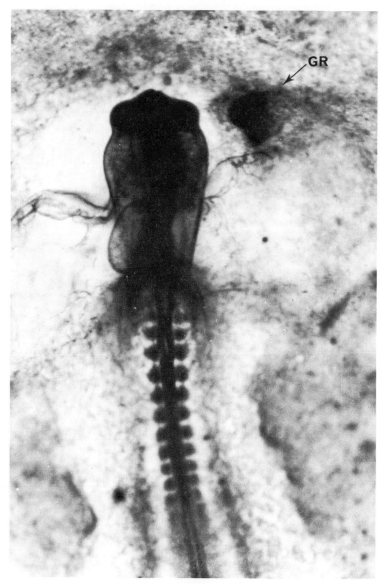

Figure 13   The implant (GR) and the host embryo at the end of the experiment.
×40.

Table 25

Relationship between the frequency of morphogenetic
displacement of minimum deviation hepatomas and their growth rate

Tumour	Mean generation time (GT) (months)	Growth rate ($1/GT$)	Morphogenetic[a] displacement (%)
Normal liver	—	—	35
9618B	9·0	0.11	50
7787	8·0	0·125	54
9633	5·1	0·19	61
7793	4·5	0·22	61
7794A	3·6	0·27	63
5123C	2·0	0·5	62

[a]The correlation between growth rate and frequency of morphogenetic displacement
was statistically highly significant with r (correlation coefficient) $= 0·959$ and
$P<0·001$.
From Sherbet *et al.* (1970).

acites cells which had a roughly similar charge density to γ-globulin-treated
HeLa cells showed roughly comparable morphogenetic displacement (Table
26). Chicken homografts show 100% MD. However, if their surface charge
is reduced by treatment with cationic substances, the frequency of morphogenetic displacement falls (Sherbet *et al.*, 1970). In astrocytomas also the
faster growing grade III and IV tumours not only possessed higher surface
charge densities, but also showed higher morphogenetic displacement than

Table 26

Relationship between surface charge density and frequency of
morphogenetic displacement of grafts

Implant	No. of implants made	Frequency of morphogenetic displacement %	Surface negative charge density $\times 10^{-13}$ cm^{-2}
HeLa cells	21	58	0·3
HeLa (γ-globulin treated)	11	82	0·7
Yoshida ascites sarcoma	23	100	0·7

From Sherbet *et al.* (1970) and Sherbet (1978).

grade I and II astrocytomas (Table 27). The phenomenon of morphogenetic displacement, therefore, appears to be dependent upon the growth characteristics and the associated surface charge properties of the implanted tissue.

Table 27

Relationship between growth rate, surface charge, and morphogenetic displacement of astrocytomas

Tumour	Generation time[a] (days)	$1/GT^a$	Surface charge[b] $\times 10^{-4} \mu m^{-2}$	Morphogenetic[c] displacement (%)
Astrocytoma Grades I and II	10·9	0·09	15·9	22
Astrocytoma Grades III and IV	7·8	0·13	18·1	35

[a]Generation time (*GT*) is the average doubling time of the tumours in culture. $1/GT$ gives the rate of growth. From Sherbet *et al.* (1977).
[b]From Sherbet and Lakshmi (1974a).
[c]Sherbet and Lakshmi (unpublished data).

The histogenetic responses   A most exciting feature of the tumour cell-embryonic cell interaction is the ability of the tumour cells to induce the "histogenetic response". This describes the induction of reponses from the cellular germ layer from which the tumour itself originated. Endoderm-derived tumours such as hepatomas have been found to induce proliferative responses from the embryonic endoderm (EPR) (Fig. 14) but they rarely, if at all, induce reaction in the embryonic ectoderm (Sherbet *et al.*, 1969; 1970). Besides this specificity, the frequency of occurrence of the endodermal response was found to be closely related to the karyotype deviation of the tumours. The greater the karyotype deviation, the greater was the endodermal response (Sherbet *et al.*, 1970; Table 24).

Mareel *et al.* (1973, 1974) have investigated the effects of normal and neo-plastic tissues on the endodermal cells of early chick embryos. Their results are at variance with those obtained in our own laboratory. Thus, the major observation of Mareel and colleagues is that if an incision is made in the hypoblast of the embryo and normal cells are then introduced into the space between the epiblast and hypoblast, the hypoblast regenerates in the normal way and heals up the defect. If neoplastic cells are present, they inhibit this process of regeneration. Mareel *et al.* (1974) state that the reason why in our laboratory this effect was not described is due to differences in the techniques employed in the implantation of tumour cells. In Waddington's (1932) technique, following an incision in the endoderm the latter is separated locally from the ectoderm (epiblast) and the cells to be

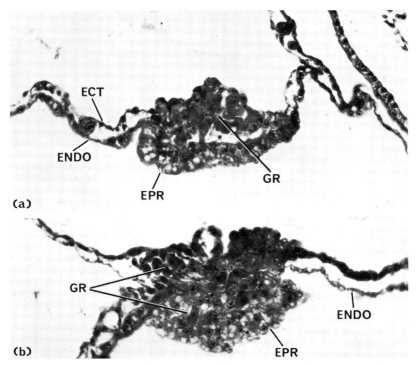

Figure 14 Implant of Morris hepatoma (GR). Note the endodermal proliferation (EPR). ENDO is the unreacted endoderm and ECT the unreacted ectoderm. × 330 (approx.). From Sherbet *et al.* (1970).

tested are inserted into the pocket and therefore may not have an opportunity to exert any influence on the process of hypoblast regeneration. In our experiments, we have occasionally noticed the absence of healing of the incision made with the result that cells spill out of the embryo. None the less, this was merely due to mechanical pressure of the graft, dependent mainly on the volume of the implant. The only way to confirm the findings of Mareel *et al.* would be to use cell-free extracts of normal and tumour tissue to see if they affect the regeneration of the endodermal layer. The basic difference in the effects on the endoderm is, in fact, more than merely technical. In all our experiments, the tumour tissues produce an excessive proliferation of endodermal cells, often accompanied by distinctive cellular arrangement (Sherbet *et al.*, 1970), while the inhibition of regeneration described by Mareel and colleagues must indeed depend primarily on an inhibition of cellular proliferation.

We also observed that the hepatoma implants induced excessive blood cell formation in close association with the implant. It is known that induction of blood cell formation is a function of the embryonic endoderm (Sherbet *et al.*, 1970; Sherbet and Lakshmi, 1971). Therefore, this may indicate the acquisition of embryonic properties by the hepatoma cells. The ability was closely associated with an extra chromosome in group 4-10. This extra chromosome appears in a majority of the minimum deviation hepatomas. This may indicate a linkage of genes responsible for blood island induction and neoplastic transformation, on a chromosome of group 4-10 (Sherbet and Lakshmi, 1971). It appears, therefore, that there is a close and intrinsic relationship between the production of the endodermal histogenetic response and the neoplastic process.

On the other hand, human astrocytomas and breast cancers, both ectoderm-derived tumours, have been found to induce reponses predominantly from the embryonic ectoderm. The responses were intense and were induced frequently (Figs 15 and 16). The induced structures usually bear much similarity to neural tissue in its characteristic palisaded cellular arrangement (Fig. 17). Often these induced structures undergo distinctive morphogenesis into neural tube-like structures (Sherbet and Lakshmi, 1974d, 1978a). Astrocytic and breast tumours are the only neoplasms which have induced the ectodermal response in a series of tumours of various histological origins that we have investigated to date. Palayoor and Batra (1971) observed that mammary carcinomas of C3H mice were able to induce neuroid reactions from the ectoderm in experiments similar to ours.

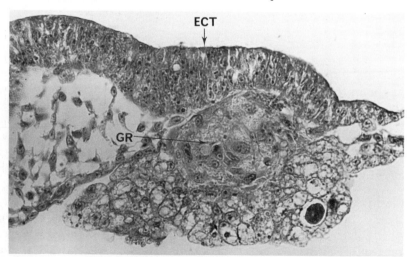

Figure 15   Ectodermal response induced by a mammary carcinoma (GR). Note the neural tissue-like ectodermal thickening over the graft (ECT). × 330 (approx.).

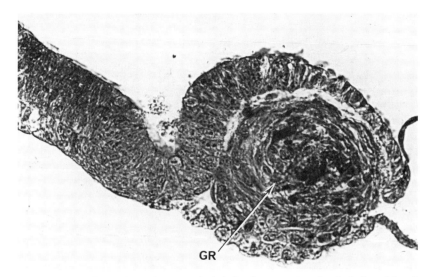

Figure 16 The formation of a neural cleft in the neural palisade induced by the graft (GR.) × 330 (approx.).

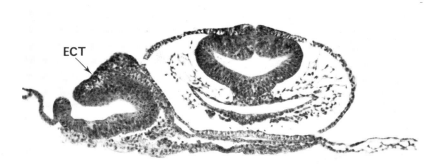

Figure 17 A secondary neural structure (ECT) produced by a Hensen's node "organizer" graft. The graft is not seen in the section. × 70 (approx.).

There is now ample evidence which suggests that the induction of histogenetic responses may be a characteristic property of neoplasms (Table 28). The nature of these histogenetic mechanisms still remains to be elucidated. Nevertheless, one can draw valid inferences from homologous interactions occurring in embryogenesis. The induction of differentiation of neural tissue by implantation of neural tissue (Mangold and Spemann, 1927; Waddington, 1933), and the induction of limb buds by implanted limb buds

Table 28

Histogenetic specificities of embryonic responses

Tumour	Ectodermal response	Endodermal response	Reference
Ectodermal			
Human astrocytoma	+	±	Sherbet and Lakshmi (1974d)
Human carcinoma of the breast	+	+	Sherbet and Lakshmi (1978a)
C3G (J) mice mammary adenocarcinoma	+	—	Palayoor and Batra (1971)
Mesodermal			
HeLa (human carcinoma of the cervix)	—	—	
Yoshida ascites sarcoma (rat)	±	—	Sherbet and Lakshmi (1970)
Landschütz ascites carcinoma (murine)	—	—	
Benzpyrene-induced sarcoma (rat)	—	—	
Leukemic bone marrow	±	—	Toivonen and Saxén (1957)
Endodermal			
Minimum-deviation hepatoma (rat)	—	+	Sherbet *et al.* (1969, 1970)
Dimethylaminoazobenzene-induced hepatoma (rat)	—	+	Sherbet and Lakshmi (1974c)

From Sherbet and Lakshmi (1978).

(Hertwig, 1925, 1927) are well-known instances of "homogenetic inductions". The homogenetic inductions are, in fact, very closely associated with the state of differentiation of the implanted tissue. Competent embryonic ectoderm is capable of inducing neural tissue differentiation only when it has itself been induced to differentiate in that direction. This histogenetic response produced by astrocytomas and breast tumours is compatible with the epigenetic model for neoplasia proposed by Sherbet (1974b) and may reflect the acquisition of embryonic characteristics by dedifferentiation accompanied by the ability to synthesize substances which can alter the path of differentiation of the ectoderm. Inappropriate synthesis of substances is not unusual in neoplasms. Tumours are often accompanied by paraneoplastic syndromes of endocrinopathy. Not only has ectopic production of hormones by some neoplasms been abundantly documented (Hall, 1974), but it has also become apparent that this ability may be closely related to the state of differentiation of the neoplasm (Sherbet, 1974b). (*see also* pp. 100-109).

Some circumstantial evidence for the production of histogenetic response by ectopic products which may be associated with breast tumours may be discussed here. In the 1960s, investigations in the author's laboratory demonstrated that follicle-stimulating hormone possesses considerable power to induce the differentiation of neural tissue from competent chick embryonic ectoderm (Sherbet, 1962, 1963; Sherbet and Mulherkar, 1963, 1965; Sherbet and Lakshmi, 1967a, 1968a, 1974b). In view of the impressive ability of breast carcinoma to induce neural tissue differentiation, it is of considerable interest that the α-subunit shared by the pituitary glycoprotein hormones, FSH, TSH and LH, and HCG has been shown to be present in breast tumour cultures (Cove *et al.*, 1979b), and also demonstrated to occur in breast carcinoma tissues (Walker, 1978). The possibility exists, therefore, that the neural tissue differentiation induced by breast carcinomas could be due to the α-subunit of the glycoprotein hormones. Incidentally, this could also justify to some extent the use of the ability of tumours to induce histogenetic effects as a basis for determining the degree of deviation of the tumour tissue from normality, since the state of differentiation of a neoplasm could be judged indisputably by the spectrum of ectopic products that it synthesizes.

The epigenetic grading procedure

Recently we described a system for the numerical grading of tumours (Sherbet and Lakshmi, 1974c). This system of grading takes into consideration the frequency and intensity of host mesodermal and histogenetic responses and the frequency of occurrence of morphogenetic displacement (Table 29).

Of each tumour to be tested, 18-24 implantations are performed and the cellular responses induced by the implants are assessed by fixing the blastodisc with the implanted tissue after they have been incubated for a further 16-18 h. The embryos are then sectioned and stained. The frequency and intensity of responses are recorded and scored as given in Table 29. The total score gives the epigenetic grade (EGG) for the tumour. In this system of scoring, the higher the EGG the greater would be the malignancy of the tumour under investigation.

The total time taken for the EGG test is approximately 5 days after the biopsy material or the excised tumour is received in the laboratory. This compares favourably with the time taken for histopathological assessment.

Table 29

Scoring system for epigenetic grading of tumours

Type of response	Frequency (%) Degree (+)	Score
Host mesodermal response	75-100	1
	50- 74	2
	25- 49	3
	0- 24	4
Morphogenetic displacement	75-100	3
	50- 74	2
	31- 49	1
	0- 30	0
Histogenetic responses	75-100	3
a. Ectodermal response, frequency	50- 74	2
b. Endodermal response, frequency	25- 49	1
	0- 24	0
a. Ectodermal response, degree	+	1
b. Endodermal response, degree	2 +	2
	3 +	3

From Sherbet and Lakshmi (1974c).

Correlation between epigenetic grade and malignancy

EGG test of Morris minimum-deviation hepatomas

Since the epigenetic grade reflects a number of important biological characteristics of tumours, it may be expected that the grading will also reflect the malignancy of tumours. The possibility of such a correlation was examined in the series of minimum-deviation hepatomas. In the opening paragraph of this book malignancy was defined in biological terms as the ability of a tumour to grow progressively free of homeostatic control, invade, form distant metastases and kill the host. We therefore attempted a correlation between the EGG of the minimum-deviation hepatomas and their metastatic ability in and survival times of Buffalo strain rats after implantation of the various tumours. The relevant data are given in Table 30. Both the grade 5 hepatomas (9618B and 9633) showed no metastases at all. Of the grade 6, however, 2 out of 3 tumours showed a few metastases, but the grade 7 hepatoma was found to have produced several large metastases. Compatible with their metastatic ability was survival time. The average survival time of the animals bearing the grade 7 hepatoma was roughly one-third of that of the lower grade hepatomas (7793 and 7794A).

Table 30

Epigenetic grades of minimum-deviation hepatomas and their relationship to degree of malignancy

Tumour	Epigenetic grade	Time after first transplantation (months)	Metastases[a]	Survival time (days)
Normal liver	1	—	—	
9618B	5	34	0	—
9633	5	38	0	—
7793	6	91	+ +	200
7794A	6	92	+	180
7787	6	94	+	
5123C	7	154	+ +	69

[a]0 = no metastases, + few metastases, + + many large metastases.
From Sherbet and Lakshmi (1974c).

A third feature of some significance was a clear correlation between the epigenetic grade of the tumours and the length of time they had been maintained by serial transplantation since they were induced by administration of a carcinogen. It is known that the malignant potential of a tumour may not be achieved in the life-time of the host which carries the tumour (Foulds, 1958). If the tumour is transplanted at the death of the host, it would continue its progression towards greater malignancy. In other words, the longer a tumour has been maintained by serial transplantation, the more malignant it will become. This phenomenon of progressive increase in malignancy is clearly reflected in the epigenetic grading of the minimum deviation hepatomas.

EGG test of metastasizing and non-metastazing lymphomas of the hamster

This ample reflection of malignancy in the EGG test has been further confirmed in two lymphomas of the hamster. One of these lymphomas (ML) is able to form metastases while the second lymphoma (NML) has no metastatic ability at all. Both lymphomas have roughly comparable growth rates, and present identical histology. In the EGG test, however, the behaviour of the two tumours was completely at variance. The major differences were found to be in the frequency and intensity of the histo-genetic ectodermal response and in the host mesodermal response. As a result, the metastasizing lymphoma was found to be of EGG 15, while the non-metastasizing tumour was only EGG 6 (Table 31). Thus, epigenetic grading clearly highlights the differences in the malignancy of the two tumours (Sherbet *et al.*, 1980). It may be pointed out that in terms of epigenetic grading the non-metastasizing lymphoma is comparable with cystic hyperplasia of the breast and meningiomas (*see* pp. 189-191).

The ability of the EGG test to distinguish a metastasizing tumour from a tumour which has no metastatic ability may be of considerable predictive value.

Table 31

EGG test of metastasizing (ML) and non-metastasizing (NML) lymphomas of the hamster

Ectodermal response		
frequency	ML 80%	NML 18%
degree	2+	+
Endodermal response		
frequency	50%	41%
degree	2+	+
Host mesodermal response	22%	57%
Morphogenetic displacement	70%	47%
Epigenetic grade (EGG)	15	6

From Sherbet *et al.* (1980).

EGG test of human astrocytic tumours and breast cancers

It appears, therefore, that epigenetic grading offers a reliable measure of malignancy. In order to examine the applicability of the EGG test to human malignancies, we have recently examined the relationship between epigenetic grades of a series of astrocytic tumours and the post-operative clinical course of the disease.

The clinical data of the patients investigated, and the histological and epigenetic grades of the tumours are given in Table 32. Although the majority of the tumours examined belonged to Kernohan (histological grades) III and IV, the post-operative survival times of the patients showed a wide variation. On the other hand, the epigenetic grades appeared to be related more closely to the survival times of the patients.

The data in Table 32 also show that some of the patients with glioma of the same epigenetic grade showed different survival times. For instance, patients 173 and 187, 170 and 186, and 189 and 205 showed wide differences in their post-operative survival, despite the fact that their neoplasms were of comparable epigenetic grades of malignancy. It may be noted, however, that in each set of cases there is also a disparity in the ages of the patients.

Clinical data of patients, and histological and epigenetic grades of the astrocytic tumours[a]

Patient	Age (years)	Nature of operation	Post-operative treatment	Histological grade	EGG	Post-operative survival time (months)
173	28	Partial	Dex DXT	Gliosis with small areas of low malignancy glioma	5	15·8
187	70	Biopsy	Dex DXT	Grade III	5	8·5
191	53	Partial	DXT	Grade IV, glioblastoma multiforme	6	10·2
218	69	Partial	DXT	Grade II, gemistocytic and fibrillary astrocytoma	7	8·0
186[b]	61	Partial	Dex	Grade IV, completely necrotic neoplasm	9	3·3
170	55	Partial	Dex	Grade IV	9	5·7
223	59	Partial	DXT	Grade III, necrotic tumour	11	4·0
205	46	Partial	Dex	Grade III, fronto-temporal infiltrating astrocytoma	12	4·5
189	26	Partial	Dex DXT	Grade IV	12	9·5
224	57	Partial	Dex	Grade IV, glioblastoma multiforme	14	2·0
207[c]	56	Biopsy	None	Grade III	6	1·5
177[d]	42	Partial	Dex DXT	Poorly differentiated oligodendroglioma with areas of protoplasmic astrocytoma	11	>28·0

Dex: Dexamethasone; DXT: Deep x-ray therapy.
[a]Part of this data is from Sherbet and Lakshmi (1974c).
[b]This tumour was reported as grade 8 in an earlier publication (Sherbet and Lakshmi, 1974c).
[c]The tumour had not been excised from the patient, nor was he on dexamethasone or deep x-ray therapy after the tumour was biopsied. This may explain the low survival.
[d]The residual tumour was a low malignancy astrocytoma.

Statistical analysis has revealed that the survival times of patients correlated highly significantly ($r = 0.656$; $P < 0.025$) with the log (age × epigenetic grade). Similar statistical treatment showed no correlation ($r = 0.461$, $P > 0.1$) between Kernohan grading and survival time. The correlation was analysed using Spearmann's rank correlation. According to Pearson $r = 2 \sin ((r/6)R)$, where r is the correlation coefficient and R is Spearmann's coefficient of rank correlation. There was no relationship between ages of the patients and their survival time.

The analysis of correlation of EGG with prognosis, therefore, took into account the ages of the patients. This analysis revealed that survival time is inversely proportional to the log(EGG × age). The correlation is highly significant $(0.025 > P > 0.01)$. A similar statistical treatment showed that there was no significant relationship between the survival times and Kernohan grade × age. It is important also to note that the post-operative survival time was not a function of the age of the patients alone. On account of the poor prognosis for astrocytic tumours, we have been able to confirm in this way that the epigenetic grading test accurately determines the degree of malignancy of tumours.

We have also examined a short series of human carcinoma of the breast. Six breast tumours, though histologically carcinomas, were found to belong to grades between 9 and 15 in the EGG test (Sherbet and Lakshmi, 1978, 1979b). Although the increasing malignancy of the tumours seemed to be reflected in descriptive histology (Table 33), histology on its own would probably predict a roughly similar course in all these cases. But the EGG tests indicate otherwise.

Table 33

Epigenetic grades of some human breast tumours and their histology

Tumour	EGG[a]	Histology[b]
BAI	4	Cystic hyperplasia with some areas of epitheliosis
MCP	9	Trabecular and tubular mucus-secreting adenocarcinoma with a light infiltrate of lymphocytes, plasma cells and histiocytes in the fibrous stroma
MCF	11	Scirrhous carcinoma with slight lymphocytic reaction, chronic inflammation but no growth in 7 lymph nodes
MCD	13	Poorly differentiated adenocarcinoma with poor lymphocyte response. Lymph nodes free of tumour
BAS	13	Poorly differentiated adenocarcinoma with lymphatic infiltration. Lymph nodes free of tumour
AME	14	Invasive carcinoma. Tumour with cellular area of anastomosing trabeculae of spheroidal cells with fibrous reaction of scirrhous adenocarcinoma. No lymphocytic response
HOR	15	Poorly differentiated finely trabecular carcinoma incompletely contained by fibrous reaction with lymphatic permeation

[a]Determined as described in Table 29.
[b]Histological data were obtained from the Department of Morbid Anatomy, University College Hospital Medical School, London.
From Sherbet and Lakshmi (1978a).

Epigenetic grading and metatstatic potential

The ability of some tumours to invade and form metastases is an intrinsic property of the neoplastic cells. Although the expression of such malignant behaviour may be influenced, and possibly controlled, by the host, it may be helpful in determining the form of treatment and subsequent management of patients if it were possible to determine the potential of the primary tumour to disseminate and form distant metastases.

The methods available for assessing metastatic potential may be described as inadequate. Therefore it was felt desirable to examine if epigenetic grading provided any clues to the metastatic potential of a primary tumour. Sherbet and Lakshmi (1981b) recently described such a correlation. For the purposes of simplifying the grading method, only the histogenetic responses were taken into account. Three tumour models were considered in this analysis. These were the Morris minimum-deviation hepatomas, a metastasizing and a non-metastasizing form of a hamster lymphoma, and human mammary tumours.

It may be seen from Fig. 18 that, in the hepatomas and the lymphosarcomas, tumours which produced histogenetic scores of 3 or less apparently possessed no metastatic ability. On the other hand, tumours which

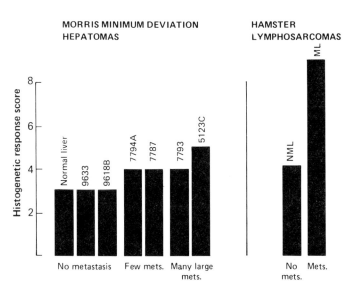

Figure 18 Correlation between histogenetic score and metastatic potential of Morris minimum-deviation hepatomas and hamster lymphosarcomas. From Sherbet and Lakshmi (1981b).

were grade 4 or higher did possess this ability. (It may be pointed out here that the non-metastasizing lymphosarcoma (NML) was found to be grade 3 when tested as whole tissue but grade 4 when the EGG tests were carried out with cell suspension of > 95% viable cells prepared from the solid tumour. The metastasizing lymphosarcoma was grade 7 and grade 9 when tested as whole tissue and as purified viable cells respectively.)

In the human mammary tumours again, the fibro-epithelial hyperplasias produced histogenetic scores ranging between 0 and 3, while the histologically proven carcinomas induced histogenetic responses ranging between 3 and 10. At the lower end of the scale (grades 3-6), the patients were disease-free for 4-7 years following mastectomy. In contrast, three patients whose tumours had induced grade 8 and 10 histogenetic responses died of disseminated disease about 3 years after mastectomy had been performed. One patient with grade 7 tumour has had a recurrent carcinoma (Fig. 19).

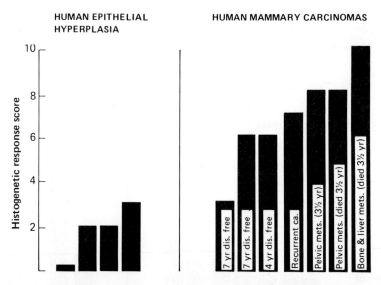

Figure 19 Correlation between histogenetic grade and metastatic potential in human carcinomas of the breast. The epithelial hyperplasia is a benign condition. From Sherbet and Lakshmi (1981b).

On reviewing the epigenetic grading of a variety of tumour models, it has become apparent that the epigenetic spectrum of malignancy can be subdivided into three groups with increasing degrees of malignancy as follows: group I (EGG grades 3-5), group II (grades 6-7) and group III (grades 8-15). It may be seen from the distribution of neoplasms on the epigenetic scale

(Fig. 20) that group I contains non-metastatic tumours, reactive gliosis, and meningiomas and cystic hyperplasias of the breast. Group III contains malignant tumours such as the metastatic hamster lymphosarcoma, human astrocytomas of Kernohan grades III-IV and carcinomas of the breast. Group II forms a narrow intermediate zone composed of non-malignant as well as lowly malignant tumours.

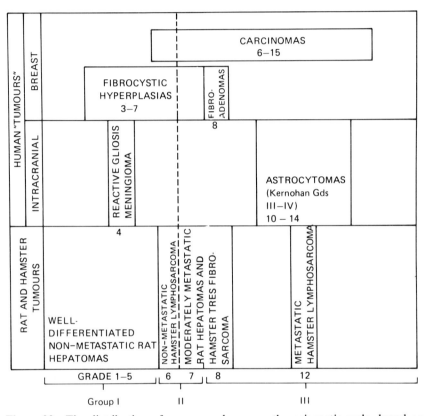

Figure 20 The distribution of some neoplasms on the epigenetic scale, based on various publications from the author's laboratory. The epigenetic data relating to tumours of the breast are from unpublished investigations by Dr M. S. Lakshmi in collaboration with Professor A. L. Latner, Professor I. D. A. Johnston, Mr R. G. Wilson and Dr G. V. Sherbet.

Since carcinomas of the breast occupy a very broad zone of the EGG scale, we recently examined their epigenetic grades in relation to their metastatic ability. Of the carcinomas in group I, 67% were localized tumours and 33% had disseminated. In contradistinction, only 33% of carcinomas in group II were localized and the rest showed dissemination to regional lymph nodes. Of the carcinomas in group III, 73% had disseminated to regional lymph nodes or had produced bony metastases. The remainder, although localized, produced little or no stromal reaction, indicating a poor immunological response by the host. This may be consistent with the degree of anaplasia and high epigenetic grading (Table 34).

Table 34

Relationship between EGG and metastatic spread of carcinomas of the breast

EGG group	No. of patients	% Distribution according to EGG		
		No lymph nodes involved	Lymph nodes involved	Distant metastases
I	6	67	—	33
II	3	33	67[a]	
IIIA	8	38[b]	50	12
B	3	—	—	100

Group I: EGG 3-5; II: EGG 6 and 7; IIIA: EGG 8-12 and IIIB: EGG 13-18.
[a]Histological reports did not report occurence of metastatic tumour in the lymph nodes, but these tumours were not localized and described as infiltrative carcinomas.
[b]The tumours showed poor or no lymphocytic infiltration, i.e. poor immune response from the host.

It may be said in conclusion that the distribution of neoplasms on the epigenetic scale not only consolidates the view that epigenetic grading reflects the degree of malignancy, but also that the EGG scale is applicable to animal and human tumours alike.

Cell surface proteins and epigenetic grading

The cell surface subserves a spectrum of biological functions in diverse phenomena such as cell differentiation, morphogenesis, cellular locomotion, cellular recognition and allied processes, and needless to say in the various stages of tumour development, invasion and metastasis. These functions have been discussed from time to time in other sections of this book and also previously (Sherbet, 1978).

The concept that the degree of malignancy may be reflected in the structure and the composition of the outer zones of the cell membrane has provided a sound basis for a variety of investigations into the biology and biochemistry of the cell surface. The evidence presented in the foregoing discussion has provided firm indication that the intensity of the cellular responses from the embryonic tissues induced by neoplastic tissues, especially the histogenetic responses, reflects the degree of malignancy and metastatic potential of the tumour. It was natural, therefore, to inquire if the histogenetic responses were a result of surface interactions between embryonic and tumour cells. The possibility that surface macromolecules could be participating in these interactions was obvious from experiments which revealed that the occurrence of the responses was related to the surface negative charge present on the tumour cells (Sherbet *et al.*, 1970). But these clues were not followed up at the time, and although cellular responses of this kind have also been reported by other investigators (Palayoor and Batra, 1971; Camon, 1976), no attempts have yet been made to elucidate the possible mechanisms that might be involved in the cellular interactions and the subsequent production of response by the embryonic cells.

In a recent investigation, we have examined the histogenetic responses produced by the hamster TRES fibrosarcoma and have attempted to see if the production of the responses is dependent upon the pattern of proteins expressed on the tumour cell surface. Latner and Sherbet (1979) had previously shown that incubation of TRES fibrosarcoma cells with aprotinin, a wide-spectrum proteinase inhibitor, altered the surface properties of the tumour cells. For instance, a 2 h incubation of TRES cells in the presence of aprotinin not only increased the net surface charge, but also rendered the cells less agglutinable by Con A and less adhesive to Con A-linked plates. An examination of the kinetics of adhesion revealed that after treatment with aprotinin, a class of receptors which had a lower affinity to Con A were predominantly expressed on the surface of the cells. Such a change would be expected if aprotinin prevented the loss of surface components by inhibiting cellular proteinases. The pattern of proteins expressed was in fact different in the treated and untreated control cells (Fig. 21). Qualitatively, there were a host of complex changes. Quantitative changes were mainly in components of average molecular weights of 115K and 48K, where increases of between 25 and 50% were observed. There was also a small (about 10%) reduction in components of approximately 95K.

Aprotinin-treated TRES and hamster lymphosarcomas both show a reduction in their ability to induce histogenetic responses (*see* Table 35 for data relating to TRES cells). The association of this loss with alterations to surface protein patterns appears to support the view that the induction of histogenetic responses may involve protein and/or glycoprotein components of the cell surface, possibly also complex processes of recognition by the embryonic cells of neoplastic cells implanted in their midst.

We have some evidence now that the degree of induction of histogenetic responses is in fact related to the extent of expression of a specific protein(s)

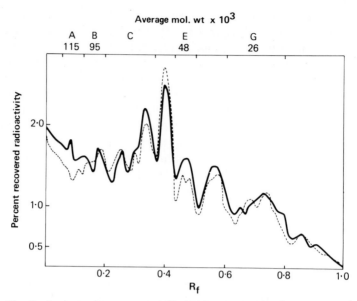

Figure 21   Surface protein patterns of TRES fibrosacroma cells, control (······) and aprotinin-treated (——). From Lakshmi *et al.* (1982).

on the cell surface. This evidence was obtained from a small series of human breast tumours which were initiated in tissue culture, their cell surface proteins labelled by lactoperoxidase-catalysed radio-iodination, and the proteins separated by electrophoresis on polyacrylamide gels (Wildridge and Sherbet, 1981). At the same time, the tumour tissue was tested by epigenetic grading (Sherbet and Lakshmi, 1978a). The relevant data obtained from these experiments are given in Table 36, from which it may be seen that the greater the ratio of protein(s) of average molecular weight of 265K and 233K the lower was the histogenetic score produced by the tumour in the EGG test. A statistical analysis revealed that the histogenetic score was inversely proportional to the ratio of 265K and 233K component(s) detected on the surface of the cells. This evidence not only confirms the involvement of surface protein in EGG tests, but raises the possiblity that the 233K proteins could serve as markers for malignancy.

Sensitivity of the EGG test

The sensitivity of the EGG test may be judged in terms of its ability to distinguish between, and respond differently to, discrete yet minute differences in the deviations from normality of the test cells. The EGG system is able to distinguish between the experimentally induced minimum-

Table 35

Effects of aprotinin on the histogenetic responses induced by TRES fibrosarcoma cells

Histogenetic response[a]	TRES control cells	Aprotinin-treated TRES cells[b]					
		0.15 TIU ml^{-1}[c]	P[d]	0.25 TIU ml^{-1}	P	0.35 TIU ml^{-1}	P[d]
No. of implants	12	14		16		30	
Ect R_f %	45	86	<0·05	0	<0·025	0	<0·005
Ect R^0	+	+		0		0	
End R_f %	82	71	N.S.	0	<0·005	33	<0·05
End R^0	+	+		0		+	

[a] Ect—End R_f %: histogenetic response frequency; Ect—End R^0: histogenetic response intensity.
[b] Cells incubated for 2 h at specified concentration.
[c] TIU: trypsin inactivator units.
[d] N.S.: not statistically significant.
Lakshmi *et al.* (1982).

Table 36

Relationship between the relative expression of surface proteins
265K/233K and histogenetic scores of some human breast tumours

Patient	% [125]I incorporation[a] 265K/233K	Histogenetic score
BAI	4·29	0
MCP	2·55	3
VG	2·30	5
MAT	2·0	5
MCF	1·67	6
BAS	2·88	8
AME	1·37	9
HOR	1·6	10

[a]Cell surface proteins were labelled with ^{125}I using lactoperoxidase-mediated radioiodination method. The proteins were then seperated by polyacrylamide gel electrophoresis. The values given in column 2 represent ratios of percentage of recovered count in proteins of mol. wt of 265K and 233K. The correlation between histogenetic grading and the ratio of incorporation of ^{125}I into 265K and 233K components was significant ($r = 0.775$, $P < 0.025$).
From Wildridge and Sherbet (1981), Sherbet and Lakshmi (1978a, 1981b) and Lakshmi *et al.* (1982).

deviation tumours which differ from one another in slight variations in growth rates and differentiation. Even the very slow-growing hepatoma 9633, a well-differentiated tumour and with no metastatic ability, could be distinguished from the normal liver implants from which the tumour could be said to differ in the main in its slightly higher growth rate. The sensitivity of the system is also indicated by the low EGG of cystic hyperplasia of the breast and the non-malignant meningiomas; both of these were of epigenetic grade 4 (Sherbet and Lakshmi, 1978). In the same vein, one case of gliosis (non-malignant cellular proliferation and modulation of glial tissue) was EGG 5. This is in sharp contrast with malignant tumours which were epigenetically graded 9-15 in the mammary tumour series, and 6-14 in tumours of the astrocytic series (Tables 32 and 33).

Applications of the EGG test

The value of any new assay system ought to be judged on its technical simplicity and potential use in scientific endeavour. The EGG test is simple in conception and practice, yet it exploits some of the fundamental features of, and intrinsic specificities in, the interactions between embryonic and tumour cells. In short, the EGG test is simple, specific and sensitive.

The test has been criticized as being empirical. Its empirical nature, i.e. being based on experiment rather than on theory, does not in any way detract from its intrinsic worth. Most science is empirical: observation and experiments brought together within a theoretical concept—which can then be retested by experiment or by its ability to accommodate new observations. The scepticism with which any new system is received is understandable. In the 1920s, the histological method of grading was considered by some as a futile exercise. Reiman (1929) expressed utter disbelief that a microscopic examination of a section of the tumour could predict the biological course of the disease.

The most encouraging aspect of the assay is the intrinsic specificity of the cellular reponses. The histogenetic response, which is the response in the embryonic germ layer corresponding with the embryological origin of the tumour, may be considered to be of some signficance. Investigations into the mechanisms by which these histogenetic responses are produced could lead to a greater understanding of epigenetic mechanisms and their possible operation in the various aspects of neoplastic development.

The EGG test may be of some use in experimental cancer research, e.g. as in the periodical testing of laboratory cell lines for possible spontaneous neoplastic transformation , in viral and chemical carcinogenesis and in the testing of antitumour compounds. To this latter area, some work in the author's laboratory is currently being directed.

The epigenetic grading test may find its most rewarding application in the clinical management of cancer patients. In several forms of cancer, especially cancer of the breast, the form of treatment is closely linked with the clinical stage of the disease, and, as pointed out by Mansfield (1976), one is posed with the dilemma of deciding whether to follow conservative forms of treatment or to adopt more radical procedures.

Zelen (1968) identified four distinct time histories in breast cancer. In one of these, where the tumour shows no extension to axillary lymph nodes and favourable nuclear differentiation, early diagnosis accompanied by simple or radical mastectomy can result in increased survival. In a second time history with no nodal involvement but with an unfavourable state of nuclear differentiation, neither early diagnosis nor a radical mastectomy alters the survival time. In the third and fourth time histories, where the axillary nodes are involved, again early diagnosis and radical mastectomy do not alter the length of survival. In other words, three subgroups can be recognized even in patients who may be predicted to have good prognosis on the basis of favourable clinical criteria, viz. (a) limited potential disease, i.e. limited metastatic potential, (b) moderately aggressive disease that has limited but potential metastatic ability, and (c) aggressive disseminated disease (*see* Henderson and Carellos, 1980).

Tobias (1980) has discussed this problem in a recent article and has asked: "What is the smallest surgical procedure that can usefully be performed?" He states further that "this is not by any means an academic question, since even simple mastectomy is a highly disfiguring operation . . . " for approximately one-fifth of all patients undergoing mastectomy develop associated psychological and/or sexual problems (Maguire, 1979).

Fisher (1979) believes that breast cancer is a systemic disease from the inception of neoplasia. This view was based on a clinical trial of the National Surgical Adjuvant Breast and Bowel Project which showed that a high proportion of patients who had undergone curative operations became treatment failures within 10 years of the operation (Fisher *et al.*, 1975). In agreement with McWhirter (1955) one might argue that if the disease is curable by surgery alone a radical operation is unlikely to be met with more success than simple mastectomy.

This concept of the biology of breast cancer would no doubt convince many clinicians of the need for developing an aid for assessing the potential of the primary tumour to disseminate and possibly form metastatic deposits. If EGG is able to estimate the metastatic potential of a tumour, as the experimental work described herein would suggest, it could serve as a useful tool in conjunction with the established methods of histological grading, and clinicopathological staging of tumours. Even then, it will be well to remember that dissemination of the tumour does not necessarily entail metastatic disease. Therefore, no assay method for measuring metastatic potential which does not take account of the host's resistance to the spread of the disease can be completely satisfactory.

Epilogue

There seems to be little need for a peroration except to express the hope that I have succeeded in demonstrating that malignancy is an intrinsic biological property of the tumour cell, and that the pattern of malignant behaviour and the phenotypic expressions of cutopic and ectopic products may be under epigenetic control. The conversion of the concept of malignancy from its abstract form into one incorporating the element of intrinsic capacity of the tumour cell has also provided a basis for believing that there exist differences in degrees of benignancy and malignancy. If one were to relate the actual potential for malignancy possessed by a tumour and the apparent potential indicated by the extent of the disease, one could infer the degree to which the host has been able to control the spread of the disease. This could provide a basis not only for determining the form of treatment and the response of the patients to such treatment but also for predicting prognosis with acceptable accuracy. The essence of these sentiments is implicit in the quoted verse with which I began this book. Although probably not appreciated by one and all, besides attempting to further the frontiers of science, the research worker hopes also to be able to contribute to the well-being of the patient as does the clinician. That this does not merely remain a pious hope requires a close and continuing collaboration between the clinician and the research scientist.

References

Abelev, G. I. (1968). *Cancer Res.* **28**, 1344.

Abelev, G. I. (1971). *Advan. Cancer Res.* **14**, 295.

Abelev, G. I. (1974). *Transplant. Rev.* **20**, 3.

Abelev, G. I., Assercritova, I. V., Karaevsky, N. A., Perova, S. D. and Perevodchikova, N. I. (1967). *Internat. J. Cancer* **2**, 551.

Abell, C. W. and Heidelberger, C. (1962). *Cancer Res.* **22**, 931.

Abercrombie, M. (1961). *Exp. Cell Res., Suppl.* **8**, 188.

Abercrombie, M. (1970a). *Eur. J. Cancer* **6**, 7.

Abercrombie, M. (1970b). *In Vitro* **6**, 128.

Abercrombie, M. (1979). *Nature* **281**, 259.

Abercrombie, M. and Ambrose, E. J. (1958). *Exp. Cell. Res.* **15**, 332.

Abercrombie, M. and Heaysman, J. E. M. (1954). *Exp. Cell Res.* **6**, 293.

Abercrombie, M. A. and Heaysman, J. E. M. (1976). *J. Natl Cancer Inst* **56**, 561.

Abercrombie, M., Heaysman, J. E. M. and Karthauser, H. M. (1957). *Exp. Cell Res* **13**, 276.

Ablin, R. J., Gonder, M. J. and Soanes, W. A. (1975). *Oncology* **32**, 127.

Abrams, H. L., Spiro, R. and Goldstein, N. (1950). *Cancer* **3**, 74.

Abramson, M., Schilling, R. W., Huang, C. C. and Salome, R. G. (1975). *Ann. Otoryngology* **84**, 158.

Adamson, E. D. and Ayers, S. E. (1979). *Cell* **16**, 953.

Adinolfi, A., Adinolfi, M. and Lessof, M. H. (1975). *J. Med Genet.* **12**, 138.

Ageeva, A. N. (1969). *Arkh. Pat. (Moscow)* **31**, 43.

Agostini, D. and Clifton, E. E. (1962). *Arch. Surg.* **84**, 449.

Albertsson, P. Å. (1971). "Partition of Cell Particles and Macromolecules", 2nd edn. Wiley-Interscience, New York.

Alexander, P. (1976). *In* "Fundamental Aspects of Metastasis", ed. Weiss, L., p. 227. North Holland Publ. Co., Amsterdam.

Alexander, P. and Eccles, S. (1975). *In* "Critical Factors in Cancer Immunology", eds Schultz, J. Leif, E., Vol. 10, p. 159. Academic Press, New York and London.

Alexander, P. and Evans, R. (1971). *Nature New Biol.* **232**, 76.

Alexander, P. and Fairley, G. H. (1967). *Br. Med. Bull.* **23**, 86.

Alexander, P., Evans, R. and Grant, C. K. (1972). *Ann. Inst. Pasteur, Paris* **122**, 645.

Allen, A. and Snow, C. (1970). *Biochem. J.* **117**, 32P.

Allison, A. C., Harrington, J. S. & Birkbeck, M. (1966). *J. Exp. Med.* **124**, 141.

Al-Sarraf, M., Baker, L., Talley, R. W., Kithier, K. and Vaitkevicius, V. K. (1979). *Cancer* **44**, 1222.

Amatruda, T. T. Jr, Mulrow, P. J., Gallagher, J. C. and Sawyer, W. H. (1963). *New Engl. J. Med.* **269**, 544.

Ambrose, E. J. and Easty, D. M. (1976a). *In* "Human Tumours in Short Term Culture", ed. Dendy, P. P., p. 45. Academic Press, London and New York.

Ambrose, E. J. and Easty, D. M. (1976b). *Differentiation* **6**, 61.

Ambrose, E. J., James, A. M. and Lowick, J. H. B. (1956). *Nature* **177**, 576.

American Joint Committee on Cancer Staging and End Result Reporting (1977). "Manual for Staging Cancer", pp. 101—4.

Anderson, N. G. and Coggin, J. H. (1974). *In* "The Cell Surface in Development", ed. Moscona, A. A., p. 297. John Wiley and Sons, New York.

Argyris, T. S. and Argyris, B. F. (1962). *Cancer Res.* **22**, 73.

Arora, P. K., Miller, H. C. and Aronson, L. D. (1978). *Nature* **274**, 589.

Ashendel, C. L. and Boutwell, R. K. (1979). *Biochem. Biophys. Res. Commun.* **90**, 623.

Atkins, D., Ibbotson, K. J., Hillier, K., Hunt, N. H., Hammonds, J. C. and Martin, T. J. (1977). *Br. J. Cancer* **36**, 601.

Attallah, A. M. and Strong, D. M. (1979). *Internat. Arch. Allergy Appl. Immunol.* **60**, 101.

Attallah, A. M., Needy, C. F., Noguchi, P. D. and Elisberg, B. L. (1979). *Internat. J. Cancer* **24**, 49.

Ausprunk, D. H. and Folkman, J. (1977). *Microvascular Res.* **14**, 53.

Aver, I. O. and Kress, H. G. (1977). *Cell. Immunol.* **30**, 173.

Azzopardi, J. G. and Whittaker, R. S. (1969). *J. Clin. Pathol.* **22**, 718.

Azzopardi, J. G. and Williams, E. D. (1968). *Cancer* **22**, 274.

Babai, F. (1976). *J. Ultrastr. Res.* **56**, 287.

Badger, A. M., Merluzzi, V. J., Mannick, J. A. and Cooperband, S. R. (1977). *J. Immunol.* **118**, 1228.

Bagshawe, K. D., Golding, P. R. and Orr, A. H. (1969). *Br. Med. J.* **3**, 733.

Baldwin, R. W. & Pimm, M. V. (1973). *Internat. J. Cancer* **12**, 420.

Baldwin, R. W. and Robins, R. A. (1976). *Br. Med. Bull.* **32**, 118.

Balls, M. (1962). *Cancer Res.* **22**, 1142.

Banwo, O., Versey, J. and Hobbs, J. E. (1974). *Lancet,* **i**, 643.

Barski, G. and Belehradek, J. Jr. (1965). *Exp. Cell Res.* **37**, 464.

Barski, G. and Youn, J. K. (1969). *J. Natl. Cancer Inst.* **43**, 111.

Barton, P. and Labauge, R. (1961). *Presse Méd.* **69**, 2635.

Bartter, F. C. and Schwartz, W. B. (1967). *Amer. J. Med.* **42**, 790.

Baserga, R. and Saffiotti, U. (1955). *Arch. Pathol.* **59**, 26.

Bastida, E., Ordinas, A. and Jamieson, G. A. (1981). *Nature* **291**, 661.

Bautzmann, H., Holtfreter, J., Spemann, H. and Mangold, O. (1932). *Naturwissenschaften* **20**, 971.

Beard, J. (1902). *Lancet,* **i**, 1758.

Becker, C. G. and Harpel, P. C. (1976). *J. Exp. Med,* **144**, 1.

Becker, L. E., Narayan, O. and Johnson, R. T. (1976). *Canad. J. Neurol. Sci,* **3**, 105.

Begent, R. H. J., Tucker, D. F. and Keen, J. (1980). *Br. J. Cancer* **41**, 481.

Bennett, A., McDonald, A. M., Simpson, J. S. and Stamford, I. F. (1975). *Lancet* **i**, 1218.

Bennett, A., Charlier, E. M., McDonald, A., Simpson, J. S. and Stamford, I. F. (1976). *Prostaglandins* **11**, 461.

Bennett, A., Del Tacca, M., Stamford, I. F. and Zebro, T. (1977). *Br. J. Cancer* **35**, 881.

Bennett, A., Carter, R. L., Stamford, I. F. and Tanner, N. S. B. (1980). *Br. J. Cancer* **41**, 204.

Bennett, H. S., Luft, J. H. and Hampton, J. C. (1959). *Amer, J. Physiol.* **196**, 381.

Ben-Sasson, Z., Weiss, D. W. and Doljanski, F. (1974). *J. Natl Cancer Inst.* **52**, 405.

Benyesh-Melnick, M. and Butel, J. S. (1974). *In* "The Molecular Biology of Cancer", ed. Busch, H., p. 403. Academic Press, New York and London.

Berenblum, I. and Shubik, P. (1947a). *Br. J. Cancer* **1**, 379.

Berenblum, I. and Shubik, P. (1947b). *Br. J. Cancer* **1**, 383.

Berenblum, I. and Shubik, P. (1949a). *Br. J. Cancer* **3**, 109.

Berenblum, I. and Shubik, P. (1949b). *Br. J. Cancer* **3**, 384.

Berkarda, F. B., O'Souza, J. P. and Bakemeier, R. F. (1974). *Proc. Amer. Assoc. Cancer Res* **15**, 19.

Berlin, N. I. (1974). *Ann. N.Y. Acad. Sci.* **230**, 209.

Bernacki, R. J. and Kim, U. (1977). *Science* **195**, 577.

Bernard, P. J., Weiss, L. and Ratcliffe, T. (1969). *Exp. Cell Res.* **54**, 293.

Berson, S. and Yalow, R. (1966). *Science* **154**, 907.

Bertalanffy, F. D. (1969). *Recent Results Cancer Res.* **17**, 136.

Berwald, Y. and Sachs, L. (1963). *Nature* **200**, 1182.

Berwald, Y. and Sachs, L. (1965). *J. Natl Cancer Inst.* **35**, 641.

Bhattacharya, M., Chatterjee, S. K. and Barlow, J. J. (1976). *Cancer Res.* **36**, 2096.

Bhisey, A. N. and Freed, J. J. (1971). *Exp. Cell Res.* **64**, 430.

Bielschowsky, F., Bielschowsky, M. and D'Ath, E. F. (1968). *Proc. Univ. Otago Med. Sch.* **46**, 31.

Birkbeck, M. S. C. and Carter, R. L. (1972). *Internat. J. Cancer* **9**, 249.

Bishop, J. M. (1981). *Cell* **23**, 51.

Bjornsson, S., Preisler, H. and Pavelic, Z. (1978). *Br. J. Cancer* **38**, 703.

Black, P. H. (1980). *Advan. Cancer Res.* **32**, 75.

Blackman, M. R., Weintraub, B. D., Rosen, S. W., Kourides, I. A., Steinwascher, K. and Gail, M. H. (1980). *J. Natl Cancer Inst.* **65**, 81.

Blandau, R. J. (1949). *Anat. Rec.* **104**, 331.

Bloom, H. J. G. (1950). *Br. J. Cancer* **4**, 259.

Bloom, H. J. G. (1956). *Br. J. Radiol.* **29**, 488.

Bloom, H. J. G. (1965). *Proc. Roy. Soc. Med.* **51**, 122.

Bloom, H. J. G. and Field, J. R. (1971). *Cancer* **28**, 1580.

Bloom, H. J. G. and Richardson, W. W. (1957). *Br. J. Cancer* **11**, 359.

Bloom, H. J. G., Richardson, W. W. and Field, J. R. (1970). *Br. Med. J.* **3**, 181.

Bloom, S. R. and Polak, J. M. (1980). *Clinics Endocrinol. Metabol.* **9**, 285.

Blythman, H. E., Casellas, P., Gros, D., Gros, P., Jansen, F. K., Paolucci, B. P. and Vidal, H. (1981). *Nature* **290**, 145.

Bockman, R. S. and Myers, W. P. L. (1977). In "Cancer Invasion and Metastasis: Biologic Mechanisms and Therapy", eds Day, S. B., Stansly, P., Laird Myers, W. P. and Garattini, S., p. 431. Raven Press, New York.

Bode, V. C. and Dziadek, M. A. (1979). *Devlop. Biol.* **73**, 272.

Bodell, P., (1974). *Ann. N.Y. Acad. Sci.* **230**, 6.

Boeryd, B. (1965). *Acta Pathol. Microbiol. Scand.* **65**, 395.

Boggust, W. A., O'Meara, R. A. and Fullerton, W. W. (1968). *Eur. J. Cancer* **3**, 467.

Bomford, R. and Olivotto, M. (1974). *Internat. J. Cancer* **14**, 226.

Bondy, P. K. (1977). *In* "Aspects of Cancer Management: Carcinoma of the Bronchus", ed. Calman, K. C. p. 9. M.C.S. Publications, Kent.

Bonner, J. T. (1960). *Amer. Sci.* **48,** 514.

Bosmann, H. B. and Hilf, R. (1974). *FEBS Letters* **44,** 313.

Bosmann, H. B., Bieber, G. F., Brown, A. E., Case, K. R., Gersten, D. M., Kimmerer, T. W. and Lione, A. (1973). *Nature* **246,** 487.

Bowen, J. G. and Kulatilake, A. E. (1979). *Br. J. Cancer* **40,** 806.

Bower, B. F. and Gordon, G. S. (1965). *Ann. Rev. Med.* **16,** 83.

Bower, B. F. and Mason, D. M. (1964). *Clin. Res.* **12,** 121.

Bower, B. F., Mason, D. M. and Forsham, P. H. (1964). *New Engl. J. Med.* **271,** 934.

Boyd, A. L. and Orme, T. W. (1975). *Internat. J. Cancer* **16,** 526.

Boyd, V. A. L. and Butel, J. S. (1972). *J. Virol.* **10,** 399.

Brackman, P., Snyder, J., Henderson, E. S. and Astrup, T. (1970). *Br. J. Haematol.* **18,** 135.

Brahma, S. K. (1966). *J. Embryol. Exp. Morphol.* **16,** 203.

Bramis, J. P., Messer, J., Nacchiero, M. and Dreiling, D. A. (1978). *Amer. J. Gastroenterol.* **69,** 565.

Bramwell, M. E. and Harris, H. (1978a). *Proc. Roy. Soc. B.* **201,** 87.

Bramwell, M. E. and Harris, H. (1978b). *Proc. Roy. Soc. B.* **203,** 93.

Bray, M. A., Gordon, D. and Morley, J. (1974). *Br. J. Pharmacol.* **52,** 453.

Brechot, C., Pourcel, C., Louise, A., Rain, B. and Tiollais, A. (1980). *Nature* **286,** 533.

Bredin, H. C., Daly, J. J. and Prout, G. R. (1975). *J. Urol.* **113,** 487.

Breedis, C. (1951). *Cancer Res.* **11,** 239.

Brem, S. Gullino, P. M. and Medina, D. (1977). *Science* **195,** 880.

Bretscher, M. S. (1973). *Science* **181,** 622.

Brinster, R. L. (1974). *J. Exp. Med.* **140,** 1049.

Broders, A. C. (1920). *J. Amer. Med. Assoc.* **74,** 656.

Brookes, R. V., Dupre, J., Gogate, A. N., Mills, I. H. and Prunty, F. T. G. (1963). *J. Clin. Endocrinol.* **23,** 725.

Brooks, D. E., Seaman, G. V. F. and Walter, H. (1971). *Nature, New Biol.* **234,** 61.

Brown, J. M. (1973a). *Cancer Res.* **33,** 1217.

Brown, J. M. (1973b). *Br. J. Radiol.* **46,** 613.

Brown, J. P., Woodbury, R. G., Hart, C. E., Hellström, I. and Hellström, K. E. (1981). *Proc. Natl. Acad. Sci. USA* **78,** 539.

Brown, P. J., Tsai, T. and Gajdusek, D. C. (1975). *Amer. J. Epidemiol.* **102,** 331.

Brown, W. H. (1928). *Lancet* **ii,** 1022.

Brunson, K. W., Beattie, G. and Nicolson, G. L. (1978). *Nature* **272,** 543.

Bubenik, J., Perlmann, P., Helmstein, K. and Moberger, G. (1970). *Internat. J. Cancer* **5,** 310.

Buck, C. A., Glick, M. C. and Warren, L. (1971). *Science* **172,** 169.

Bunting, J. S., Hemstead, E. H. and Kremer, J. K. (1976). *Clin. Radiol.* **27,** 9.

Burger, M. (1969). *Proc. Natl Acad. Sci. U.S.A.* **62,** 994.

Burger, M. (1970). *Nature* **227,** 170.

Burger, M. (1973). *Fed. Proc.* **32,** 91.

Burgess, E. A. and Sylvén, B. (1962). *Cancer Res.* **22,** 581.

Burnet, F. M. (1964). *Br. Med. Bull.* **20,** 154.

Burnet, F. M. (1967). *Lancet* **ii,** 1171.

Burnet, F. M. (1970). *Prog. Exp. Tumor Res.* **13,** 1.

Burnet, F. M. (1971). *Transplant. Rev.* **7**, 3.

Burtin, P. (1978). *Ann, Immunol. (Inst. Pasteur)* **129C**, 185.

Butler, T. P. and Gullino, P. M. (1975). *Cancer Res.* **35**, 512.

Bystryn, J. C. (1977). *J. Natl Cancer Inst.* **59**, 325.

Calman, K. C. and Paul, J. (1978). "An Introduction to Cancer Medicine", p. 78. Macmillan, London.

Camerini, E. and Zavanella, T. (1968). *Il Cancro* **21**, 379.

Camiolo, S. M., Markus, G., Evers, J. L., Hobika, G. H., De Pasquala, J. L. and Beckley, S. (1981). *Internat. J. Cancer* **27**, 191.

Camon, J. (1976). Morphological behaviour of human tumours implanted into chick embryos. Ph. D. Thesis (in Spanish), University of Zaragoza.

Campbell, F. R. (1977). *J. Natl Cancer Inst.* **58**, 369.

Carlson, B. M. (1974). *In* "Neoplasia and cell differentiation", ed. Sherbet, G. V. p. 60. Karger AG, Basle.

Carlsson, R. N. K. and Ingvarsson, B. I. (1979). *Develop. Biol.* **73**, 1.

Carlsson, S. (1973). *Acta Chir. Scand.* **139**, 499.

Carr, I., McGinty, F. & Norris, P. (1976). *J. Pathol.* **118**, 91.

Carrel, S., Sordat, B. and Merenda, C. (1976). *Cancer Res.* **36**, 3978.

Carter, R. L. (1978a). *In* "Secondary Spread of Cancer", ed. Baldwin, R. W., p. 1. Academic Press, London and New York.

Carter, R. L. (1978b). *In* "Secondary Spread of Cancer", ed. Baldwin, R. W., p. 53. Academic Press, London and New York.

Carter, R. L. (1978c). *Invest. Cell. Pathol.* **1**, 275.

Carter, R. L. and Gershon, R. K. (1966). *Amer. J. Pathol.* **49**, 637.

Carter, S. B. (1967). *Nature* **213**, 256.

Cash, J. D., Woodfield, D. G., Das, P. C. and Allan, A. G. E. (1969). *Br. Med. J.* **2**, 576.

Cassai, E., Rotola, A., Meneguzzi, G., Milanesi, G., Garsia, S., Remotti, G. and Rizzi, G. (1981a). *Eur. J. Cancer* **17**, 685.

Cassai, E., Rotola, A., DiLuca, D., Manservigi, R., Meneguzzi, G., Milanesi, G. and Califano, A. (1981b). *Eur. J. Cancer* **17**, 695.

Castleman, B., Scully, R. E. and McNeely, B. U. (1972). *New Engl. J. Med.* **286**, 713.

Chakraborty, P. R., Ruiz-Opazo, N., Shouval, D. and Shafritz, D. A. (1980). *Nature* **286**, 531.

Chambers, A. F., Hill, R. P. and Ling, V. (1981). *Cancer Res.* **41**, 1368.

Champion, H. R. and Wallace, I. W. J. (1971). *Br. J. Cancer* **25**, 441.

Chan, S. Y. and Pollard, M. (1980). *J. Natl Cancer Inst.* **64**, 1121.

Chase, P. S. (1972). *Cell Immunol.* **5**, 544.

Chatterjee, S. K. and Kim, U. (1978). *J. Natl Cancer Inst.* **61**, 151.

Chatterjee, S. K., Bhattacharya, M. and Barlow, J. J. (1979). *Cancer* **39**, 1943.

Chen, T. T. and Mealey, J. Jr (1972). *Cancer Res.* **32**, 558.

Chew, E. and Wallace, A. C. (1976). *Cancer Res.* **36**, 1904.

Chew, E. C., Josephson, R. L. and Wallace, A. C. (1976). *In* "Fundamental Aspects of Metastasis", ed. Weiss, L., p. 121. North Holland Publ. Co., Amsterdam.

Child, J. A., Späti, B., Illingworth, S., Bernard, D., Corbett, S., Simmons, A. V., Stone, J., Worthy, T. S. and Cooper, E. H. (1980). *Cancer* **45**, 318.

Chmielewska, J., Poggi, A., Janik, P., Latallo, Z. S. and Donati, M. B. (1980). *Eur. J. Cancer* **16**, 919.

Christman, J. K., Acs, S., Silagi, S., Newcome, E. W. and Silverstein, S. (1974). *J. Cell Biol.* **63**, 61a.

Chu, T. M. and Nemoto, T. (1973). *J. Natl Cancer Inst.* **51**, 1119.

Cikes, M., Beth, E., Giraldo, G., Acheson, N. and Hirt, B. (1977). *In* "Origins of Human Cancer", p. 1009. Cold Spring Harbor Lab., Cold Spring Harbor.

Clark, S. S., and Srinivasan, V. (1973). *J. Urol.* **109**, 444.

Clifton, E. E. and Grossi, C. E. (1955). *Cancer* **8**, 1146.

Cochrane, C. G., Revak, S. D. and Wuepper, K. D. (1973). *J. Exp. Med.* **138**, 1546.

Cohnheim, J. (1875). *Virchows Arch.* **65**, 64.

Coman, D. R. and Sheldon, W. F. (1946). *Amer. J. Pathol.* **22**, 821.

Concannon, J. P., Dalbow, M. H. and Frich, J. C. (1973). *Radiology* **108**, 191.

Contractor, S. F. and Davies, H. (1973). *Nature* **243**, 284.

Cook, G. M. W. and Jacobson, W. (1968). *Biochem. J.* **107**, 549.

Coombes, R. C. (1978). *Cancer Topics* **2**, 4.

Coombes, R. C., Powles, T. J. and Gazet, J. C. (1977). *Lancet* **ii**, 132.

Coombes, R. C., Hillyard, C., Greenberg, P. B. and McIntyre, I. (1974). *Lancet* **i**, 1080.

Cooperband, S., Bondevik, H., Schmid, K. and Mannick, J. A. (1968). *Science* **159**, 1243.

Copley, A. L. and Witte, S. (1976). *Thromb. Res.* **8**, 251.

Corey, L., Stamm, W. E., Feorino, P. M., Bryan, J. A., Weseley, F., Gregg, M. B. and Solangi, K. (1975). *New Engl. J. Med.* **293**, 1273.

Cove, D. H., Woods, K. L., Smith, S. C. H., Burnett, D., Leonard, J., Grieve, R. J. and Howell, A. (1979a). *Br. J. Cancer* **40**, 710.

Cove, D. H., Smith, S. C. H., Walker, R. and Howell, A. (1979b). *Eur. J. Cancer* **15**, 693.

Crawford, L. V., Lane, D. P., Denhardt, D. T., Harlow, E. E., Nicklin, P. M., Osborn, K. and Pim, D. C. (1980). *Cold Spring Harb. Symp. Quant. Biol.* **44**, 179.

Crocker, J. F. S. and Vernier, R. L. (1972). *J. Paediat.* **80**, 69.

Currie, G. A. and Alexander, P. (1974). *Br. J. Cancer* **29**, 72.

Currie, G. A. and Basham, C. (1972). *Br. J. Cancer* **26**, 427.

Currie, G. A. and Basham, C. (1975). *J. Exp. Med.* **142**, 1600.

Currie, G. A. and Gage, J. O. (1973). *Br. J. Cancer* **28**, 136.

Curtis, A. S. G. (1969). *J. Embryol. Exp. Morphol.* **22**, 305.

Cushing, H. (1932). *Bull. Johns Hopkins Hosp.* **50**, 137.

Dabbous, M. K., Roberts, A. N. and Brinkley, B. (1977). *Cancer Res.* **37**, 3537.

Daniel, M. R. (1970). *Br. J. Cancer* **24**, 712.

Dao, T. L., Ip, C. and Patel, J. (1980). *J. Natl Cancer Inst.* **65**, 529.

Darai, G. and Munk, K. (1976). *Internat. J. Cancer* **18**, 469.

Das, M. R. and Mink, M. M. (1979). *Cancer Res.* **39**, 5106.

Davey, G. C., Currie, G. A. and Alexander, P. (1976). *Br. J. Cancer* **33**, 9.

David, J. R. (1975). *In* "The Phagocytic Cell in Host Resistance", eds. Bellanti, J. A. and Dayton, D. H., p. 143. Raven Press, New York.

Davies, P. and Allison, A. C. (1976). *In* "Lysosomes in Biology and Medicine", eds Dingle, J. T. and Dean, R. T., p. 61. North-Holland Publ. Co., Amsterdam.

De Baetselier, P., Katzav, S., Gorelik, E., Feldman, M. and Segal, S. (1980). *Nature* **288**, 179.

De Cosse, J. J., Gossens, C. L., Kuzma, J. F. and Unsworth, B. R. (1973). *Science* **181**, 1057.

Defendi, V., Lehman, J. and Kraemer, P. (1963). *Virology* **19**, 592.

Deichman, G. I. and Kluchureva, T. E. (1966). *J. Natl Cancer Inst.* **36**, 647.

Del Regato, J. A. (1977). *Seminars Oncol.* **4**, 33.

De Lustig, E. S. (1968). *In* "Cancer Cells in Culture", ed. Katsuta, H., p. 135. University of Tokyo Press, Tokyo.

De Lustig, E. S. and De Matrajt, H. A. (1961). *Rev. Soc. Argent. Biol.* **37**, 180.

De Lustig, E. S. and Lustig, L. (1964). *Rev. Soc. Argent. Biol.* **40**, 207.

Deman, J. J. and Bruyneel, E. A. (1974). *Exp. Cell Res.* **89**, 206.

Denk, H., Tappeiner, G., Eckerstorfer, R. and Holzner, J. H. (1972). *Internat. J. Cancer* **10**, 262.

Dennert, G. (1980). *Nature* **287**, 47.

Den Otter, W., Evans, R. and Alexander, P. (1972). *Transplantation* **14**, 220.

De Thé, G., Gesser, A., Day, N. E., Tukei, P. M., Williams, E. H., Beri, D. P., Smith, P. G., Dean, A. G. Bornkamm, G. W., Feorino, P. and Henle, W. (1978). *Nature* **274**, 756.

De Vore, D. P., Houchens, D. P., Ovejara, A. A., Dill, G. S. and Hutson, T. B. (1980). *Exp. Cell Biol.* **48**, 367.

Dewey, M. J. and Mintz, B. (1978). *Develop. Biol.* **66**, 55.

Diener, E. and Feldman, M. (1972). *Transplant Rev.* **8**, 76.

Dilman, V. M. (1966). *Internat. J. Cancer* **1**, 239.

Dingemans, K. P. (1974). *J. Natl Cancer Inst.* **53**, 1813.

Di Persio, L., Dingle, S., Michael, J. G. and Pesce, A. J. (1980). *Exp. Cell Biol.* **48**, 429.

Donati, M. B., Mussoni, L., Poggi, A., De Gaetano, G. and Garattini, S. (1978). *Eur. J. Cancer* **14**, 343.

Dorsey, K. J. and Roth, S. (1973). *Develop Biol.* **33**, 249.

Dosogne-Guérin, M., Stolarczyk, A. and Borkowski, A. (1978). *Eur. J. Cancer* **14**, 525.

Dougherty, R. M. (1976). *J. Gen. Virol.* **33**, 61.

Dreesman, G. R., Burek, K., Adam, E., Kaufman, R. H., Melnick, J. L., Powell, K. L. and Purifoy, D. J. M. (1980). *Nature* **283**, 591.

Dresden, M. H., Heilman, S. A. and Schmidt, J. D. (1972). *Cancer Res.* **32**, 993.

Dunn, C. J., Koh, M. S., Willoughby, D. A. and Giroud, G. P. (1977). *J. Pathol.* **122**, 201.

Dunn, T. B. (1954). *J. Natl Cancer Inst.* **14**, 1281.

Durand, R. E. (1975a). *Br. J. Radiol.* **48**, 556.

Durand, R. E. (1975b). *Proc. Internat. Symp. Cancer Therapy Hyperthermia and Radiation,* Washington D.C., American College of Radiology, p. 101.

Durand, R. E. (1976a). *Cell Tissue Kinet.* **9**, 403.

Durand, R. E. (1976b). *Radiology* **119**, 217.

Easty, D. M. and Easty, G. C. (1974). *Br. J. Cancer* **29**, 36.

Easty, G. C. (1974). *In* "Neoplasia and Cell Differentiation", ed. Sherbet, G. V., p. 189. Karger AG, Basle.

Easty, G. C. and Easty, D. M. (1973). *In* "Chemotherapy of Cancer Dissemination and Metastasis", eds. Garattini, S. and Franchi, G., p. 45. Raven Press, New York.

Easty, G. C., Easty, D. M. and Tchao, R. (1969). *Eur. J. Cancer* **5**, 287.

Eaves, G. J. (1973). *J. Pathol.* **109**, 233.

Eccles, S. A. and Alexander, P. (1974a). *Nature* **250**, 667.

Eccles, S. A. and Alexander, P. (1974b). *Br. J. Cancer* **30**, 42.

Eckhart, W., Dulbecco, R. and Burger, M. M. (1971). *Proc. Natl Acad. Sci. U.S.A.* **68**, 283.

Edman, J. C., Gray, P., Valenzuela, P., Rall, L. B. and Rutter, W. J. (1980). *Nature* **286**, 531.

Edwards, J. G., Dysart, J. M., Edgar, D. H. and Robson, R. T. (1979). *J. Cell. Sci.* **35**, 307.

Eichwald, E. J. and Chang, H. Y. (1951). *Cancer Res.* **11**, 811.

Eisenstein, R., Sorgente, N., Soble, L. W., Miller, A. W. and Kuettner, K. E. (1973). *Amer. J. Pathol.* **73**, 765.

Eisenstein, R., Kuettner, K. E., Neopolitan, C., Soble, L. W. and Sorgente, N. (1975). *Amer. J. Pathol.* **81**, 337.

Ellison, M. L., Ambrose, E. J. and Easty, G. C. (1969). *Exp. Cell Res.* **55**, 198.

Ellison, M. L., Lamb, D., Rivett, J. and Neville, A. M. (1977). *J. Natl Cancer Inst.* **59**, 309.

Englesberg, E. J., Irr, J., Power, J. and Lee, N. (1965). *J. Bacteriol.* **90**, 946.

Englesberg, E. J., Squires, C. and Meronk, F. Jr (1969). *Proc. Natl Acad. Sci. U.S.A.* **62**, 1100.

Enterline, H. T. and Coman, D. R. (1950). *Cancer Res.* **3**, 1033.

Epstein, M. A. (1978a). *Nature* **274**, 270.

Epstein, M. A. (1978b). *In* "Nasopharyngeal Carcinoma: Aetiology and Control", eds De Thé, G., Ito, Y. and Davis, W., p. 333. IARC, Lyon.

Epstein, M. A. and Achong, B. G. (1977). *Ann. Rev. Microbiol.* **31**, 421.

Epstein, M. A. and Achong, B. G. (1979). *In* "The Epstein—Barr Virus", eds Epstein, M. A. and Achong, B. G., p. 321. Springer, Berlin.

Ertl, N. and Immich, H. (1968). *Exp. Pathol. (Jena)* **2**, 270.

Evans, A. S., Rothfield, N. F. and Niederman, J. C. (1971). *Lancet* **i**, 167.

Evans, A. S., Dolan, M. F., Sobocinski, P. Z. and Quinn, F. A. (1974). *Cancer Res.* **34**, 538.

Evans, M. J. (1972). *J. Embryol. Exp. Morphol.* **28**, 164.

Evans, R. (1972). *Transplantation* **14**, 468.

Evans, R. (1973). *Br. J. Cancer* **28**, Suppl. 19.

Evans, R. and Alexander, P. (1970). *Nature* **228**, 620.

Evans, R. and Alexander, P. (1972). *Nature* **236**, 168.

Evans, R. and Lawler, E. M. (1980). *Internat. J. Cancer* **26**, 831.

Ewing, J. (1940). "Neoplastic Disease", Saunders, Philadelphia.

Fenyö, E. M., Klein, E., Klein, G. and Swiech, K. (1968). *J. Natl Cancer Inst.* **40**, 69.

Feraci, R. P. (1974). *Surgery* **76**, 649.

Fidler, I. J. (1973a). *Nature New Biol.* **242**, 148.

Fidler, I. J. (1973b). *Eur. J. Cancer* **9**, 223.

Fidler, I. J. (1974a). *Cancer Res.* **34**, 491.

Fidler, I. J. (1974b). *Cancer Res.* **34**, 1074.

Fidler, I. J. (1975). *Cancer Res.* **35**, 219.

Fidler, I. J. (1978). *Cancer Res.* **38**, 2651.

Fidler, I. J. and Hart, I. R. (1981). *Eur. J. Cancer* **17**, 487.

Fidler, I. J. and Nicolson, G. L. (1976). *J. Natl Cancer Inst,* **57**, 1199.

Fidler, I. J., Gersten, D. M. and Hart, I. R. (1978). *Advan. Cancer Res.* **28**, 149.

Finch, B. W. and Ephrussi, B. (1967). *Proc. Natl Acad. Sci. U.S.A.* **57**, 615.

Fisher, B. (1979). *New Engl. J. Med.* **301**, 326.

Fisher, B. and Fisher, E. R. (1965). *Science* **152**, 1397.

Fisher, B. and Fisher, E. R. (1966). *Surg. Gynaecol. Obstet.* **122**, 791.

Fisher, B. and Slack, N. H. (1970). *Surg. Gynaecol. Obstet.* **131**, 79.

Fisher, B., Slack, N. and Katrych, D. (1975). *Surg. Gynaecol. Obstet.* **140**, 528.

Fisher, E. R. and Fisher, B. (1967). *Arch. Pathol.* **83**, 321.

Fisher, E. R. and Fisher, B. (1976). *Int. J. Radiat. Oncol. Biol. Phys.* **1**, 96.

Fisher, E. R., Gregorio, R. M., Fisher, B., Redmond, C., Vellios, F. and Sommers, S. C. (1975). *Cancer* **36**, 1.

Fisher, J. W. and Birdwell, B. J. (1961). *Acta Haematol.* **26**, 224.

Fisher, R. A. and Yates, Y. B. (1974). "Statistical Tables for Biological, Agricultural and Medical Research". Oliver and Boyd, Edinburgh.

Fitzpatrick, F. A. and Stringfellow, D. W. (1979). *Proc. Natl Acad. Sci. U.S.A.* **76**, 1765.

Flannery, G. R., Chalmers, R. J., Rolland, J. M. and Nairn, R. C. (1973). *Br. J. Cancer* **28**, 118.

Flores, M., Marti, J. H., Grosser, N., MacFarlane, J. K. and Thompson, D. M. P. (1977). *Cancer* **39**, 494.

Fogel, M., Gorelik, E., Segal, S. and Feldman, M. (1979). *J. Natl Cancer Inst.* **62**, 585.

Foley, E. J. (1953). *Cancer Res.* **13**, 835.

Folkman, J. (1974a). *Cancer Res.* **34**, 2109.

Folkman, J. (1974b). *Advan. Cancer Res.* **19**, 331.

Folkman, J. (1975). *In* "Cancer, A Comprehensive Treatise", ed. Becker, F. F., p. 355. Plenum Press, New York.

Folkman, J. and Haudenschild, C. (1980). *Nature* **288**, 551.

Folkman, J. and Tyler, K. (1977). *In* "Cancer Invasion and Metastasis: Biologic Mechanisms and Therapy", eds Day, S. B., Laird Myers, W. P., Stansley, P., Garattini, S. and Lewis, M. G., p. 95. Raven Press, New York.

Folkman, J., Merler, E., Abernathy, C. and Williams, G. (1971). *J. Exp. Med.* **133**, 275.

Foote, F. W. (1959). *In* "Cancer of the Breast", ed. Parsons, W. H., p. 59. Blackwell, Oxford.

Foote, F. W. Jr and Stewart, F. W. (1946). *Surgery* **19**, 74.

Foulds, L. (1949). *Br. J. Cancer* **3**, 345.

Foulds, L. (1954). *Cancer Res.* **14**, 327.

Foulds, L. (1958). *In* "Cancer", ed. Raven, R. W., Vol. 2, p. 27. Butterworths, London.

Foulds, L. (1963). *In* "Biological Organisation at the Cellular and Supercellular Level", ed. Harris, R. J. C., p. 229. Academic Press, London.

Foulds, L. (1969). "Neoplastic Development", Vol. 1, Academic Press, London and New York.

Foulds, L. (1975). "Neoplastic Development", Vol. 2. Academic Press, London and New York.

Franks, L. M., Riddle, P. N. and Seal, P. (1969). *Exp. Cell Res.* **54**, 157.

Freedman, L. S., Edwards, D. N., McConnell, E. M. and Downham, D. Y. (1979). *Br. J. Cancer* **40**, 44.

Freedman, V. H., Brown, A. L., Klinger, H. P. and Shin, S. (1976). *Exp. Cell Res.* **98**, 143.

Fried, W., Plzak, L., Jacobson, L. O. and Goldwasser, E. (1956). *Proc. Soc. Exp. Biol. (N.Y.).* **92**, 203.

Fujimoto, S. and Tada, T. (1978). *In* "Cancer Immunotherapy and its Immunological Basis", ed. Yamamura, Y., p. 11. University Park Press, Baltimore.

Fujimoto, S., Greene, M. and Sehon, A. H. (1975). *Immunol. Commun.* **4**, 201.

Fujimoto, S., Greene, M. and Sehon, A. H. (1976a). *J. Immunol.* **116**, 791.

Fujimoto, S., Green, M. and Sehon, A. H. (1976b). *J. Immunol.* **116**, 800.

Fujimoto, S., Matsuzawa, T., Nakagawa, K. and Tada, T. (1978). *Cell. Immunol.* **38**, 378.

Fukase, M. (1978). *Med. J. Kobe Univ.* **37**, 283.

Gabbiani, G., Csank-Brassert, J., Schneeberger, J. C., Kapanci, Y., Trenchev, P. and Holborow, E. J. (1976). *Amer. J. Pathol.* **83**, 457.

Galasko, C. S. B. (1976). *Nature* **263**, 507.

Galasko, C. S. B. and Bennett, A. (1976). *Nature* **263**, 508.

Gallili, U., Vanky, F., Rodriguez, L. and Klein, E. (1979). *Cancer Immunol. Immunother.* **6**, 129.

Gardner, R. L. (1968). *Nature* **220**, 596.

Gardner, S. D. (1973). *Br. Med. J.* **1**, 77.

Gardner, S. D., Field, A. M., Coleman, D. V. and Hulme, B. (1971). *Lancet* **i**, 1253.

Gasic, G. J., Gasic, T. B. and Stewart, C. C. (1968). *Proc. Natl Acad. Sci. U.S.A.* **61**, 46.

Gasic, G. J., Gasic, T. B. and Murphy, S. (1972). *Lancet* **ii**, 932.

Gasic, G. J., Gasic, T. B., Galanti, N., Johnson, T. and Murphy, S. (1973a). *Internat. J. Cancer* **11**, 704.

Gasic, G. J., Gasic, T. B. and Murphy, S. (1973b). *Proc. Amer. Assoc. Cancer Res.* **14**, 87.

Gelder, F., Reese, C. J., Moossa, A. R., Hall, T. and Hunter, R. (1978a). *Cancer Res.* **38**, 313.

Gelder, F., Reese, C., Moossa, A. R. and Hunter, R. (1978b). *Cancer* **42**, 1635.

Gerber, P. and Kirchstein, R. L. (1962). *Virology* **18**, 582.

Gershon, R. and Carter, R. L. (1970). *Nature* **226**, 368.

Gershon, R. K., Carter, R. L. and Lane, N. J. (1967a). *Amer. J. Pathol.* **51**, 1111.

Gershon, R. K., Carter, R. L. and Kondo, K. (1967b). *Nature* **213**, 674.

Gershon, R. K., Carter, R. L. and Kondo, K. (1968). *Science* **159**, 646.

Gershon, R. K., Birnhaum-Mokyr, M. and Mitchell, M. S. (1974). *Nature* **250**, 594.

Ghose, T. and Blair, A. H. (1978). *J. Natl Cancer Inst.* **61**, 657.

Gibson, M. and Halaka, A. (1978). *J. Neurol. Neurosurg. Psychiat.* **41**, 185.

Gidlund, M., Örn, A., Wigzell, H., Senik, A. and Gresser, I. (1978). *Nature* **273**, 759.

Gidlund, M., Örn, A., Pattengale, P. K., Jansson, M., Wigzell, H., and Nilsson, K. (1981). *Nature* **292**, 848.

Gilby, A. H. (1977). *In* "Aspects of Cancer Management: Carcinoma of the Bronchus", ed. Calman, K. C., p. 32. MCS Publications, Kent.

Gilby, E. D., Rees, L. H. and Bondy, P. K. (1975). *Advan. Tumour Prevent. Detect. Characterisat.* **3**, 132.

Gimbrone, M. A. and Gullino, P. M. (1976). *J. Natl Cancer Inst.* **56**, 305.

Gimbrone, M. A., Leapman, S., Cotram, R. and Folkman, J. (1973). *J. Natl Cancer Inst.* **50**, 219.

Gimbrone, M., Cotran, R. and Folkman, J. (1974). *J. Natl Cancer Inst.* **52**, 413.

Giovanella, B. C., Yim, S. O., Morgan, A. C., Stehlin, J. S. and Williams, L. J. Jr (1973). *J. Natl Cancer Inst.* **50**, 1051.

Giovanella, B. C., Stehlin, J. S. and Williams, L. J. Jr (1974). *J. Natl Cancer Inst.* **52**, 921.

Giraldi, T., Nisi, C. and Sava, G. (1977a). *Eur. J. Cancer* **13**, 1321.

Giraldi, T., Kopitar, M. and Sava, G. (1977b). *Eur. J. Cancer* **13**, 3834.

Giraldi, T., Sava, G., Kopitar, M., Brzin, J. and Turk, V. (1980). *Eur. J. Cancer* **16**, 449.

Gitlin, D. (1975). *Ann. N. Y. Acad. Sci.* **259**, 7.

Glaser, M. and Nelken, D. (1972). *Proc. Soc. Exp. Biol. Med.* **140**, 996.

Glaser, M., Cohen, I. and Nelken, D. (1972a). *J. Immunol.* **108**, 286.

Glaser, M., Ofek, I. and Nelken, D. (1972b). *Immunology* **23**, 205.

Glasgow, A. H., Cooperband, S., Occhino, J. C., Schmid, K. and Mannick, J. A. (1971). *Proc. Soc. Exp. Biol. Med.* **138**, 753.

Glaves, D. (1980). *Internat. J. Cancer* **26**, 115.

Glenister, T. W. (1961). *J. Anat.* **95**, 474.

Gold, J. (1974). *Ann. N. Y. Acad. Sci.* **230**, 103.

Gold, P. and Freedman, S. O. (1965). *J. Exp. Med.* **121**, 439.

Goldyne, M., Claesson, H. E., Lindgrom, J. A. and Hammarstrom, S. (1978). *Eur. J. Biochem.* **74**, 13.

Good, R. A. (1977). *In* "Cancer Invasion and Metastasis: Biologic Mechanisms and Therapy", eds Day, S. B., Laird Myers, W. P., Stansley, P., Garattini, S. and Lewis, M. G., p. V. Raven Press, New York.

Goodwin, J. S. Bankhurst, A. D. and Messner, R. P. (1977). *J. Exp. Med.* **146**, 1719.

Goodwin, J. S., Messner, R. P. and Peake, G. T. (1978). *J. Clin. Invest.* **62**, 753.

Gorczynski, R. M., Kilburn, D. G., Knight, R. A., Norbury, C., Parker, D. C. and Smith, J. B. (1975). *Nature* **254**, 141.

Gordon, D., Bray, M. and Morley, J. (1976). *Nature* **262**, 401.

Gordon, G. S. (1967). *In* "Current Concepts in Breast Cancer", ed. Segaloff, A., p. 132. Williams and Wilkins, Baltimore.

Gottschalk, A. (1960). *Nature* **186**, 949.

Grabar, P. (1968). *Curr. Topics Microbiol. Immunol.* **44**, 86.

Greaves, M. F.,Tursi, A., Playfair, J. H. L., Torrigiani, G., Zamir, R. and Riott, I. M. (1969). *Lancet* **i**, 68.

Greenberg, A. H. and Shen, L. (1973). *Nature New Biol.* **245**, 282.

Greenblatt, M. and Shubik, P. (1968). *J. Natl Cancer Inst.* **41**, 111.

Greene, H. S. N. (1941). *J. Exp. Med.* **73**, 461.

Greene, H. S. N. (1952). *Cancer* **5**, 24.

Greene, H. S. N. and Harvey, E. K. (1968). *Amer. J. Pathol.* **53**, 483.

Greene, M. I., Dorf, M. E., Pierres, M. and Benacerraf, B. (1977). *Proc. Natl Acad. Sci. U.S.A.* **74**, 5118.

Greenough, R. B. (1925). *J. Cancer Res.* **9**, 453.

Griffiths, J. D. (1960). *Ann. Roy. Coll. Surg. Engl.* **27**, 14.

Griffiths, J. D. and Salsbury, A. J. (1965). "Circulating Cancer Cells", C. C. Thomas, Springfield, Illinois.

Grinwich, K. D. and Plescia, D. J. (1977). *Prostaglandins* **14**, 1175.

Grobstein, C. (1957). Exp. Cell Res. **13**, 575.

Gropp, C., Egbring, R. and Havemann, K. (1980). *Eur. J. Cancer* **16**, 679.

Gross, L. (1970). "Oncological Viruses", 2nd edn, p. 831. Pergamon Press, Oxford and London.

Grosser, N. and Thomson, D. M. P. (1975). *Cancer Res.* **35**, 2571.

Grosser, N. and Thomson, D. M. P. (1976). *Internat. J. Cancer* **18**, 58.

Gurchot, C. (1975). *Oncology* **31**, 310.

Gurdon, J. B. (1962). *Develop. Biol.* **4**, 256.

Gurdon, J. B. and Laskey, R. A. (1970). *J. Embryol. Exp. Morphol.* **24**, 227.

Gurney, C. W. (1960). *Trans. Assoc. Amer. Phys.* **73**, 103.

Guy, D. (1979). "Surface macromolecules: A comparison of primary cancers and their metastases". Ph.D. Thesis, University of Newcastle upon Tyne, England.

Guy, D., Latner, A. L. and Turner, G. A. (1977). *Br. J. Cancer* **36**, 166.

Guy, D., Latner, A. L., Sherbet, G. V. and Turner, G. A. (1980). *Br. J. Cancer* **42**, 915.

Haagensen, C. D. (1933). *Amer. J. Cancer* **19**, 285.

Haagensen, C. D. (1974). *Surgery* **76**, 685.

Haas, H. G. (1964). *Praxis (Bern)* **18**, 610.

Hagmar, B. (1970). *Acta Pathol. Microbiol. Scand. A.* **78**, 131.

Hagmar, B. (1972a). *Eur. J. Cancer* **8**, 17.

Hagmar, B. (1972b). *Arch. Pathol. Microbiol. Scand. A.* **80**, 357.

Hakim, A. A. (1980). *Exp. Cell Biol.* **48**, 445.

Hall, T. C. (1969). *Cancer J. Clinicians* **18**, 322.

Hall, T. C. (1974). *Ann. N. Y. Acad. Sci.* **203**, 5.

Hall, T. C. and Nathanson, L. (1969). The paraneoplastic syndromes. *Cancer J. Clinicians* **18**, 322.

Haller, O., Kiessling, R., Orn, A., Karre, K., Nelsson, K. and Wigzell, H. (1977). *Internat. J. Cancer* **20**, 93.

Halliday, W. S. and Miller, S. (1972). *Internat. J. Cancer* **9**, 477.

Hallwright, G. P., North, K. A. K. and Reid, J. D. (1964). *J. Clin. Endocrinol.* **24**, 496.

Hamlin, I. M. E. (1968). *Br. J. Cancer* **22**, 383.

Hammond, D. and Winnick, S. (1974). *Ann. N. Y. Acad. Sci.* **230**, 219.

Handler, A. H. (1956). *Fed. Proc.* **15**, 517.

Hara, Y., Steiner, M. and Baldini, M. G. (1980). *Cancer Res.* **40**, 1217.

Harik, S. I. and Sutton, C. H. (1979). *Cancer Res.* **39**, 5010.

Harris, H. (1971). *Proc. Roy. Soc. London* **179**, 1.

Harshbarger, J. C. (1965-78). Activities reports of Registry of Tumours in Lower Animals, National Museum of Natural History, Smithsonian Institute, Washington D.C.

Hart, I. R. (1979). *Amer. J. Pathol.* **97**, 587.

Hart, I. R. and Fidler, I. J. (1978). *Cancer Res.* **38**, 3218.

Hart, I. R. and Fidler, I. J. (1980). *Cancer Res.* **40**, 2281.

Hart, I. R., Talmadge, J. E. and Fidler, I. J. (1981). *Cancer Res.* **41**, 1281.

Harvin, J. S. and Smith, J. R. (1968). *Amer. Surg.* **34**, 555.

Hashimoto, K., Yamanishi, Y., Maeyens, E., Dabbous, M. K. and Kanzaki, T. (1973). *Cancer Res.* **33**, 2790.

Haskill, R. S., Yamamura, Y. and Radov, L. (1975). *Internat. J. Cancer* **16**, 798.

Hatcher, V. B., Wertheim, M. S., Rhel, C. Y., Tsien, G. and Burk, P. (1976). *Biochim. Biophys. Acta* **451**, 499.

Hatter, B. G. and Soehnlen, B. (1974). *Science* **184**, 1374.

Hausemann, D. von (1892). *Virchows Arch. Path. Anat.* **129**, 436.

Hay, E. D. and Fishchman, D. A. (1961). *Develop Biol.* **3**, 26.

Hayman, M. J. (1981). *J. Gen. Virol.* **52**, 1.

Hedner, U. and Nilsson, J. M. (1971). *Acta Med. Scand.* **189**, 471.

Hellmann, A. J., Burrage, K. and Hellmann, K. (1970). *Br. Med. J.* **4**, 344.

Hellström, I. and Hellström, K. E. (1970). *Internat. J. Cancer* **5**, 195.

Hellström, I., Hellström, K. E., Evans, C. A., Heppner, G. H., Pierce, G. E. and Yang, J. P. S. (1969). *Proc. Natl Acad. Sci. U.S.A.* **62**, 362.

Hellström, I., Sjögren, H. O., Warner, G. A. and Hellström, K. E. (1971). *Internat. J. Cancer* **7**, 266.

Hellström, K. E. and Hellström, I. (1970). *Ann. Rev. Microbiol.* **24**, 373.

Henderson, I. C. and Canellos, G. P. (1980). *New Engl. J. Med.* **302**, 11.

Henle, W. and Henle, G. (1976). *Internat. J. Cancer* **17**, 1.

Henle, G., Henle, W. and Diehl, J. (1968). *Proc. Natl. Acad. Sci. U.S.A.* **59**,. 94.

Henle, W., Ho, H. C., Henle, G. and Hwan, H. C. (1973). *J. Natl Cancer Inst.* **51**, 361.

Hennen, G. (1966). *Arch. Int. Physiol.* **74**, 303.

Hennen, G. (1967). *J. Clinical Endocrinol. Metabol.* **27**. 610.

Henney, C. S., Kuribayashi, K., Kern, D. and Gillis, S. (1981). *Nature* **291**, 335.

Herberman, R. B. and Holden, H. T. (1978). *Advan. Cancer Res.* **27**, 305.

Herberman, R. B. and Holden, H. T. (1980). *J. Natl. Cancer Inst.* **62**, 441

Herberman, R. B. and Oldham, R. K. (1980). *Natl Cancer Inst. Monogr.* **52**, 434.

Herberman, R. B., Nunn, M. E. and Lavrin, D. H. (1975a). *Internat. J. Cancer* **16**, 216.

Herberman, R. B., Nunn, M. E., Holden, H. T. and Lavrin, D. H. (1975b). *Internat. J. Cancer* **16**, 230.

Herberman, R. B., Djeu, J. Y., Ortaldo, J. R., Bonnard, G. D. and Holden, H. T. (1978). *In* "Human Lymphocyte Differentiation: Its Application to Cancer", eds Serrou, B. and Rosenfeld, C., p. 191. Elsevier/North Holland, Amsterdam.

Herberman, R. B., Ortaldo, J. R. and Bonnard, G. D. (1979). *Nature* **277**, 221.

Hertwig, G. (1925). *Wilhelm Roux Arch. Entwickl. Mech. Org.* **105**, 294.

Hertwig, G. (1927). *Wilhelm Roux Arch. Entwickl. Mech. Org.* **111**, 292.

Hetzel, F. W., Kruuv, J., Frey, H. E. and Koch, C. J. (1973). *Radiat. Res.* **56**, 460.

Hewlett, J. S., Hoffman, G. C., Senhauser, D. A. and Battle, J. D. (1960). *New Engl. J. Med.* **262**, 1058.

Hibbs, J. B. (1974a). *Science* **184**, 468.

Hibbs, J. B. (1974b). *J. Natl Cancer Inst.* **53**, 1487.

Hilgard, P. and Maat, B. (1979). *Eur. J. Cancer* **15**, 183.

Hilgard, P. and Thornes, R. D. (1976). *Eur. J. Cancer* **12**, 755.

Hilgard, P., Schulte, H., Wetzig, G., Schmitt, G. and Schmidt, C. G. (1977). *Br. J. Cancer* **35**, 78.

Hirai, H. and Miyaji, T. (eds) (1973). "Alpha-fetoprotein and Hepatoma", Gann. Monograph, Cancer Res. Vol. 14.

Hirata, Y., Matsukura, S., Imura, H., Nakamura, M. and Tanaka, A. (1976). *J. Clin. Endocrinol. Metabol.* **42**, 33.

Hirshaut, Y., Glade, P., Vieira, L. O. B., Ainbenda, E., Dvorak, B. and Stilzbach, L. E. (1970). *New Engl. J. Med.* **283**, 502.

Hodges, G. M. (1981). *In* "Regulation of Growth in Neoplasia", ed. Sherbet, G. V., p. 52. Karger A.G., Basle.

Hoffman, H. C. and Marty, R. (1972). *Amer. J. Surg.* **124**, 194.

Holden, H. T., Haskill, J. S., Kirchner, H. and Haberman, K. B. (1976). *J. Immunol.* **117**, 440.

Hollinshead, A. C., Chuang, C. Y., Cooper, E. H. and Catalona, W. J. (1977). *Cancer* **40**, 2993.

Holtfreter, J. (1938). *Roux Arch. Entwickl. Mech. Org.* **138**, 163.

Holub, D. A. and Katz, F. H. (1961). *Clin. Res.* **9**, 194.

Holyoke, E. D. and Ichihashi, H. (1966). *J. Natl Cancer Inst.* **36**, 1049.

Holyoke, E. D., Frank, A. L. and Weiss, L. (1972a). *Internat. J. Cancer* **9**, 258.

Holyoke, D., Reynoso, G. and Chu, T. M. (1972b). *Ann. Surg.* **176**, 559.

Holyoke, E. D., Chu, T. M., Evans, J. T. and Mittelman, A. (1979). *In* "Biological Basis for Cancer Diagnosis", ed. Fox, M., p. 151. Pergamon Press, Oxford.

Hong, S. L., Cynkin, R. P. and Levine, L. (1976). *J. Biol. Chem.* **251**, 776.

Hong, S. L., Wheless, C. M. and Levine, L. (1977). *Prostaglandins* **13**, 271.

Hoover, H. C. Jr, Jones, D. and Ketcham, A. S. (1976). *Surgery* **79**, 625.

Horton, J. E., Raisz, L. G., Simmons, H. A., Oppenheim, J. J. and Mergenhagen, S. E. (1972). *Science* **177**, 793.

Horton, J. E., Oppenheim, J. J., Mergenhagen, S. E. and Raisz, L. G. (1974). *J. Immunol.* **113**, 1278.

Hsu, C. C. and Lo Gerfo, P. (1972). *Proc. Soc. Exp. Biol. Med.* **139**, 575.

Huang, D. P., Ho, J. H., Henle, W. and Henle, G. (1974). *Internat. J. Cancer* **14**, 580.

Huberman, E. and Sachs, L. (1966). *Proc. Natl Acad. Sci. U.S.A.* **56**, 1123.

Huddlestone, J. R., Merigan, T. C. Jr and Oldstone, M. B. A. (1979). *Nature* **282**, 417.

Huggins, J. W., Chestnut, R. W., Durham, N. N. and Carraway, K. L. (1976). *Biochim. Biophys. Acta* **426**, 630.

Hultborn, K. A. and Törnberg, B. (1960). *Acta Radiol.*, Suppl. **196**, 91.

Humes, J. L. and Strausser, H. R. (1974). *Prostaglandins* **5**, 183.

Humes, J. L., Bonney, R. J., Pelus, L., Dahlgren, M. E., Sadowski, S. J., Kuehl, F. A. and Davies, P. (1977). *Nature* **269**, 149.

Hung, W., Blizzard, R. M., Migeon, C. J., Camacho, A. M. and Nyhan, W. L. (1963). *J. Paediat.* **63**, 895.

Husby, G., Hoagland, P. M., Strickland, R. G. and Williams, R. C. (1976). *J. Clin. Invest.* **57**, 1471.

Hutton, J. J., Coleman, M. S., Keneklis, T. P. and Bollum, F. J. (1978). *In* "Biological Basis for Cancer Diagnosis", ed. Fox, M., p. 165. Pergamon Press, Oxford.

Hynes, R. O. (1973). *Proc. Natl Acad. Sci. U.S.A.* **70**, 3170.

Hynes, R. O. (1979). *In* "Surface of Normal and Malignant Cells", ed. Hynes, R. O. John Wiley, London.

Illmensee, K. and Mintz, B. (1976). *Proc. Natl Acad. Sci. U.S.A.* **73**, 549.

Imura, H. (1980). *Clinics in Endocrinol. Metabol.* **9**, 235.

Imura, H., Nakai, Y., Nakao, K., Oki, S., Matsukura, S., Hirata, Y., Fukase, M., Hattori, M., Yoshimi, H. and Sueoka, S. (1978). *Proteins, Nucleic Acid and Enzymes* **23**, 641.

Inch, W. R., McCredie, J. A. and Sutherland, R. M. (1970). *Growth* **34**, 271.

Ioachim, H. L. (1976). *J. Natl Cancer Inst.* **57**, 465.

Ioachim, H. L., Dorsett, B., Sabbath, M. and Keller, S. (1972). *Nature, New Biol.* **237**, 215.

Ioachim, H. L., Keller, S. E., Dorsett, B. H. and Pearse, A. (1974). *J. Exp. Med.* **139**, 1382.

Ioachim, H. L., Dorsett, B. and Paluch, E. (1976a). *Cancer* **38**, 2296.

Ioachim, H. L., Pearse, A. and Keller, S. (1976b). *Cancer Res.* **36**, 2854.

Ioachim, H. L., Pearse, A. and Keller, S. E. (1977). *In* "Cancer Invasion and Metastasis", eds. Day, S. B., Laird Myers, W. P., Stansly, P., Garattini, S. and Lewis, M. G., p. 333. Raven Press, New York.

Isenberg, G., Rathke, P. C., Hülsman, N., Franke, W. W. and Wohlfarth-Botterman, K. E. (1976). *Cell Tissue Res.* **166**, 427.

Ishikawa, A. and Aizawa, T. (1973). *J. Gen. Virol.* **21**, 227.

Ishizaka, S., Otani, S. and Morisawa, S. (1977). *J. Immunol.* **118**, 1213.

Ivarsson, L. and Rudenstam, C. (1975). *Br. J. Cancer* **32**, 502.

Iwasaki, T. (1915). *J. Pathol. Bacteriol.* **20**, 85.

Jagarlamoody, S. M., Aust, J. C., Tew, R. H. and McKahnn, R. H. (1971). *Proc. Natl Acad. Sci. U.S.A.* **68**, 1346.

Javadpour, N. (1979). *Semin. Oncology* **6**, 37.

Jonasson, J., Povey, S. and Harris, H. (1977). *J. Cell Sci.* **24**, 217.

Jondal, M. and Klein, G. (1975). *Biomedicine* **23**, 163.

Jones, A. C. (1981). *Cancer Topics* **3**, 86.

Jones, D. S., Wallace, A. C. and Fraser, E. E. (1971). *J. Natl Cancer Inst.* **46**, 493.

Jones, P. A. E., Miller, F. M., Worwood, M. and Jacobs, A. (1973). *Br. J. Cancer* **27**, 212.

Kahan, B. W. and Ephrussi, B. (1970). *J. Natl Cancer Inst.* **44**, 1015.

Kalser, M. H., Barkin, J. S., Redlhammer, R. N. and Heal, A. H. (1978). *Cancer* **42**, 1468.

Kaluš, M. and Klement, V. (1966). *Folia Biol.* **12**, 468.

Kaluš, M. and O'Neal, R. M. (1968). *Arch. Pathol.* **86**, 52.

Kaluš, M., Ghidoni, J. J. and O'Neal, R. M. (1968). *Cancer* **22**, 507.

Kamrin, B. B. (1958). *Ann. N.Y. Acad. Sci.* **73**, 848.

Kamrin, B. B. (1959). *Proc. Soc. Exp. Biol. Med.* **100**, 58.

Kaplan, A. P. and Austen, K. F. (1971). *J. Exp. Med.* **133**, 696.

Kaplan, G. and Seljelid, R. (1977). *In* "Macrophage and Cancer", eds Keith, J., McBride, B, and Stuart, A., p. 347. Econoprint, Edinburgh.

Karlsson, B. W. (1970). *Comp. Biochem. Physiol.* **34**, 535.

Karlsson, B. W., Berstrand, C. G., Ekelund, H. and Lindberg, T. (1972). *Acta Paediat. Scand.* **61**, 133.

Karpatkin, S., Pearlstein, E., Salk, P. L. and Yogeeswaran, G. (1981). *Ann. N.Y. Acad. Sci.* **370**, 101.

Kefalides, N. A. (1971). *Biochem. Biophys. Res. Commun.* **45**, 226.

Kefalides, N. A. (1973). *Internat. Rev. Connect. Tissue Res.* **6**, 63.

Keller, A. R., Kaplan, H. S., Lukes, R. J. and Rappaport, II. (1968). *Cancer* **22**, 487.

Keller, R. (1976). *J. Natl Cancer Inst.* **57**, 1355.

Kellner, B. and Sugar, J. (1967). *In* "Endogenous Factors Influencing Host-Tumour Balance", eds Wissler, R. W., Dao, T. L. and Wood, Jr S., p. 239. University of Chicago Press, Chicago.

Kemp, R. B., Jones, B. M., Cunningham, I. and James, M. C. M. (1967). *J. Cell Sci.* **2**, 333.

Kerbel, R. S. and Davies, A. J. S. (1974). *Cell* **3**, 105.

Kerbel, R. S. and Pross, H. F. (1976). *Internat. J. Cancer* **18**, 432.

Kerbel, R. S., Pross, H. F. and Elliott, E. V. (1975). *Internat. J. Cancer* **15**, 918.

Kerbel, R. S., Twiddy, R. R. and Robertson, D. M. (1978). *Internat. J. Cancer* **22**, 583.

Kernohan, J. W., Mabon, R. F., Svien, H. J. and Adson, A. W. (1949). *Proc. Mayo Clinic* **24**, 71.

Kessel, D., Sykes, E. and Henderson, M. (1977). *J. Natl Cancer Inst.* **59**, 29.

Khudoley, V. V. and Picard, J. J. (1980). *Internat. J. Cancer* **25**, 679.

Kibbey, W. E., Bronn, D. G. and Minton, J. P. (1978). *Lancet* **i**, 101.

Kiessling, R. and Haller, O. (1978). *Contemp. Topics Immunobiol.* **8**, 171.

Kiessling, R., Klein, E. and Wigzell, H. (1975). *Eur. J. Immunol.* **5**, 112.

Kim, U., Baumler, A., Carruthers, C. and Bielat, K. (1975). *Proc. Natl Acad. Sci. U.S.A.* **72**, 1012.

Kinsey, D. L. (1960). *Cancer* **13**, 674.

Kirchner, H., Chused, T. M., Herberman, R. B., Holden, H. T. and Larvin, D. H. (1974). *J. Exp. Med.* **139**, 1473.

Kiricuta, I., Todurutiu, C., Muresian, T. and Risca, R. (1973). *Cancer* **31**, 1392.

Klagsbrun, M., Knighton, D. and Folkman, J. (1976). *Cancer Res.* **36**, 110.

Klein, A. S., Kim, U. and Shin, S. (1978). *J. Cell. Biol.* **79**, A90 (Abs. C1-140).

Klein, G., Giovanella, B. C., Lindahl, T., Fialkow, P. J., Singh, S. and Stehlin, J. S. (1974). *Proc. Natl Acad. Sci. U.S.A.* **71**, 4737.

Kleinerman, J. and Liotta, L. (1977). *In* "Cancer Invasion and Metastasis: Biologic Mechanisms and Therapy", eds Day, S. B., Laird Myers, W. P., Stansley, P., Garattini, S. and Lewis, M. G., p. 135. Raven Press, New York.

Kleinsmith, L. J. and Pierce, G. B. (1964). *Cancer Res.* **24**, 1544.

Kohn, J., Orr, A. H., McElwain, R. J., Bentall, M. and Peckham, M. J. (1976). *Lancet* **ii**, 433.

Kolenich, J. J., Manson, E. G. and Flynn, A. (1972). *Lancet* **ii**, 714.

Koono, M., Ushijima, J. and Hayashi, H. (1974). *Internat. J. Cancer* **13**, 105.

Korst, D. R., Frenkel, E. P., Cousineau, L. and Muirhead, E. E. (1962). *In* "Erythropoiesis", eds Jacobson, L. O. and Doyle, M., p. 374. Grune and Stratton, New York.

Kovach, A. G. B., Foldi, M., Szlanka, I., Ecker, A. and Hamori, M. (1965). *Arzneim. Forsch.* **19**, 610.

Krebs, B., Turchi, P., Bonet, C., Schneider, M., Lalanne, C. M. and Nemer, N. (1977). *Eur. J. Cancer* **13**, 375.

Kripke, M. L., Budmen, M. B. and Fidler, I. J. (1977). *Cell Immunol.* **30**, 341.

Kucera, L. S. and Gusdon, J. P. (1976). *J. Gen. Virol.* **30**, 257.

Kung, J. T., Brooks, S. B., Jakway, J. P., Leonard, L. J. and Talmage, D. W. (1977). *J. Exp. Med.* **146**, 665.

Kurman, R. J., Scardino, P. T., McIntire, K. R., Waldman, T. A. and Javadpour, N. (1977). *Cancer* **40**, 2136.

Kuroda, Y. (1974). *Exp. Cell Res.* **84**, 351.

Lack, C. H. and Rogers, A. J. (1958). *Nature* **182**, 948.

Laki, K., Tyler, H. M. and Yancey, S. T. (1966). *Biochem. Biophys. Res. Commun.* **24**, 776.

Lakshmi, M. S. (1970). *Advan. Cancer Res.* **13**, 133.

Lakshmi, M. S. and Sherbet, G. V. (1974). *In* "Neoplasia and Cell Differentiation", ed. Sherbet, G. V., p. 380. Karger AG, Basle.

Lakshmi, M. S., Latner, A. L. and Sherbet, G. V. (1982). *Exp. Cell Biol.* **50**, (In press).

Lang, W. E., Jones, P. A. and Benedict, W. F. (1975). *J. Natl Cancer Inst.* **54**, 173.

Lash, J. W. (1963). *In* "Cytodifferentiation and Macromolecular Synthesis", ed. Locke, M., p. 35. Academic Press, New York and London.

Latner, A. L. and Sherbet, G. V. (1979). *Exp. Cell Biol.* **47**, 392.
Latner, A. L. and Turner, G. A. (1974). *J. Cell Sci.* **14**, 203.
Latner, A. L. and Turner, G. A. (1978). *Exp. Cell Biol.* **46**, 298.
Latner, A. L., Longstaff, E. and Lunn, J. M. (1971). *Br. J. Cancer* **25**, 568.
Latner, A. L., Longstaff, E. and Pradhan, K. (1973a). *Br. J. Cancer* **27**, 460.
Latner, A. L., Longstaff, E. and Turner, G. A. (1973b). *Br. J. Cancer* **27**, 218.
Latner, A. L., Turner, G. A. and Lamin, M. M. (1976). *Oncology* **33**, 12.
Lauder, I., Aherne, W., Stewart, J. and Sainsbury, R. (1977). *J. Clin. Pathol.* **30**, 563.
Laurence, D. J. R. and Neville, A. M. (1972). *In* Endocrinology—Proc. III Internat. Symp., ed. Taylor, S. p. 225. Heinemann, London.
Laurence, D. J. R., Stevens, U., Bettelheim, R., Darcy, D., Leese, C., Turberville, C., Alexander, P., Johns, E. W. and Neville, A. M. (1972). *Br. Med. J.* **3**, 605.
Lee, J. C. and Ihle, J. N. (1977). *J. Immunol.* **118**, 928.
Leighton, J. (1951). *J. Natl Cancer Inst.* **12**, 545.
Leighton, J. (1963). *Natl Cancer Inst. Monogr.* **11**, 157.
Leighton, J. (1967). "The Spread of Cancer", Academic Press, New York and London.
Leighton, J. (1970). *In* "Carcinoma of the Colon and Antecedent Epithelium", ed. Burdette, W. C., p. 103. Thomas, Springfield, Illinois.
Leighton, J., Kline, I., Belkin, M. and Tetenbaum, Z. (1956). *J. Natl Cancer Inst.* **16**, 1353.
Leighton, J., Kline, I., Belkin, M. and Orr, H. C. (1957). *Cancer Res.* **17**, 336.
Leighton, J., Kalla, R. L., Turner Jr, J. M. and Fennell, R. H. (1960). *Cancer Res.* **20**, 575.
Leighton, J., Justh, G., Esper, M. and Kronenthal, R. L. (1967). *Science* **155**, 1259.
Leighton, J., Mark, R. and Justh, G. (1968). *Cancer Res.* **28**, 286.
Leighton, J., Mansukhani, S. and Fetterman, G. H. (1972). *Eur. J. Cancer* **8**, 281.
Leone, V. (1953). *Tumori* **39**, 420.
Le Serve, A. W. and Hellman, K. (1972). *Br. Med. J.* **1**, 597.
Levine, L. (1977). *Nature,* **268**, 447.
Levine, L. and Hassida, A. (1977). *Biochem. Biophys. Res. Commun.* **79**, 477.
Levine, L., Hinkle, P. M., Voelkel, E. F. and Tashjian, A. H. (1972). *Biochem. Biophys. Res. Commun.* **47**, 888.
Levy, R., Hurwitz, E., Maron, R., Arnon, R. and Sela, M. (1975). *Cancer Res.* **35**, 1182.
Liddle, G. W. (1960). *J. Clin. Endocrinol.* **20**, 1539.
Likhite, V. V. (1974). *Internat. J. Cancer* **14**, 684.
Lindahl, P., Gresser, I., Leary, P. and Tovey, M. (1976). *Proc. Natl Acad. Sci. U.S.A.* **73**, 1284.
Linzer, D. I. H., Maltzman, W. and Levine, A. J. (1980). *Cold Spring Harbor Symposium Quant. Biol.* **44**, 215.
Liotta, L. A., Klinerman, J. and Saidel, G. H. (1974). *Cancer Res.* **34**, 997.
Liotta, L. A., Klinerman, J. and Saidel, G. M. (1976). *Cancer Res.* **36**, 889.
Liotta, L. A., Abe, S., Gheron, R. P. and Martin, G. R. (1979a). *Proc. Natl Acad. Sci. U.S.A.* **76**, 2268.
Liotta, L. A., Garbisa, S., Tryggvason, K., Gheron, R. P. and Martin, G. R. (1979b). *Amer. Assoc. Cancer Res. 17th Ann. Meeting,* p. 235.
Liotta, L. A., Tryggvason, K., Garbisa, S., Hart, I., Foltz, C. M. and Shafie, S. (1980). *Nature* **284**, 67.

Lipscomb, H. S., Wilson, C., Retiene, K., Matsen, F. and Ward, D. N. (1968). *Cancer Res.* **28,** 378.

Lipsett, M. B., Odell, W. D., Rosenberg, L. E. and Waldmann, T. A. (1964). *Ann. Intern. Med.* **61,** 733.

Loewenstein, M. S., Rittgers, R. A., Kupchik, H. Z. and Zamcheck, N. (1981). *J. Natl Cancer Inst.* **66,** 803.

Logroscino, D. C., Ciaccia, A. and Merelli, B. (1967). *Riv. Pathol. Clin. Sper.* **8,** 365.

Lohmann-Matthes, M. L., Schleich, A., Schantz, G. and Schirrmacher, V. (1980). *J. Natl Cancer Inst.* **64,** 1413.

Lomnitzer, R., Rabson, A. R. and Koornhof, H. J. (1976). *Clinical Exp. Immunol.* **24,** 42.

Lord, E. M., Penney, D. P., Sutherland, R. M. and Cooper, J. A. Jr (1979). *Virchow's Arch. B. Cell. Pathol.* **31,** 103.

Lotzova, E. and Richie, E. R. (1977). *J. Natl Cancer Inst.* **58,** 1171.

Luben, R. A., Mundy, G. R., Trummel, C. L. and Raisz, L. G. (1974). *J. Clin. Invest.* **53,** 1473.

Lucke-Huhle, J. and Dertinger, H. (1977). *Eur. J. Cancer* **13,** 23.

Lupulescu, A. (1978). *J. Natl Cancer Inst.* **61,** 97.

Maat, B. (1980). *Br. J. Cancer* **41,** 313.

McBride, W. H., Tauch, S. and Marmion, B. P. (1975). *Br. J. Cancer* **32,** 558.

MacCarty, W. C. (1922). *Ann. Surg.* **76,** 9.

MacCarty, W. C. and Blackford, J. M. (1912). *Ann. Surgery* **4,** 810.

McCormick, P. J., Keys, B. J., Pucci, C. and Millis, A. J. T. (1979). *Cell,* **18,** 173.

McDivitt, R. W., Stewart, F. W. and Berg, J. W. (1968). *In* "Atlas of Tumour Pathology", pp. 57-61. Armed Forces Institute of Pathology, Washington, D.C.

McDougall, J. K., Galloway, D. A. and Fenoglio, C. M. (1980). *Internat. J. Cancer* **25,** 1.

McFadzean, A. J. S. and Yeung, T. T. (1956). *Arch. Intern. Med.* **98,** 720.

MacFarlane, I. A., Barnes, D., Howat, J. M. T., Swindell, R., During, P., Beardwell, C. G., Bush, H. and Sellwood, R. A. (1980). *Br. J. Cancer* **42,** 645.

Machowka, W. W. and Schegaloff, S. B. (1935). *Roux. Arch. Entwickl. Mech.* **133,** 694.

McIlhenny, A. and Hogan, B. L. M. (1974). *Biochem. Biophys. Res. Commun.* **60,** 348.

McIntire, K. R., Bogel, C. L., Princler, G. L. and Patel, I. R. (1972). *Cancer Res.* **32,** 1941.

McIntire, K. R., Waldman, T. A., Moertel, C. G. and Go, V. L. W. (1975). *Cancer Res.* **35,** 991.

McKinney, R. and Singh, B. (1977). *Oral. Surg.* **44,** 875.

Macnab, J. C. M. (1974). *J. Gen. Virol.* **24,** 143.

McNutt, N. S. (1976). *Lab. Invest.* **35,** 132.

MacSween, J. M., Warner, N. L., Bankhurst, A. D. and MacKay, I. R. (1972). *Br. J. Cancer* **26,** 356.

McWhirter, R. (1955). *Br. J. Radiol.* **28,** 128.

Maguire, P. (1979). *Cancer Topics* **2,** 6.

Major, E. O. and Di Mayorca, G. (1973). *Proc. Natl Acad. Sci. U.S.A.,* **70,** 3210.

Malech, H. L. and Lentz, T. L. (1974). *J. Cell Biol.* **60,** 473.

Mangold, O. and Spemann, H. (1927). *Wilhelm Roux Arch. Entwickl. Mech. Org.* **111**, 341.

Mannick, J. A. and Schmid, K. (1967). *Transplantation* **5**, 1231.

Mansfield, C. M. (1976). "Early Breast Cancer", Exp. Biol. Med. Mongr. 5, eds. Wolsky, A., Pizarello, D. J., Sherbet, G. V. and Steiner, J. Karger AG, Basle and New York.

Mantovani, A. (1978). *Internat. J. Cancer* **22**, 741.

Marcus, D. M. and Zinberg, N. (1975). *J. Natl Cancer Inst.* **55**, 791.

Marczynska, B., McPherson, L., Wilbanks, G. D., Tsurumoto, D. M. and Deinhardt, F. (1980). *Exp. Cell Biol.* **48**, 114.

Mareel, M., Vakaet, L. and De Ridder, L. (1968). *Eur. J. Cancer* **4**, 249.

Mareel, M., Vakaet, L. and De Ridder, L. (1973). *J. Natl Cancer Inst.* **51**, 809.

Mareel, M., Vakaet, L., De Ridder, L., Debrabander, M., Bozzi, A. and Deman, J. (1974). *J. Natl Cancer Inst* **53**, 1351.

Mariani, G., Carmellini, M., Bonaguidi, F., Benelli, M. A. and Toni, M. G. (1980). *Eur. J. Cancer* **16**, 1009.

Markert, C. L. (1968). *Cancer Res.* **28**, 1908.

Marti, J. H. and Thomson, D. M. P. (1976). *Br. J. Cancer* **34**, 116.

Martinez-Palomo, A. (1970). *Internat. Rev. Cytol.* **29**, 29.

Martinez-Palomo, A. and Braislovsky, C. (1968). *Virology* **34**, 379.

Marynen, P., Van der Schueren, B., Van Leuven, F. and Cassiman, J. J. (1981). *Cell Biol. Int. Rep.* **5** (Suppl. A), 39.

Maslow, D. E. and Mayhew, E. (1975). *J. Natl Cancer Inst.* **54**, 1097.

Maslow, D. E. and Weiss, L. (1978). *J. Cell Sci.* **29**, 271.

Maslow, D. E. and Weiss, L. (1979). *Internat. J. Cancer* **24**, 450.

Maslow, D. E., Mayhew, E. and Minowada, J. (1976). *Cancer Res.* **36**, 2707.

Mavligit, G., Cohen, J. L. and Sherwood, L. M. (1971). *New Engl. J. Med.* **285**, 154.

Mavligit, G. M., Stickey, S. E., Cabanillas, F. F., Keating, M. I., Tourtellutte, W. W., Schold, S. C. and Freireich, E. J. (1980). *New Engl. J. Med.* **303**, 718.

May, P., Kress, M., Lange, M. and May, E. (1980). *Cold Spring Harbor Symp. Quant. Biol.* **44**, 189.

Meador, C. K., Liddle, G. W.,. Island, D. P., Nicholson, W. E., Lucas, C. P., Nuckton, J. G. and Leutscher, J. A. (1962). *J. Clin. Endocrinol.* **2**, 693.

Melick, R. A., Martin, T. J. and Hicks, J. D. (1972). *Br. Med. J.* **2**, 204.

Meltzer, M., Stevenson, M. and Leonard, E. (1977). *Cancer Res.* **37**, 721.

Mihalev, A., Tzingilev, D. and Sirakov, L. M. (1976). *Neoplasma* **23**, 103.

Milgrom, F., Humphrey, L. J., Tönder, O., Yasuda, J. and Witebsky, F. (1968). *Int. Arch. Allergy* **33**, 478.

Milhaud, G., Calmette, C., Taboulet, J., Julienne, A. and Moukhtar, M. S. (1974). *Lancet* **i**, 462.

Miller, J. A. and Miller, E. (1971). *J. Natl Cancer Inst.* **47**, V.

Mintz, B. and Cronmiller, C. (1978). *Proc. Natl Acad. Sci. U.S.A.* **75**, 6247.

Mintz, B. and Illmensee, K. (1975). *Proc. Natl Acad. Sci. U.S.A.* **72**, 3585.

Miyaji, H., Morris, H. P. and Wagner, B. P. (1968). *Methods Cancer Res.* **4**, 153.

Mizell, M. (1960). *Anat. Rec.* **137**, 382.

Mizell, M. (1961). In *Proc. Frog Kidney Adenocarcinoma Conference*, eds. Duryce, W. R. and Warner, L., p. 65.

Mizell, M. (1965). *Amer. Zool.* **5**, 215.

Mondal, S. and Heidelberger, C. (1970). *Proc. Natl Acad. Sci. U.S.A.* **65**, 219.

Moore, M. and Potter, M. R. (1980). *Br. J. Cancer* **41**, 378.
Moore, M., White, W. J. and Potter, M. R. (1980). *Internat. J. Cancer* **25**, 565.
Morgan, J. E. and Bleehan, N. M. (1981). Br. J. Cancer **43**, 384.
Morley, J. (1974). *Prostaglandins* **8**, 315.
Morris, H. P. and Wagner, B. P. (1968). *Methods Cancer Res.* **4**, 125.
Moscona, A. A. (1957). *Proc. Natl Acad. Sci. U.S.A.* **43**, 184.
Moscona, A. A. (1961). *Exp. Cell Res.* **22**, 455.
Motlik, K., Kucheland, O. and Horky, K. (1968). *Cs. Pat.* **4**, 202.
Mowbray, J. F. (1963). *Transplantation* **1**, 15.
Mowbray, J. F. and Hargrave, D. C. (1966). *Immunology* **11**, 413.
Mundy, G. R., Raisz, L. G., Cooper, R. A., Schechter, G. P. and Salmon, S. E. (1974). *New Engl. J. Med.* **291**, 1041.
Munk, K. and Darai, C. (1973). *Nature New Biol.* **241**, 268.
Munson, P. L., Tashjian, A. H. Jr and Levine, L. (1965). *Cancer Res.* **25**, 1062.
Murgita, R. A. and Tomasi, T. B. (1975a). *J. Exp. Med.* **141**, 269.
Murgita, R. A. and Tomasi, T. B. (1975b). *J. Exp. Med.* **141**, 440.
Murphy, G. P., Mirand, E. A., Johnston, G. S., Gibbons, R. P., Jones, R. L. and Scott, W. W. (1967). *Johns Hopkins Med. J.* **120**, 26.
Murray, J. C., Liotta, L., Rennard, S. I. and Martin, G. R. (1980). *Cancer Res.* **40**, 347.
Mustard, J. F., Movat, H. Z., McMorine, D. R. C. and Senyi, A. (1965). *Proc. Soc. Exp. Biol. Med.* **119**, 988.
Myers, W. P. L., Tashima, C. K. and Rothschild, E. O. (1966). *Med. Clin. N. Amer.* **50**, 763.
Nachman, R. L., Weksler, B. and Ferris, B. (1970). *J. Clin. Invest.* **49**, 274.
Nachman, R. L., Weksler, B. and Ferris, B. (1972). *J. Clin. Invest.* **51**, 549.
Nadler, W. H. and Wolfer, J. A. (1929). *Arch. Intern. Med.* **44**, 700.
Najjar, V. A. and Nishioka, K. (1970). *Nature* **228**, 672.
Nakanishi, S., Inoue, A., Kita, T., Numa, S., Chang, A. C. Y., Cohen, S. N., Nunberg, J. and Schimkl, R. T. (1978). *Proc. Natl Acad. Sci. U.S.A.* **75**, 6021.
Naor, D. (1979). *Advan. Cancer Res.* **29**, 45.
Nayak, N. C. and Mital, I. (1977). *Amer. J. Pathol.* **86**, 359.
Needham, J. (1950). "Biochemistry and Morphogenesis". Oxford University Press, Oxford and London.
Needham, J., Waddington, C. H. and Needham, D. M. (1933). *Nature* **132**, 239.
Needham, J., Waddington, C. H. and Needham, D. M. (1934). *Proc. Roy. Soc. Ser. B.* **114**, 393.
Neel, B. G., Hayward, W. S., Robinson, H. L., Fang, J. and Astrin, S. M. (1981). *Cell* **23**, 323.
Nelken, D. (1973). *J. Immunol.* **110**, 1161.
Nelken, D. and Glaser, M. (1972). *Transplantation* **14**, 268.
Nelson, D. S. (ed.) (1976). "Immunobiology of Macrophages", Academic Press, New York and London.
Nelson, K., Pollack, S. B. and Hellström, K. E. (1975a). *Internat. J. Cancer* **15**, 806.
Nelson, K., Pollack, S. B. and Hellström, K. E. (1975b). *Internat. J. Cancer* **16**, 539.
Neville, A. M. and Cooper, E. H. (1976). *Ann. Clin. Biochem.* **13**, 283.
Neville, D. M. (1968). *Biochim. Biophys. Acta* **154**, 540.
Nevo, A., deVries, A. and Katchalsky, A. (1955). *Biochim. Biophys. Acta* **17**, 536.
New, D. A. T. (1955). *J. Embryol. Exp. Morphol.* **3**, 326.

Newlands, E. S., Dent, J., Kardana, A., Searle, F. and Bagshawe, K. D. (1976). *Lancet* **ii**, 744.

Ng, A. B. P. and Atkin, N. B. (1973). *Br. J. Cancer* **28**, 322.

Nicolson, G. L. (1977). *In* "Cancer Invasion and Metastasis: Biological Mechanisms and Therapy", eds Day, S. B., Laird Myers, W. P., Stansly, P., Garattini, S. and Lewis, M. G., p. 163. Raven Press, New York.

Nicolson, G. L. (1981). *Br. Soc. Cell Biol. Conference* (Abstract), Nottingham.

Nicolson, G. L. and Winkelhake, J. L. (1975). *Nature* **255**, 230.

Nicolson, G. L., Birdwell, C. R., Brunson, K. W. and Robbins, J. C. (1976a). *J. Supramol. Struct., Suppl.* **1**, 237.

Nicolson, G. L., Birdwell, C. R., Brunson, K. W. and Robbins, J. C. (1976b). *In* "Membranes and Neoplasia: New Approaches and Strategies", ed. Marchesi, V. T., p. 237. Liss, New York.

Nicolson, G. L., Winkelhake, J. L. and Nussey, A. C. (1976c). *In* "Fundamental Aspects of Metastasis", ed. Weiss, L., p. 291. North Holland Publishing Co., Amsterdam.

Nicolson, G. L., Birdwell, C. R., Brunson, K. W., Robbins, J. C., Beattie, G. and Fidler, I. J. (1977). *In* "Cell and Tissue Interactions", eds Burger, M. M. and Lash, J., p. 225. Raven Press, New York.

Nind, A. P. P., Matthews, N., Pihl, E. A., Rolland, J. M. and Nairn, R. C. (1975). *Br. J. Cancer* **31**, 620.

Nishioka, A. (1979a). *Gann* **70**, 845.

Nishioka, A. (1979b). *Br. J. Cancer* **29**, 342.

Nishioka, A., Constantopoulos, A., Satoh, P. S. and Najjar, V. A. (1972). *Biochem. Biophys. Res. Commun.* **47**, 172.

Nishioka, A., Constantopoulos, A., Satoh, P. S., Mitchell, W. M. and Najjar, V. A. (1973). *Biochim. Biophys. Acta* **310**, 217.

Nishioka, K., Romsdahl, M. M. and McMurtrey, M. J. (1977). *J. Surg. Oncol.* **9**, 555.

Nishizaw, E., Miller, W. L., Gorman, R. R., Bundy, G. L., Svensson, J. and Hamberg, M. (1975). *Prostaglandins* **9**, 109.

North, S. M., Dean, C. J. and Styles, J. M. (1981). *Cell Biol. Intern. Rep.* **5**, (Suppl. A), 41.

North, R., Kirsten, D. and Tuttle, R. (1976). *J. Exp. Med.* **143**, 559.

Nowell, P. C. and Morris, H. P. (1969). *Cancer Res.* **29**, 969.

Nowell, P. C., Morris, H. P. and Potter, V. R. (1967). *Cancer Res.* **27**, 1565.

Nunn, M. E., Djeu, J. Y., Glaser, M., Lavrin, D. H. and Herberman, R. B. (1976). *J. Natl Cancer Inst.* **56**, 393.

Odagiri, E., Sherrell, R. J, Mount, C. D., Nicholson, W. E. and Orth, D. N. (1979). *Proc. Natl Acad. Sci. U.S.A.* **76**, 2027.

Odell, W. D., Bates, R. W., Rivlin, R. S., Lipsett, M. D. and Hertz, R. (1963). *J. Clin. Endocrinol.* **23**, 658.

Odell, W. D., Wolfson, A. F., Yoshimoto, Y., Weitzman, R., Fisher, D. A, and Hirose, F. (1977). *Trans. Assoc. Amer. Phys.* **90**, 204.

Oehler, J. R. and Herberman, R. B. (1978). *Internat. J. Cancer* **21**, 221.

Oehler, J. R., Lindsay, L. R., Nunn, M. E., Holden, H. T. and Herberman, R. B. (1978). *Internat. J. Cancer* **21**, 210.

Ogura, T., Tsubura, E. and Yamamura, Y. (1970). *Gann* **61**, 443.

Old, L. J., Stockert, E., Boyse, E. A. and Kim, J. H. (1968). *J. Exp. Med.* **127**, 523.

O'Meara, R. A. Q. (1958). *Irish J. Med. Sci.* **394**, 474.

O'Meara, R. A. Q. (1964). *Lancet* ii, 963.

Omenn, G. S. (1970). *Ann. Intern. Med.* 72, 136.

Ossowski, L. (1979). *In* "Hormones and Cell Culture Book A", eds Sato, G. H. and Ross, R., p. 249. Cold Spring Harbor Laboratory, Cold Spring Harbor.

Ossowski, L., Quigley, J. P., Kellerman, G. M. and Reich, E. (1973a). *J. Exp. Med.* 138, 1056.

Ossowski, L., Unkeless, J. C., Tobia, A., Quigley, J. P., Rifkin, D. B. and Reich, E. (1973b). *J. Exp. Med.* 137, 112.

O'Steen, W. K. and Walker, B. E. (1961). *Anat. Rec.* 139, 547.

Ottoson, R. and Sylvén, B. (1960). *Arch. Biochem, Biophys.* 87, 41.

Otu, A. A., Russell, R. J., Wilkinson, P. C. and White, R. G. (1977). *Br. J. Cancer* 36, 330.

Ovadia, H., Hanna, N. and Nelken, D. (1975). *Eur. J. Cancer* 11, 413.

Owen, K., Gomulka, D. and Droller, M. J. (1980). *Cancer Res.* 40, 3167.

Owers, N. O. (1970). *Anat. Rec.* 166, 358.

Owers, N. O. and Blandau, R. G. (1971). *In* "Biology of the Blastocyst", ed. Blandau, R. G., p. 207. University of Chicago Press, Chicago.

Ozaki, T., Yoshida, K., Ushijima, K. and Hayashi, H. (1971). *Internat. J. Cancer* 7, 93.

Padgett, B. L. and Walker, D. L. (1976). *Progr. Med. Virol.* 22, 1.

Padgett, B. L. and Walker, D. L., ZuRhein, G. M. and Varakis, J. V. (1977). *Cancer Res.* 37, 718.

Pagano, R. E. and Takeichi, M. (1977). *J. Cell Biol.* 74, 531.

Paget, S. (1889). *Lancet* i, 571.

Pagnini, C. A., Palma, P. D. and De Laurentii, G. (1980). *Br. J. Cancer* 41, 415.

Paik, Y. K., Kimura, L., Yanagihava, E., Ochiai, H., Tam, R., Muraoka, M. and Hokama, Y. (1972). *J. Reticuloendothel. Soc.* 11, 420.

Palayoor, S. T. and Batra, B. K. (1971). *Ind. J. Exp. Biol.* 9, 300.

Papadimitriou, J. M. and Woods, A. E. (1975). *J. Pathol.* 116, 65.

Papageorgiou, P. S., Sorokin, C., Kouzoutzakoglou, K. and Glader, P. R. (1971). *Nature* 231, 47.

Papermaster, B. W., McEntire, J. E., Skisak, C. M., Robbins, C. H., Scott, J., Buchok, S. J., Smith, M. E., Miller, A. S. and Hokanson, J. A. (1978). *In* "Human Lymphocyte Differentiation: Its Application to Cancer", eds Serrou, B. and Rosenfeld, C., p. 391. North Holland Publishing Co., Amsterdam.

Parks, R. C. (1974). *J. Natl Cancer Inst.* 52, 971.

Paterson, R. (1948). "Treatment of Malignant Disease by Radium and X-rays". p. 309. Edward Arnold, London.

Patey, D. H. and Scarff, R. W. (1928). *Lancet* i, 801.

Patey, D. H. and Scarff, R. W. (1929). *Lancet* ii, 492.

Paul, J. (1978). *In* "Cell Differentiation and Neoplasia", ed. Saunders, G. F., p. 525. Raven Press, New York.

Payne, G. S., Courtneidge, S. A., Crittenden, L. B., Fadly, A. M., Bishop, J. M. and Varmus, H. E. (1981). *Cell* 23, 311.

Peckham, M. A., Nishizawa, E. E. and Mustard, J. F. (1968). *Biochem. Pharmacol.* 17, (Suppl.), 171.

Penn, I. (1977). *Tranpl. Proc.* 9, 1121.

Pessac, B. and Defendi, V. (1972). *Science* 175, 898.

Petermann, M. L. and Hogness, K. R. (1948). *Cancer* 1, 100.

Petricciani, J. C. (1977). Presented at the Lord Dowding Fund Conference, London, January 1977.

Pierres, M., Germain, R. M., Dorf, M. E. and Benacerraf, B. (1977). *Proc. Natl Acad. Sci. U.S.A.* **74**, 3975.

Piller, N. B. (1976a). *Br. J. Exp. Pathol.* **57**, 411.

Piller, N. B. (1976b). *Arzneim. Forsch.* **27**, 860.

Piller, N. B. (1977). *Lymphologie* **1**, 106.

Piller, N. B. (1978). *Br. J. Exp. Pathol.* **59**, 93.

Pimm, M. V. and Baldwin, R. W. (1975). *Internat. J. Cancer* **15**, 260.

Pimm, M. V. and Baldwin, R. W. (1977). *Internat. J. Cancer* **20**, 37.

Pimm, M. V. and Baldwin, R. W. (1978). *In* "Secondary Spread of Cancer", ed. Baldwin, R. W., p. 163. Academic Press, London and New York.

Pinaev, G., Hoorn, B. and Albertsson, P. Å. (1976). *Exp. Cell. Res.* **98**, 127.

Pitot, H. C. and Heidelberger, C. (1963). *Cancer Res.* **23**, 1694.

Plescia, O. J., Smith, A. H. and Grinwich, K. (1975). *Proc. Natl Acad. Sci. U.S.A.* **72**, 1848.

Podolsky, D. K. and Weiser, M. M. (1978). *Gastroenterology* **74**, 1140.

Poggi, A., Mussoni, L., Kornblihtt, L., Ballabio, E., Degaetano, G. and Donati, M. B. (1978). *Lancet* **i**, 163.

Polverini, P. J., Cotran, R. S., Gimbrone, Jr, M. A. and Unanue, E. R. (1977). *Nature* **269**, 804.

Poole, A. R. (1973). *In* "Lysosomes in Biology and Pathology", ed Dingle, J. T., Vol. 2, p. 303. North Holland Publishing Co., Amsterdam.

Portolani, M., Borgatti, M., Corallini, A., Cassai, E., Grossi, M. P., Barbanti-Brodano, G. and Passati, L. (1978). *J. Gen. Virol.* **38**, 369.

Poste, G. (1971). *Exp. Cell Res.* **65**, 359.

Poste, G. (1973). *Exp. Cell Res.* **77**, 264.

Poste, G. (1975). *Cancer Res.* **35**, 2558.

Poste, G. (1977). *In* "Cancer Invasion and Metastasis", eds Day, S. B., Stansly, P., Laird Myers, W. P., Garattini, S. and Lewis, M. G., p. 19. Raven Press, New York.

Poste, G. and Nicolson, G. (1980). *Proc. Natl Acad. Sci. U.S.A.* **77**, 399.

Potter, M., Rahey, J. L. and Pilgrim, H. I. (1957). *Proc. Soc. Exp. Biol. Med.* **94**, 327.

Potter, V. R. (1961). *Cancer Res.* **21**, 1331.

Potter, V. R. and Watanabe, M. (1968). In *Proc. Internat. Conf. Leukemia—Lymphoma*, ed. Zarafonetis, C. J. D., p. 33. Lea and Fabiger, Philadelphia.

Poupon, M. F., Kolb, J. P. and Lespinats, G. (1976). *J. Natl Cancer Inst.* **57**, 1241.

Powles, T. J., Easty, G. C., Easty, D. M. and Neville, A. M. (1973a). *Lancet* **ii**, 100.

Powles, T. J., Easty, G. C., Easty, D. M., Bondy, P. K. and Neville, A. M. (1973b). *Nature New Biol.* **245**, 83.

Powles, T. J., Leese, C. L. and Bondy, P. K. (1975). *Br. Med. J.* **2**, 164.

Powles, T. J., Dowsett, M., Easty, D. M., Easty, G. C. and Neville, A. M. (1976). *Lancet* **i**, 608.

Powles, T. J., Easty, G. C., Easty, D. M., Dowsett, M. and Neville, A. M. (1977). *In* "Cancer Invasion and Metastasis: Biologic Mechanisms and Therapy", eds Day, S. B., Laird Myers, W. P., Stansly, P., Garattini, S. and Lewis, M. G., p. 425. Raven Press, New York.

Prehn, R. T. and Main, J. M. (1957). *J. Natl Cancer Inst.* **18**, 769.

Price, M. R. and Stoddart, R. W. (1976). *Biochem. Soc. Trans.* **4**, 673.

Pritchard, D. G., Todd, C. W. and Egan, M. L. (1978). *Methods Cancer Res.* **14**, 55.

Proctor, J. W., Auclair, B. G. and Lewis, M. G. (1976). *Eur. J. Cancer* **12**, 203.

Proctor, J. W., Auclair, B. G. and Rudenstam, C. M. (1977). *Internat. J. Cancer* **18**, 255.

Puccetti, P. and Holden, H. T. (1979). *Internat. J. Cancer* **23**, 123.

Puissant, M. and Benvenista, M. (1971). *Progr. Med. (Paris)* **99**, 239.

Purdom, L., Ambrose, E. J. and Klein, G. (1958). *Nature* **191**, 1586.

Purves, L. R., Branch, W. R., Geddes, E. W., Manso, C. and Portugal, M. (1973). *Cancer* **31**, 578.

Quan, P. C. and Burtin, P. (1978). *In* "Human Lymphocyte Differentiation: Its Application to Cancer", eds Serrou, B. and Rosenfeld, C., p. 387. Elsevier and North Holland Publ. Co., Amsterdam.

Quagliata, F., Lawrence, W. J. M. and Phillips-Quagliata, J. M. (1973). *Cell Immunol.* **6**, 457.

Quigley, J. P. (1976). *J. Cell Biol.* **71**, 472.

Rabinovitch, M. and DeStefano, M. J. (1974). *Exp. Cell Res.* **88**, 153.

Rae-Venter, B. and Reid, L. M. (1980). *Cancer Res* **40**, 95.

Ran, M. and Witz, I. P. (1970). *Internat. J. Cancer* **6**, 361.

Ran, M. and Witz, I. P. (1972). *Internat. J. Cancer* **9**, 242.

Rao, V. S. and Bonavida, B. (1976). *Cancer Res.* **36**, 1384.

Rao, V. S. and Bonavida, B. (1977). *Cancer Res.* **37**, 3385.

Rapp, F. and Duff, R. (1973). *Cancer Res.* **33**, 1527.

Rashid, S. A., Cooper, E. H., Axon, A. T. R. and Eaves, G. (1980). *Biomedicine* **33**, 112.

Ratcliffe, J. G., Scott, A. P., Bennett, H. P. J., Lowry, P. J., McMartin, C., Strong, J. A. and Walbaum, P. R. (1973). *Clin. Endocrinol.* **2**, 51.

Ray, P. K. and Chatterjee, S. (1975). *Experientia* **31**, 1075.

Raz, A., McLellan, W. L., Hart, I., Bucana, C. D., Hoyer, L. C., Sela, B. M., Dragsten, P. and Fidler, I. J. (1980a). *Cancer Res.* **40**, 1645.

Raz, A., Bucana, C. D., McLellan, W. L. and Fidler, I. J. (1980b). *Nature* **284**, 363.

Reading, C. L., Belloni, P. N. and Nicolson, G. L. (1980). *J. Natl Cancer Inst.* **62**, 1241.

Reddi, N. K. and Holland, J. F. (1976). *Proc. Natl Acad. Sci. U.S.A.* **73**, 2308.

Reich, E. (1974). *In* "Control of Proliferation in Animal Cells", eds Clarkson, B. and Baserga, R., p. 351. Cold Spring Harbor Laboratory, Cold Spring Harbor.

Reid, L. M., Minato, N., Gresser, I., Holland, J., Kadish, A., and Bloom, B. R. (1981). *Proc. Natl Acad. Sci. U.S.A.* **78**, 1171.

Reiman, S. P. (1929). *Arch. Pathol.* **8**, 803.

Reitherman, R., Flanagan, S. D. and Barondes, S. H. (1973). *Biochim. Biophys. Acta* **297**, 193.

Renger, H. C. and Basilico, C. (1972). *Proc. Natl Acad. Sci. U.S.A.* **69**, 109.

Renger, H. C. and Basilico, C. (1973). *J. Virol.* **11**, 702.

Retik, A. B., Arons, M. S., Ketcham, A. S. and Mantel, N. (1962). *J. Surg. Res.* **2**, 49.

Reynoso, G., Chu, T. M., Guinan, P. and Murphy, G. P. (1972). *Cancer* **30**, 1.

Richmond, J. J. (1959). *In* "Cancer" ed. Raven, R. W., p. 375. Butterworths, London.

Rifkin, D., Loeb, J. N., Moore, E. and Reich, E. (1974). *J. Exp. Med.* **139**, 1317.
Risely, G. P. and Sherbet, G. V. (1981). *Cell Biol. Intern. Rep.* **5**, (Suppl. A), 47.
Robb, J. A., Smith, H. S. and Scher, C. D. (1972). *J. Virol.* **9**, 969.
Roberts, J. L., Phillips, M., Rosa, P. A. and Herbert, E. (1978). *Biochemistry* **17**, 3609.
Robertson, D. M. and Williams, D. C. (1969). *Nature* **221**, 259.
Roblin, R., Hammond, M. E., Bensky, N. D., Dvorak, A. M., Dvorak, H. F. and Black, P. H. (1977). *Proc. Natl Acad. Sci. U.S.A.* **74**, 1570.
Roder, J. C. and Duwe, A. K. (1979). *Nature* **278**, 451.
Roder, J. C., Ahrlund-Richter, L. and Jondal, M. (1979). *J. Exp. Med.* **150**, 471.
Roder, J. C., Haliotis, T., Klein, M., Korec, S., Jett, J. R., Ortaldo, J., Herberman, R. B., Katz, P. and Fauci, A. S. (1980). *Nature* **284**, 553.
Rolland, P. H., Martin, P. M., Jacquimies, J., Rolland, A. M. and Toga, M. (1980). *J. Natl Cancer Inst.* **64**, 1061.
Röller, M., Owen, S. P. and Heidleberger, C. (1966). *Cancer Res.* **26**, 626.
Romsdahl, M. D., Chu, E. W., Hume, R. and Smith, R. R. (1961). *Cancer* **14**, 883.
Roos, E., Dingemans, K. P., Van de Paverk, I. V. and Van den Bergh Wearman, M. (1977). *J. Natl Cancer Inst.* **58**, 399.
Rosato, F. E. and Seltzer, M. H. (1969). *Amer. J. Surg.* **118**, 61.
Rose, S. M. and Rose, F. C. (1952). *Cancer Res.* **12**, 1.
Rose, S. M. and Wallingford, H. M. (1948). *Science* **107**, 457.
Rosen, S. W. and Weintraub, B. D. (1974). *New Engl. J. Med.* **290**, 1441.
Ross, E. J. (1972). *Br. Med. J.* **1**, 735.
Rosse, W. F., Waldeman, T. A. and Cohen, P. (1963a). *Amer. J. Med.* **34**, 76.
Rosse, W. F., Berry, R. J. and Waldmann, T. A. (1963b). *J. Clin. Invest.* **42**, 124.
Rostedt, I. (1968). *Scand. J. Lab. Invest.* **21**, (Suppl. 101), 49.
Rostedt, I. (1971). *Ann. Med. Exp. Biol. Fenn.* **49**, 186.
Rous, P. and Kidd, J. G. (1941). *J. Exp. Med.* **73**, 365.
Rubens, L. N. (1955). *J. Exp. Zool.* **128**, 29.
Rubens, L. N. and Balls, M. (1964a). *J. Morphol.* **115**, 225.
Rubens, L. N. and Balls, M. (1964b). *J. Morphol.* **115**, 239.
Ruckley, C. V., Das, P. C., Leitch, A. G., Donaldson, A. A., Copland, W. A., Redpath, A. T., Scott, P. and Cash, J. D. (1970). *Br. Med. J.* **4**, 395.
Ruco, L. P. and Meltzer, M. S. (1977). *J. Immunol.* **119**, 889.
Rudnick, P. and Odell, W. D. (1971). *New Engl. J. Med.* **284**, 405.
Rundell, K., Hearing, P. and Yang, Y. C. (1980). *Cold Spring Harbor Symp. Quant. Biol.* **44**, 211.
Rungger-Brändle, E. and Gabbiani, G. (1980). *Eur. J. Cancer* **16**, 12.
Ruoslahti, E., Pihko, H. and Seppälä, M. (1974). *Transpl. Rev.* **20**, 38.
Russel, B. R. (1980). *Sci. Report Imperial Cancer Res. Fund* **3**, 341.
Russel, D. H. (1971). *Nature New Biol.* **233**, 144.
Russel, D. H. and Levy, C. C. (1971). *Cancer Res.* **31**, 248.
Russel, D. H. and Russel, S. D. (1975). *Clin. Chem.* **21**, 860.
Rutter, W. J., Wessels, N. K. and Grobstein, C. (1964). *Natl Cancer Inst. Monogr.* **13**, 51.
Saba, T. and Antikatzides, T. G. (1975). *Br. J. Cancer* **32**, 471.
Sabin, A. B. and Koch, M. A. (1963). *Proc. Natl Acad. Sci. U.S.A.* **50**, 407.
Sachs, B. A. (1965). *Bull. N.Y. Acad. Med.* **41**, 1069.
Sachtleben, P., Gsell, R. and Mehrishi, J. N. (1972). *Vox Sang.* **25**, 519.

Saito, D., Sawamura, M., Umezawa, K., Kanai, Y., Furihata, C., Matshushima, T. and Sugimura, T. (1980). *Cancer Res.* **40**, 2539.

Salomon, J. C., Chassoux, D. and Yao, C. S. (1980). In *Proc. EORTC Conf. on Metastasis*, London, Abs. 4.3.

Salsbury, A. J. (1975). *Cancer Treatment Rev.* **2**, 55.

Salsbury, A. J., Burrage, K. and Hellmann, K. (1970). *Br. Med. J.* **4**, 344.

Sambrook, J., Westphal, H., Srinivasan, P. R. and Dulbecco, R. (1968). *Proc. Natl Acad. Sci. U.S.A.* **60**, 1288.

Sanders, F. K. and Burford, B. O. (1967). *Nature* **213**, 1171.

Santoro, M. G., Philpott, G. W. and Gaffe, B. M. (1976). *Nature* **263**, 777.

Saxén, L. and Toivonen, S. (1962). "Primary Embryonic Induction", Logos/ Academic Press, London and New York.

Schenk, P. (1975). *Krebsforschung* **84**, 241.

Scher, C. D., Haudenschild, C. and Klagsbrun, M. (1976). *Cell* **8**, 373.

Scherneck, S., Lübbe, L., Geissler, E., Nisch, G., Rudolph, M., Wählte, H., Weickmann, F. and Zimmermann, W. (1979a). *Zbl. Neurochir.* **40**, 121.

Scherneck, S., Rudolph, M., Geissler, E., Vogel, F., Lübbe, L., Wählte, H., Nisch, G., Weickmann, F. and Zimmermann, W. (1979b). *Internat. J. Cancer* **24**, 523.

Schirrmacher, V. (1979). *Internat. J. Cancer* **24**, 80.

Schirrmacher, V. and Jacobs, W. (1979). *J. Supramolec. Str.* **11**, 105.

Schirrmacher, V., Shantz, G., Clauer, K., Komitowski, D., Zimmermann, H. P. and Lohmann-Matthes, M. L. (1979a). *Internat. J. Cancer* **23**, 233.

Schirrmacher, V., Bosslet, K., Shantz, G., Clauer, K. and Hübsch, D. (1979b). *Internat. J. Cancer* **23**, 245.

Schleich, A. (1967). *Eur. J. Cancer* **3**, 243.

Schleich, A. (1973). *In* "Chemotherapy of Cancer Dissemination and Metastasis", eds Garattini, S. and Franchi, G., p. 51. Raven Press, New York.

Schleich, A. (1976). *In* "Human Tumours in Short Term Culture", ed. Dendy, P. P., p. 55. Academic Press, London and New York.

Schmidt, M. and Good, R. A. (1975). *J. Natl Cancer Inst.* **5**, 81.

Schnebli, H. P. (1974). *In* "Proteinase Inhibitors", eds. Fritz, H., Tschesche, H., Greene, L. J. and Trutscheit, E., p. 615. Springer, Berlin.

Schnebli, H. P. and Burger, M. M. (1972). *Proc. Natl Acad. Sci. U.S.A.* **69**, 3825.

Schonfeld, A., Babbett, D. and Gundersen, K. (1961). *New Engl. J. Med.* **265**, 231.

Schor, A. M., Schor, S. L. and Kumar, S. (1979). *Internat. J. Cancer* **24**, 225.

Schor, A. M., Schor, S. L., Weiss, J. B., Brown, R. A., Kumar, S. and Phillips, P. (1980). *Br. J. Cancer* **41**, 790.

Schultz, R. M., Papamattheakis, J. D. and Chirigos, M. A. (1977a). *Science* **197**, 674.

Schultz, R. M., Papamattheakis, J. D., Leutzeler, J. and Chirigos, M. A. (1977b). *Cancer Res.* **37**, 3338.

Schwartz, M. K. (1976). *Cancer* **37**, 542.

Schwartz, W. B., Bennett, W., Curelop, S. and Bartter, F. C. (1957). *Amer. J. Med.* **23**, 529.

Scott, M. T. (1974). *J. Natl Cancer Inst.* **53**, 855.

Scott, R. B. and Bell, E. (1965). *Science* **147**, 405.

Sefton, B. M. and Rubin, H. (1970). *Nature* **227**, 843.

Segal, S., Gorelik, E., Isakov, N. and Feldman, M. (1980). In *Proc. EORTC Metastasis Conference*, London, Abs. 4.2.

Seibert, F. B., Seibert, M. V., Atno, A. J. and Campbell, H. W. (1947). *J. Clin. Invest.* **26**, 90.

Seilern-Aspang, F. and Kratochwil, K. (1962). *J. Embryol. Exp. Morhol.* **10**, 337.

Seilern-Aspang, F. and Kratochwil, K. (1963a). *Arch. Geschwultforsch.* **21**, 293.

Seilern-Aspang, F. and Kratochwil, K. (1963b). *Wien. Klin. Wschr.* **19**, 337.

Seilern-Aspang, F. and Kratochwil, K. (1963c). *Acta Biol. Med. Germ.* **10**, 443.

Seilern-Aspang, F. and Kratochwil, K. (1965). *In* "Regeneration in Animals and Related Problems", ed. Kiortsis, V. and Tramusch, H. A. L., p. 452. North-Holland Publ. Co., Amsterdam.

Seilern-Aspang, F. and Weissberg, M. (1963). *Acta Biol. Med. Germ.* **10**, 439.

Seilern-Aspang, F., Honus, E. and Kratochwil, K. (1963a). *Acta Biol. Med. Germ.* **11**, 281.

Seilern-Aspang, F., Honus, E. and Kratochwil, K. (1963b). *Acta Biol. Med. Germ.* **10**, 447.

Sell, H. T. and Wepsic, S. (1975). *In* "The Liver, the Molecular Biology of its Diseases", ed. Becker, F., p. 773. Marcel Dekker, New York.

Sell, S., Nichols, M., Becker, F. F. and Leffeit, H. L. (1974). *Cancer Res* **34**, 865.

Sendo, F., Aoki, T., Boyse, E. A. and Buofo, C. K. (1975). *J. Natl Cancer Inst.* **55**, 603.

Seyberth, H. W., Segre, G. V., Morgan, J. L., Sweetman, B. J., Potts, J. T. and Oates, J. A. (1975). *New Engl. J. Med.* **293**, 1278.

Seyberth, H. W., Raisz, L. G. and Oates, J. A. (1978). *Ann. Rev. Med.* **29**, 23.

Shah, K. V., Daniel, R. W. and Worszawski, S. (1973). *J. Infect. Dis.* **128**, 784.

Shah, K. V., Daniel, R. W. and Strandber, J. D. (1975). *J. Natl Cancer Inst.* **54**, 945.

Shanbag, V. P. and Axelsson, C. G. (1975). *Eur. J. Biochem.* **60**, 17.

Sharin, A. T., Delwiche, R., Zamchek, N., Lokich, J. J. and Frei, E. (1974). *Cancer* **33**, 1239.

Shearman, P. J., Gallatin, W. M. and Longnecker, B. M. (1980). *Nature* **286**, 267.

Sheil, A. G. (1977). *Tranpl. Proc.* **9**, 1133.

Shellam, G. R. (1977). *Internat. J. Cancer* **19**, 225.

Shellam, G. R. and Hogg, N. (1977). *Internat. J. Cancer* **19**, 212.

Sheppard, J. R. (1972). *Nature New Biol.* **236**, 14.

Sherbet, G. V. (1962). *Naturwissenschaften* **49**, 471.

Sherbet, G. V. (1963). *J. Embryol. Exp. Morphol.* **11**, 227.

Sherbet, G. V. (1966). *Progr. Biophys. Mol. Biol.* **16**, 89.

Sherbet, G. V. (1970). *Advan. Cancer Res.* **13**, 97.

Sherbet, G. V. (1974a). *In* "Neoplasia and Cell Differentiation", ed. Sherbet, G. V., pp. XII-XIV. Karger, Basle and New York.

Sherbet, G. V. (1974b). *Ann. N. Y. Acad. Sci.* **230**, 516.

Sherbet, G. V. (1978). "The Biophysical Characterisation of the Cell Surface", Academic Press, London and New York.

Sherbet, G. V. (ed.) (1981). "Regulation of Growth in Neoplasia". S. Karger AG, Basle.

Sherbet, G. V. and Lakshmi, M. S. (1967a). *Nature* **215**, 1089.

Sherbet, G. V. and Lakshmi, M. S. (1967b). *Experientia* **23**, 969.

Sherbet, G. V. and Lakshmi, M. S. (1968a). *Nature* **217**, 1257.

Sherbet, G. V. and Lakshmi, M. S. (1968b). *Br. Empire Cancer Campaign Ann. Report* p. 57.

Sherbet, G. V. and Lakshmi, M. S. (1968c). *Br. Empire Cancer Campaign Ann. Report* p. 61.

Sherbet, G. V. and Lakshmi, M. S. (1969a). *Experientia* **25**, 481.

Sherbet, G. V. and Lakshmi, M. S. (1969b). *Experientia* **25**, 1130.

Sherbet, G. V. and Lakshmi, M. S. (1970). *Oncology* **24**, 58.

Sherbet, G. V. and Lakshmi, M. S. (1971) *Oncology* **25**, 558.

Sherbet, G. V. and Lakshmi, M. S. (1973). *Biochim. Biophys. Acta* **298**, 50.

Sherbet, G. V. and Lakshmi, M. S. (1974a). *Oncology* **29**, 335.

Sherbet, G. V. and Lakshmi, M. S. (1974b). *Differentiation* **2**, 51.

Sherbet, G. V. and Lakshmi, M. S. (1974c). *J. Natl Cancer Inst.* **52**, 681.

Sherbet, G. V. and Lakshmi, M. S. (1974d). *J. Natl Cancer Inst.* **52**, 687.

Sherbet, G. V. and Lakshmi, M. S. (1976). *In* "Molecular Base of Malignancy", eds Deutsch, E., Moser, K., Rainer, H. and Stacher, A., p. 5. Georg Thieme, Stuttgart.

Sherbet, G. V. and Lakshmi, M. S. (1978a). *Eur. J. Cancer* **14**, 415.

Sherbet, G. V. and Lakshmi, M. S. (1978b). *Exp. Cell Biol.* **46**, 82.

Sherbet, G. V. and Lakshmi, M. S. (1979a). *Exp. Cell Biol.* **47**, 61.

Sherbet, G. V. and Lakshmi, M. S. (1979b). *In* "The Year Book of Cancer", eds. Clark, R. L., Cumley, R. W. and Hickey, R. S., p. 424. Year Book Medical Publishers Inc., Chicago.

Sherbet, G. V. and Lakshmi, M. S. (1981a). *Exp. Cell Biol.* **49**, 267.

Sherbet, G. V. and Lakshmi, M. S. (1981b). *In* "Metastasis: Clinical and Experimental Aspects", eds Hellmann, K., Hilgard, P. and Eccles, S., p. 38. Martinus Nijhoff Publ., The Hague.

Sherbet, G. V. and Mulherkar, L. (1963). *Roux Arch. Entwickl. Mech.* **154**, 506.

Sherbet, G. V. and Mulherkar, L. (1965). *Roux Arch. Entwickl. Mech.* **155**, 701.

Sherbet, G. V., Lakshmi, M. S. and Morris, H. P. (1969). *Br. Empire Cancer Res. Campaign Ann. Report* p. 109.

Sherbet, G. V., Lakshmi, M. S. and Morris, H. P. (1970). *J. Natl Cancer Inst.* **45**, 419.

Sherbet, G. V., Lakshmi, M. S. and Rao, K. V. (1972). *Exp. Cell Res.* **70**, 113.

Sherbet, G. V., Lakshmi, M. S. and Coakham, H. B. (1974). *Internat. Res. Commun. System* **2**, 1485.

Sherbet, G. V., Lakshmi, M. S. and Haddad, S. K. (1977). *J. Neurosurg.* **47**, 864.

Sherbet, G. V., Lakshmi, M. S. and Guy, D. (1980). *Eur. J. Cancer* **16**, 561.

Sherbet, G. V., Lakshmi, M. S., Risely, G. P., Shah, S. A. and Tindle, M. E. (1982). *Experientia.* In press.

Sheremetieva, E. A. (1965). *J. Exp. Zool.* **158**, 101.

Sherman, M. I., Strickland, S. and Reich, E. (1976). *Cancer Res.* **36**, 4208.

Sherwood, L. M., O'Riordan, J. L. H., Aurbach, G. D. and Potts, J. T. Jr (1967). *J. Clin. Endocrinol.* **27**, 140.

Shih, C., Padhy, L. C., Murray, M. and Weinberg, R. A. (1981). *Nature,* **290**, 261.

Shimosato, Y., Kameya, T., Nagai, K., Hiroshi, S., Koide, T. and Nomura, T. (1976). *J. Natl Cancer Inst.* **56**, 1251.

Shiu, R. P. C., Pouyssegur, J. and Pastan, I. (1977). *Proc. Natl Acad. Sci. U.S.A.* **74**, 3840.

Shivas, A. A. and Finlayson, N. D. C. (1965). *Br. J. Cancer* **19**, 486.

Shuster, J., Freedman, S. O. and Gold, P. (1977). *Amer. J. Clin. Pathol.* **68**, 679.

Siciliano, M. J., Bordelon, M. R. and Humphrey, R. M. (1978). *In* "Cell Differentiation and Neoplasia", ed. Saunders, G. F., p. 509. Raven Press, New York.

Sidky, Y. A. and Auerbach, R. (1976). *Science* **192**, 1237.

Sigot-Luizard, M. F. (1974). *In* "Neoplasia and Cell Differentiation", ed. Sherbet, G. V., p. 350. Karger AG, Basle.

Sikovics, J. G. and Györkey, F. (1973). *J. Med.* **4**, 282.

Silva, O. L., Becker, K. I., Primack, A., Doppman, J. and Snider, R. H. (1974). *Eur. J. Cancer* **5**, 331.

Sindelas, W. F., Tralka, T. S. and Ketcham, A. S. (1975). *J. Surg. Res.* **18**, 137.

Sisskin, E. E., Weinstein, J. B., Evans, C. H. and Di Paolo, J. A. (1980). *Internat. J. Cancer* **33**, 331.

Sistrunk, W. E. and MacCarty, W. C. (1922). *Ann. Surgery* **75**, 61.

Sivak, A. and Van Duuren, B. L. (1969). *Cancer Res.* **29**, 624.

Sjögren, H. O., Hellström, I., Bansal, S. C. and Hellström, K. E. (1971). *Proc. Natl Acad. Sci. U.S.A.* **68**, 1372.

Slaughter, D. and Triplett, E. (1975a). *Cell Differentiation* **4**, 11.

Slaughter, D. and Triplett, E. (1975b). *Cell Differentiation* **4**, 23.

Slayter, H. S. and Coligan, J. E. (1975). *Biochemistry* **14**, 2323.

Smith, G. V. S. and Bartlett, M. K. (1929). *Surgery Gynec. Obstet.* **48**, 314.

Smith, I. E. (1981). *Cancer Topics* **3**, 412.

Smith, J., Silver, M., Ingerman, C. and Kocsis, J. (1976). *J. Thromb. Res.* **5**, 291.

Smith, J. B. and Willis, A. L. (1971). *Nature New Biol.* **231**, 235.

Smith, J. W., Steiner, A. L. and Parker, C. W. (1971). *J. Clin. Invest.* **50**, 442.

Snodgrass, M., Harris, T., Geeraets, R. and Kaplan, A. (1977). *J. Reticuloendothel. Soc.* **22**, 149.

Snyderman, R. and Pike, M. (1976). *In* "The Macrophage in Neoplasia", ed. Fink, M., p. 49. Academic Press, New York and London.

Snyderman, R., Pike, M., Blaylock, B. and Weinstein, P. (1976). *J. Immunol.* **116**, 585.

Solomon, J. B. (1964). *Folia Biol. (Prague)* **10**, 268.

Sorgente, N., Knettner, K. E., Soble, L. W. and Eisenstein, R. (1975). *Lab. Invest.* **32**, 217.

Späti, B., Child, J. A., Kerruish, S. M. and Cooper, E. H. (1980). *Acta Haematol.* **64**, 79.

Spemann, H. (1938). "Embryonic Development and Induction". Yale University Press, New Haven.

Spemann, H. and Mangold, H. (1924). *Roux' Arch. Entwickl. Mech. Org.* **100**, 599.

Staab, H. J., Anderer, F. A., Stumpf, E. and Fischer, R. (1980). *Br. J. Cancer* **42**, 26.

Stackpole, C. W. (1981). *Nature* **289**, 798.

Steigbeigel, N., Oppenheim, J., Fishman, l. M. and Carbone, P. (1964). *New Engl. J. Med.* **271**, 345.

Steinberg, M. S. (1970). *J. Exp. Zool.* **173**, 395.

Steinberg, M. S. (1978). *In* "Cell-Cell Recognition", ed. Curtis, A.S.G., p. 25. Cambridge University Press, Cambridge and London.

Steinberg, M. S., Armstrong, P. B. and Granger, R. E. (1973). *J. Memb. Biol.* **13**, 97.

Stein-Werblowsky, R. (1978). *Br. J. Exp. Pathol.* **59**, 386.

Stein-Werblowsky, R. (1980). *Experientia* **36**, 108.

Stevens, D. A. (1973). *Natl Cancer Inst. Monogr.* **36**, 55.

Steward, E. M., Nixon, D., Zamcheck, N. and Aisenberg, A. (1974). *Cancer* **33**, 1246.

Stitleler, R. D., Proctor, J. W., Yamamura, Y. and Mansell, P. W. A. (1978). *J. Reticuloendothel. Soc.* **24**, 687.

Stjernswärd, J. and Douglas, P. (1977). *In* "Cancer Invasion and metastasis: Biologic Mechanisms and Therapy", eds Day, S. B., Laird Myers, W. B., Stansly, P., Garattini, S. and Lewis, M. G., p. 319. Raven Press, New York.

Stoddart, R. W., Collins, R. D. and Jacobson, W. (1974). *Biochem. Soc. Trans.* **2**, 481.

Stoker, M. G. P. and Rubin, H. (1967). *Nature* **215**, 171.

Stossel, T. P. (1975). *Seminars Haematol.* **12**, 83.

Strauch, L. (1971). *In* "Rheumatoid Arthritis—pathogenic Mechanisms and Consequences in Therapeutics", eds Müller, W., Harwerth, H. G. and Fehr, K., p. 157. Academic Press, London and New York.

Strauch, L. (1972). *In* "Tissue Interactions in Carcinogenesis", ed. Tarin, D., p. 399. Academic Press, London and New York.

Sträuli, P. and Weiss, L. (1977). *Eur. J. Cancer* **13**, 1.

Strausser, H. R. and Humes, J. L. (1975). *Internat. J. Cancer* **15**, 724.

Strickland, S., Reich, E. and Sherman, M. I. (1976). *Cell* **9**, 231.

Stringfellow, D. A. and Fitzpatrick, F. A. (1979). *Nature* **282**, 76.

Stuhimiller, G. M. and Seigler, H. F. (1977). *J. Natl Cancer Inst.* **58**, 215.

Stutman, O. (1973). *Transplan. Proc.* **5**, 969.

Stutman, O. (1975). *Advan. Cancer Res.* **22**, 261.

Suddith, R. L., Kelly, P. J., Hutchinson, H. T., Murray, E. A. and Haber, B. (1975). *Science* **190**, 682.

Sugarbaker, E. V. and Cohen, A. M. (1972). *Surgery* **72**, 155.

Sugarbaker, E. V., Cohen, A. M. and Ketcham, A. S. (1971). *Ann. Surg.* **174**, 161.

Suomalainen, P. and Toivonen, S. (1939). *Ann. Acad. Sci. Fenn. Ser. A.* **53**, 1.

Sutherland, R. M. and Durand, R. E. (1972). *Internat. J. Radiat. Biol.* **22**, 613.

Sutherland, R. M. and Durand, R. E. (1973). *Internat. J. Radiat. Biol.* **23**, 235.

Sutherland, R. M., Inch, W. R., McCredie, J. A. and Kruuv, J. (1970). *Internat. J. Radiat. Biol.* **18**, 491.

Sutherland, R. M., McCredie, J. A. and Inch, W. R. (1971). *J. Natl Cancer Inst.* **46**, 113.

Sutherland, R. M., Howell, R. L. and Stroude, E. C. (1976). *Radiat. Res.* **67**, 617.

Sutherland, R. M., MacDonald, J. R. and Howell, R. L. (1977). *J. Natl Cancer Inst.* **58**, 1849.

Sutherland, R. M., Eddy, H. A., Bareham, B., Reich, K. and Vanantwerp, D. (1979). *Internat. J. Radiat. Oncol. Biol. Phys.* **5**, 1225.

Svien, H. J., Mabon, R. F., Kernohan, J. W. and Adson, A. W. (1949). *Proc. Mayo Clinic* **24**, 54.

Sylvén, B. (1968). *Eur,. J. Cancer* **4**, 463.

Sylvén, B. and Bois, I. (1960). *Cancer Res.* **20**, 831.

Tada, T., Taniguchi, M. and David, C. S. (1977). *Cold Spring Harbor Symp. Quant. Biol.* **41**, 119.

Takahashi, M. and Yamanishi, K. (1974). *Virology* **61**, 306.

Takami, H. and Nishioka, K. (1980). *Br. J. Cancer* **41**, 751.

Takemoto, K. K., Todaro, G. J. and Habel, K. (1968). *Virology* **35**, 1.

Takemoto, K. K., Robson, A. S., Mullarky, M. F., Blease, R. M., Garon, C. F. and Nelson, D. (1974). *J. Natl Cancer Inst.* **53**, 1205.

Tanaka, K., Nicholson, W. E. and Orth, D. N. (1978). *J. Clin. Invest.* **62**, 94.

Taniyama, T. and Holden, H. T. (1979). *Internat. J. Cancer* **24**, 151.

Tao, T. W., Matter, A., Vogel, K. and Burger, M. M. (1979). *Internat. J. Cancer* **23**, 854.

Tashjian, A. H. (1978). *Cancer Res.* **38**, 4138.

Tashjian, A. H., Levine, L. and Munson, P. L. (1964). *J. Exp. Med.* **119**, 467.

Tashjian, A. H., Voelkel, E. F., Levine, L. and Goldhaber, P. (1972). *J. Exp. Med.* **136**, 1329.

Tashjian, A. H., Voelkel, E. F., Goldhaber, P. and Levine, L. (1974). *Fed. Proc.* **33**, 81.

Taylor, A. C., Levy, B. M. and Simpson, J. W. (1970). *Nature* **228**, 366.

Taylor, G. W. and Nathanson, I. T. (1939). *Surg. Gynec. Obstet.* **69**, 484.

Tchao, R., Schleich, A. B., Frick, M. and Mayer, A. (1980). *In* "Metastasis Clinical and Experimental Aspects", eds Hellmann, K., Hilgard, P. and Eccles, S., p. 28. Martinus Nijhoff, The Hague.

Tegtmeyer, P. (1972). *J. Virol.* **10**, 591.

Temin, H. M. (1974). *Cancer Res.* **34**, 2835.

Theofilopoulos, A. N., Andrews, B. S., Urist, M. M., Morton, D. L. and Dixon, F. J. (1977). *J. Immunol.* **119**, 657.

Theologides, A. (1974). *Ann. N.Y. Acad. Sci.* **230**, 14.

Thomas, A. N., Loken, H. F., Gordon, G. S. and Goldman, L. (1960). *Surg. Forum* **11**, 70.

Thomson, A. W. and Fowler, E. F. (1977). *Transplantation* **24**, 397.

Thomson, A. W., Pugh-Humphreys, R. G. P., Tweedie, D. J. and Horne, C. H. W. (1978). *Experientia* **34**, 528.

Thomson, D. M. P. (1975). *Internat. J. Cancer* **15**, 1016.

Thomson, D. M. P., Eccles, S. and Alexander, P. (1973a). *Br. J. Cancer* **28**, 6.

Thomson, D. M. P., Sellons, V., Eccles, S and Alexander, P. (1973b). *Br. J. Cancer* **28**, 377.

Thomson, D. M. P., Steele, K. and Alexander, P. (1973c). *Br. J. Cancer* **27**, 27.

Thunold, S., Tönder, O. and Larsen, O. (1973). *Acta Pathol. Microbiol. Scand. (A) (Suppl.)*, **236**, 97.

Tickle, C., Crawley, A. and Goodman, M. (1978). *J. Cell Sci.* **31**, 293.

Tickle, C., Crawley, A. and Roscoe, J. P. (1979). *J. Cell Sci.* **37**, 143.

Tiedemann, H. (1968). *J. Cell Physiol.* **72** (Suppl. 1), 129.

Ting, C. C. and Rogers, M. J. (1977). *Nature* **266**, 727.

Tobey, R. A. and Campbell, E. W. (1965). *Virology* **27**, 11.

Todaro, G. J., Green, H. and Goldberg, B. D. (1964). *Proc. Natl Acad. Sci. U.S.A.* **51**, 66.

Toivonen, S. and Saxén, L. (1957). *J. Natl Cancer Inst.* **19**, 1095.

Toivonen, S. and Wartiovaara, J. (1976). *Differentiation* **5**, 61.

Toivonen, S., Tarin, D. and Saxén, L. (1976). *Differentiation* **5**, 49.

Tom, B. H., Rutzky, L. P., Oyasu, R., Tomita, J. T., Goldenberg, D. M. and Kahn, B. D. (1977). *J. Natl Cancer Inst.* **58**, 1507.

Tønder, O. and Thunold, S. (1973). *Scand. J. Immunol.* **2**, 207.

Toolan, H. W. (1954). *Cancer Res.* **14**, 660.

Tormey, D. C., Waalkes, T. P., Ahmann, D., Gehrke, C. W., Zumwatt, R. W., Snyder, J. and Hansen, H. (1975). *Cancer* **35**, 1095.

Tormey, D. C., Waalkes, T. P., Synder, J. J. and Simon, R. M. (1977). *Cancer* **39**, 2397.

Tough, I. C. K., Carter, D. C., Fraser, J. and Bruce, J. (1969). *Br. J. Cancer* **23**, 294.

Trevisani, A., Ferretti, E., Capuzzo, A. and Tomasi, V. (1980). *Br. J. Cancer* **41**, 341.

Trinchieri, G. and Santoli, D. (1978). *J. Exp. Med.* **147**, 1314.

Trinchieri, G., Santoli, D. and Knowles, B. B. (1977). *Nature* **270**, 611.

Trinchieri, G., Santoli, D., Dee, R. R. and Knowles, B. B. (1978). *J. Exp. Med.* **147**, 1299.

Trinkaus, J. P. (1976). *Cell Surface Rev.* **1**, 225.

Trowell, D. A. (1954). *Exp. Cell Res.* **6**, 246.

Trummel, C. L., Mundy, G. R. and Raisz, L. G. (1975). *J. Lab. Clin. Med.* **85**, 1001.

Turner, G. A., Sherbet, G. V. and Wildridge, M. (1980a). *Exp. Cell Biol.* **48**, 385.

Turner, G. A., Guy, D., Latner, A. L. and Sherbet, G. V. (1980b). *In* "Metastasis: Clinical and Experimental", eds Hellmann, K., Hilgard, P. and Eccles, S., p. 222. Martinus Nijhoff Publishers, The Hague.

UICC (1974). "TNM Classification of Malignant Tumours", 2nd edn.

Underwood, J. C. E. and Carr, I. (1972). *J. Pathol.* **107**, 157.

Unkeless, J. C., Tobia, A., Ossowski, L., Quigley, J. P., Rifkin, D. B. and Reich, E. (1973). *J. Exp. Med.* **137**, 85.

Unkeless, J. C., Dano, K., Kellerman, G. and Reich, E. (1974). *J. Biol. Chem.* **249**, 4295.

Uriel, J. (1979). *Advan. Cancer Res.* **29**, 127.

Vacquier, V. D., Epel, D. and Douglas, L. A. (1972). *Nature* **237**, 34.

Vacquier, V. D., Tegner, M. J. and Epel, D. (1973). *Exp. Cell Res.* **80**, 111.

Van Beek, W. P., Smets, L. A. and Emmelot, P. (1973). *Cancer Res.* **33**, 2913.

Van den Brenk, H. A. S. and Kelly, H. (1973). *Br. J. Cancer* **28**, 349.

Van den Brenk, H. A. S. and Kelly, H. (1974). *Br. J. Cancer* **47**, 332.

Van den Brenk, H. A. S., Stone, M. G., Kelly, H. and Sharpington, C. (1976). *Br. J. Cancer* **33**, 60.

Van der Noordaa, J. (1976). *J. Gen. Virol.* **30**, 331.

Van Nagell, J. R., Donaldson, E. S., Wood, E. G., Maruyama, Y. and Utley, J. (1977). *Cancer* **40**, 2243.

Van Nagell, J. R., Donaldson, E. S., Wood, E. G. and Parker, J. C. (1978). *Cancer* **41**, 228.

Varani, J., Orr, W. and Ward, P. A. (1979). *J. Cell Sci.* **36**, 241.

Vasiliev, J. M., Gelfand, I. M., Domina, L. V. Ivanova, O. Y., Komm, S. G. and Olshevskaja, L. V. (1970). *J. Embryol. Exp. Morphol.* **24**, 625.

Vassalli, J. D., Hamilton, J. A. and Reich, E. (1976). *Cell* **8**, 271.

Verloes, R., Atassi, G., Dumont, P. and Kanarek, L. (1978). *Eur. J. Cancer* **14**, 23.

Vincent, R. G. and Chu, T. M. (1973). *Surgery* **66**, 320.

Vlaeminck, M. N., Adenis, L., Mouton, Y. and Demaille, A. (1972]. *Internat. J. Cancer* **10**, 619.

Voelkel, E. F., Tashjian, A. H. Jr, Franklin, R., Wasserman, E. and Levine, L. (1975). *Metabolism* **24**, 973.

Vorbrodt, A. and Koprowski, H. (1969). *J. Natl Cancer Inst.* **43**, 1241.

Vorherr, H. (1974). *Oncology* **29**, 382.

Waalkes, T. P., Gehrke, C. W. and Bleyer, W. A. (1975a). *Cancer Chemother. Rep.* **59**, 721.

Waalkes, T. P., Gehrke, C. W. and Tormey, D. C. (1975b). *Cancer Chemother. Rep.* **59**, 1103.

Waalkes, T. P., Gehrke, C. W., Tormey, D. C., Wood, K. B., Kuo, K. C., Snyder, J. and Hansen, H. (1978). *Cancer* **41**, 1871.

Waddington, C. H. (1932). *Phil. Trans. Roy. Soc. B.* **221**, 179.

Waddington, C. H. (1933). *J. Exp. Biol.* **10**, 38.

Waddington, C. H. (1934). *J. Exp. Biol.* **11**, 211.

Waddington, C. H. (1936). *J. Exp. Biol.* **13**, 86.

Waddington, C. H. (1941). *J. Hered.* **32**, 268.

Waddington, C. H. (1952). "Epigenetics of Birds". Cambridge University Press, Cambridge and London.

Waddington, C. H. (1962). "New Patterns in Genetics and Development". Columbia University Press, New York.

Waddington, C. H. (1966). *Proc. Roy. Soc. London, Ser. B* **164**, 219.

Waddington, C. H. and Schmidt, G. A. (1933). *Rous' Arch. Entwickl. Mech. Org.* **128**, 522.

Wade, H. (1908). *J. Pathol. Bact.* **12**, 384.

Wakely, J. and England, M. A. (1978). *Experientia* **34**, 243.

Walker, R. A. (1978). *J. Clin. Pathol.* **31**, 245.

Wall, R. and Darnell, J. E. (1971). *Nature New Biol.* **232**, 73.

Walter, H. (1975). *Methods Cell Biol.* **9**, 25.

Walter, H. (1977). *Methods Cell Separation* **1**, 307.

Walter, H., Selby, F. W. and Garza, R. (1967). *Biochim. Biophys. Acta* **136**, 148.

Walter, H., Krob, E. J., Ascher, G. S. and Seaman, G. V. F. (1973a). *Exp. Cell Res.* **82**, 15.

Walter, H., Eriksson, G., Taube, O. and Albertsson, P. Å. (1973b). *Exp. Cell Res.* **77**, 361.

Walter, H., Miner, K. M. and Nicolson, G. L. (1981). In *2nd Internat. Conf. on Partitioning*, Sheffield, England (Abstract).

Walther, B. T., Öhman, R. and Roseman, S. (1973). *Proc. Natl Acad. Sci.* **70**, 1569.

Wang, B. S., McLoughlin, G. A., Richie, J. and Mannick, J. A. (1980). *Cancer Res.* **40**, 288.

Wang, D. Y., Bulbrook, R. D., Hayward, J. L., Hendrick, J. C. and Franchimont, P. (1975). *Eur. J. Cancer* **11**, 615.

Ward, M. A., Cooper, E. H., Turner, R., Anderson, J. A. and Neville, A. M. (1977a). *Br. J. Cancer* **35**, 170.

Ward, M. A., Cooper, E. H. and Houghton, A. L. (1977b). *Br. J. Urol.* **49**, 411.

Warren, B. A. (1974). *Thromb. Diath. Haemorrh. Suppl.* **59**, 139.

Warren, B. A. (1976). *Z. Krebsforsch* **87**, 1.

Warren, B. A. and Vales, O. (1972). *Br. J. Exp. Pathol.* **53**, 301.

Warren, B. A., Chauvin, W. J. and Phillips, J. (1977). *In* "Cancer Invasion and Metastasis: Biologic Mechanisms and Therapy", eds Day, S. B., Laird Myers, W. P., Stansly, P., Garattini, S. and Lewis, M. G., p. 185. Raven Press, New York.

Warren, L., Fuhrer, J. P. and Buck, C. A. (1972a). *Proc. Natl Acad. Sci. U.S.A.* **69**, 1838.

Warren, L., Critchley, D. and Macpherson, I. (1972b). *Nature* **235**, 275.

Warren, L., Zeidman, I. and Buck, C. A. (1975). *Cancer Res.* **35**, 2185.

Watkins, J. F. and Dulbecco, R. (1967). *Proc. Natl Acad. Sci. U.S.A.* **58**, 1396.

Watson, R. D., Smith, A. G. and Levy, J. G. (1974). *Br. J. Cancer* **29**, 183.

Weinstein, I. B., Lee, L. S., Fisher, P. B., Mufson, A. and Yamasaki, H. (1979). *J. Supramolec. Str.* **12**, 195.

Weiser, M. M., Podolsky, D. M. and Isselbacher, K. J. (1976). *Proc. Natl Acad. Sci. U.S.A.* **73**, 1319.

Weiss, A. F., Portman, R., Fischer, H., Simon, J. and Zang, K. D. (1975). *Proc. Natl Acad. Sci. U.S.A.* **72**, 609.

Weiss, L. (1963). *Exp. Cell Res.* **30**, 509.

Weiss, L. (1965). *J. Cell Biol.* **26**, 735.

Weiss, L. (1967). "The Cell Periphery, Metastasis and Other Contact-dependent Phenomena". North Holland Publishing Co., Amsterdam.

Weiss, L. (1968). *Exp. Cell Res.* **53**, 603.

Weiss, L. (1976). *Exp. Cell Res.* **86**, 223.

Weiss, L. (1977). *Internat. J. Cancer* **20**, 87.

Weiss, L. (1978). *Internat. J. Cancer* **22**, 196.

Weiss, L. and Holyoke, E. D. (1969). *J. Natl Cancer Inst.* **43**, 1045.

Weiss, L., Glaves, D. and Waite, D. (1974). *Internat. J. Cancer* **13**, 850.

Weiss, L., Subjeck, J. R. and Poste, G. (1975). *Internat. J. Cancer* **16**, 914.

Weiss, P. (1934). *J. Exp. Zool.* **68**, 393.

Weiss, P. (1947). *Yale J. Biol. Med.* **19**, 235.

Weiss, P. (1961). *Exp. Cell Res.* **8**, 260.

Wepsic, H. T. and Sell, S. (1974). *Progr. Exp. Tumour Res.* **19**, 297.

Wessels, N. K. and Wilt, F. (1965). *J. Molec. Biol.* **13**, 767.

Whitney, J. and Massey, C. (1961). *J. Clin. Endocrinol.* **21**, 541.

Whur, P. and Koppel, H. (1975). *Br. J. Cancer* **32**, 248.

Whur, P., Urquhart, C. M., Williams, D. C., Donaldson, D. and Sakula, A. (1978). *Eur. J. Cancer* **14**, 315.

Wiener, F., Klein, G. and Harris, H. (1974a). *J. Cell Sci.* **15**, 177.

Wiener, F., Klein, G. and Harris, H. (1974b). *J. Cell Sci.* **16**, 189.

Wildridge, M. and Sherbet, G. V. (1981). *Br. J. Cancer* **43**, 118.

Wildridge, M. and Sherbet, G. V. (1982). *Exp. Cell Biol.* **50**, 27.

Wilkins, D. J., Ottewill, R. H. and Bangham, A. D. (1962). *J. Theoret. Biol.* **2**, 165.

Williams-Ashman, H. G., Coppoc, G. L. and Weber, G. (1972). *Cancer Res.* **32**, 1924.

Williams, R. C. N., Lyndon, P J. and Tudway, A. J. C. (1980). *Br. J. Cancer* **42**, 85.

Willis, R. A. (1967). "Pathology of Tumours", 4th ed. Butterworths, London.

Willis, R. A. (1973). "The Spread of Tumours in the Human Body", 3rd ed. Butterworths, London.

Wilson, E. L. and Dowdle, E. (1978). *Internat. J. Cancer* **22**, 390.

Winterbauer, R. H., Elfenbein, I. B. and Ball, W. C. (1968). *Amer. J. Med.* **45**, 271.

Withers, H. R. and Milas, L. (1973). *Cancer Res.* **33**, 1931.

Witkin, S. S., Egeli, R. A., Sarkar, N. H., Good, R. A. and Day, N. K. (1979). *Proc. Natl Acad. Sci. U.S.A.* **76**, 2984.

Witkin, S. S., Sarkar, N. H., Kinne, D. W., Good, R. A. and Day, N. K. (1980). *Internat. J. Cancer* **25**, 721.

Wolf, H., Zur Hausen, H. and Becker, V. (1973). *Nature New Biol.* **244**, 245.

Wolff, Et. and Haffen, K. (1952). *Tex. Reports. Biol. Med.* **10**, 463.

Wolff, Et. and Schneider, N. (1956). *C.R. Soc. Biol.* **150**. 845.

Wolff, Et. and Schneider, N. (1957). *Arch. Anat. Micr. Morphol. Exp.* **46**, 173.

Wolff, Et. and Sigot, M. F. (1961a). *C.R. Soc. Biol.* **155**, 265.
Wolff, Et. and Sigot, M. F. (1961b). *C.R. Soc. Biol.* **155**, 960.
Wolff, Et. and Wolff, E. (1961). *J. Embryol. Exp. Morphol.* **9**, 678.
Wolff, Et., Zajdela, F. and Sigot, M. F. (1964). *C.R. Acad. Sci.* **258**, 4633.
Wolsky, A. (1974). *In* "Neoplasia and Cell Differentiation", ed. Sherbet, G. V., p. 153. Karger, Basle and New York.
Wood, G. W. and Gillespie, G. Y. (1975). *Internat. J. Cancer* **16**, 1022.
Wood, G. W. and Gollahon, K. A. (1977). *J. Natl Cancer Inst.* **59**, 1081.
Wood, G. W., Gillespie, G. Y. and Barth, R. F. (1975). *J. Immunol.* **114**, 950.
Wood, P. C., Vareba, V., Palmquist, M. and Weber, F. (1973). *J. Surg. Oncol.* **5**, 251.
Wood, S. Jr (1958). *Arch. Pathol.* **66**, 550.
Wood, S. Jr and Hilgard, P. (1972). *Lancet* ii, 1416.
Wood, S. Jr, Holyoke, E. D. and Yardley, J. H. (1956). *Proc. Amer. Assn. Cancer Res.* **2**, 157.
Wood, R. A. B. Moossa, A. R. (1977). *Br. J. Surg.* **64**, 718.
Woodbury, R. G., Brown, J. P., Yeh, M. Y., Hellström, I. and Hellström, K. E. (1980). *Proc. Natl Acad. Sci. U.S.A.* **77**, 2183.
Woodbury, R. G., Brown, J. P., Loop, S. M., Hellström, K. E. and Hellström, I. (1981). *Internat. J. Cancer* **27**, 145.
Woodruff, M. F. A. and Warner, N. L. (1977). *J. Natl Cancer Inst.* **58**, 111.
Woodruff, M. F. A., Ghaffar, A. and Whitehead, V. L. (1976). *Internat. J. Cancer* **17**, 652.
Worwood, M., Summers, M., Midler, F., Jacobs, A. and Whittaker, J. A. (1974). *Br. J. Haematol.* **28**, 27.
Wyss, F. (1967). *Triangle* **8**, 96.
Yamada, T. and Karasaki, S. (1963). *Develop. Biol.* **7**, 595.
Yamada, T. and Roesel, M. E. (1964). *J. Embryol. Exp. Morphol.* **12**, 713.
Yamaguchi, N. and Kuchino, T. (1975). *J. Virol.* **15**, 1297.
Yamanishi, Y., Dabbous, M. K. and Hashimoto, K. (1972). *Cancer Res.* **32**, 2551.
Yamanishi, Y., Maeyens, E., Dabbous, M. K., Ohyama, H. and Hashimoto, K. (1973). *Cancer Res* **33**, 2507.
Yarnell, M. M. and Ambrose, E. J. (1969a). *Eur. J. Cancer* **5**, 255.
Yarnell, M. M. and Ambrose, E. J. (1969b). *Eur. J. Cancer* **5**, 265.
Yarnell, M. M., Ambrose, E. J., Shepley, K. and Tchao, R. (1964). *Br. Med. J.* **2**, 490.
Yogeeswaran, G. and Salk, P. (1980). *In* "Metastasis: Clinical and Experimental Aspects", eds Hellmann, K., Hilgard, P. and Eccles, S., p. 422. Martinus Nijhoff, The Hague.
Yogeeswaran, G., Stein, B. and Sebastian, H. (1978). *Cancer Res.* **38**, 1336.
Yoshida, K., Yoshinaga, M. and Hayashi, H. (1968). *Nature* **218**, 977.
Yoshinaga, M., Yoshida, K., Tashiro, A. and Hayashi, H. (1971). *Immunology* **21**, 281.
Youle, R. J. and Neville, D. M. Jr (1980). *Proc. Natl Acad. Sci. U.S.A.* **77**, 5483.
Youn, J. K., LeFrançois, D. and Barski, G. (1973). *J. Natl Cancer Inst.* **50**, 921.
Yuhas, J. M., Li, A. P., Martinez, A. O. and Ladman, A. J. (1977). *Cancer Res.* **37**, 3639.
Zarling, J. M. and Kung, P. C. (1980). *Nature* **288**, 394.
Zarling, J. M., Eskra, L., Borden, E. C., Horoszewicz, J. and Carter, W. A. (1979). *J. Immunol.* **123**, 63.

Zarling, J. M., Schlais, J., Eskara, L., Green, J. J., Ts'O, P. and Carter, W. A. (1980). *J. Immunol.* **124,** 1852.

Zaunders, J., Werkmeister, J., McCarthy, W. H. and Hersey, P. (1981). *Br. J. Cancer* **43,** 5.

Zeidman, I. (1955). *Cancer Res.* **15,** 719.

Zeidman, I. (1957). *Cancer Res.* **17,** 157.

Zeidman, I. (1961). *Cancer Res.* **21,** 38.

Zeidman, I. and Buss, J. M. (1952). *Cancer Res.* **12,** 731.

Zelen, M. (1968). *Cancer Res.* **28,** 207.

Zembala, M., Mytar, B., Popiela, T. and Asherson, G. L. (1977). *Internat. J. Cancer* **19,** 605.

Zetter, B. R. (1980). *Nature* **285,** 41.

Subject Index

Acid phosphatase,
  association with tumours, 111
  in Gaucher's disease, 111
Actinomycin D,
  effect on competent state of neuro-
    ectoderm, 97
Actomyosin filaments,
  and cell locomotion, 15
Acute phase reactant proteins,
  in cancer, 112
Adenocarcinoma, human GI tract,
  collagenolytic activity of, 88
  plasminogen activator activity associ-
    ated with, 87
  relationship between metastatic dis-
    semination and CEA immune
    complexes, 66
Adenocarcinoma, human mammary,
  MuMTV sequence homology with
    nucleic acids of, 8
Adenocarcinoma, renal, Lucké,
  differentiation in regeneration field,
    146
Adhesion,
  differential adhesion of hamster
    lymphomas, 38
  fibronectin in, 165
  heterotypic adhesion and organ-
    specific metastasis, 38
  invasiveness and intercellular, 164-166
  low mol. wt. components in, 165
  of tumour cells to endothelium, 24-25,
    31,32, 38
  surface charge in intercellular, 165
Adrenocorticotropic hormone,
  in Cushing's syndrome, 100
Aetiology,
  viral, of cancer, 6-10

Alexander cell line,
  Hepatitis B virus from, 8-9
  Hepatitis B antigens in growth medium
    of, 9
Alkaline phosphatase,
  association with tumours, 111
  in non-neoplastic conditions, 111
Alpha fetoprotein (AFP),
  association with non-neoplastic con-
    ditions, 110
  frequency of incidence in cancer, 120
  histogenetic specificity of production
    of, 120
  immunosuppressive effects of, 78
  in regenerating liver, 120
  production by foetal liver, 119
  production by tumours, 110, 119-120
  role in cancer management, 119-120
Anaplasia,
  and CEA production by tumours, 119
  ectopic products and degree of, 114
  malignancy and degree of, 128-135
Ancrod,
  effects on metastasis, 26-27
Angiogenesis, see Vascularisation, hyper-
    emia
Anticoagulants,
  effects on metastasis, 26-27
Antidiuretic hormone (ADH)
  in bronchogenic carcinoma, 103
Antigenic adaptation,
  for evasion of immune surveillance,
    58-59
Antigenic modulation,
  and evasion of immune surveillance,
    66-71
  in ESb, Eb DBA2 murine lymphomas,
    67